Pharmacy Practice and Administration

Pharmacy Practice and Administration

Editor

Georges Adunlin

MDPI • Basel • Beijing • Wuhan • Barcelona • Belgrade • Manchester • Tokyo • Cluj • Tianjin

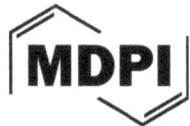

Editor
Georges Adunlin
Pharmaceutical, Social and
Administrative Sciences
Samford University,
McWhorter School of
Pharmacy
Birmingham
United States

Editorial Office
MDPI
St. Alban-Anlage 66
4052 Basel, Switzerland

This is a reprint of articles from the Special Issue published online in the open access journal *Healthcare* (ISSN 2227-9032) (available at: www.mdpi.com/journal/healthcare/special_issues/ Pharmacy_Practice_Administration).

For citation purposes, cite each article independently as indicated on the article page online and as indicated below:

LastName, A.A.; LastName, B.B.; LastName, C.C. Article Title. *Journal Name* **Year**, *Volume Number*, Page Range.

ISBN 978-3-0365-4730-5 (Hbk)
ISBN 978-3-0365-4729-9 (PDF)

© 2022 by the authors. Articles in this book are Open Access and distributed under the Creative Commons Attribution (CC BY) license, which allows users to download, copy and build upon published articles, as long as the author and publisher are properly credited, which ensures maximum dissemination and a wider impact of our publications.

The book as a whole is distributed by MDPI under the terms and conditions of the Creative Commons license CC BY-NC-ND.

Contents

Carla Perpétuo, Ana I. Plácido, Jorge Aperta, Maria Teresa Herdeiro and Fátima Roque
Profile of Prescription Medication in an Internal Medicine Ward
Reprinted from: *Healthcare* **2021**, *9*, 704, doi:10.3390/healthcare9060704 1

Anita Tuula, Daisy Volmer, Liisa Jõhvik, Ieva Rutkovska, Indre Trečiokienė and Piotr Merks et al.
Factors Facilitating and Hindering Development of a Medication Use Review Service in Eastern Europe and Iran-Cross-Sectional Exploratory Study
Reprinted from: *Healthcare* **2021**, *9*, 1207, doi:10.3390/healthcare9091207 9

Giulio Barigelletti, Giovanna Tagliabue, Sabrina Fabiano, Annalisa Trama, Alice Bernasconi and Claudio Tresoldi et al.
Analysis of the Consumption of Non-Oncological Medicines: A Methodological Study on Patients of the Ada Cohort
Reprinted from: *Healthcare* **2021**, *9*, 1121, doi:10.3390/healthcare9091121 21

Po-Feng Lee, Chung-Yi Li, Yen-Chin Liu, Chang-Ta Chiu and Wen-Hsuan Hou
Population-Based Study on the All-Cause and Cause-Specific Risks of Mortality among Long-Term Opioid Analgesics Users without Cancer in Taiwan
Reprinted from: *Healthcare* **2021**, *9*, 1402, doi:10.3390/healthcare9111402 39

Hubert Jin, Sue Yang, David Bankes, Stephanie Finnel, Jacques Turgeon and Alan Stein
Evaluating the Impact of Medication Risk Mitigation Services in Medically Complex Older Adults
Reprinted from: *Healthcare* **2022**, *10*, 551, doi:10.3390/healthcare10030551 49

Christian Kunow, Moulika Aline Bello, Laura Diedrich, Laura Eutin, Yanneck Sonnenberg and Nele Wachtel et al.
A Nationwide Mystery Caller Evaluation of Oral Emergency Contraception Practices from German Community Pharmacies: An Observational Study Protocol
Reprinted from: *Healthcare* **2021**, *9*, 945, doi:10.3390/healthcare9080945 63

Andreas Sandberg, Pauliina Ehlers, Saku Torvinen, Heli Sandberg and Mia Sivén
Regulation Awareness and Experience of Additional Monitoring among Healthcare Professionals in Finland
Reprinted from: *Healthcare* **2021**, *9*, 1540, doi:10.3390/healthcare9111540 81

Cody K. Dukes and Elizabeth A. Sheaffer
Biosensing Technology to Track Adherence: A Literature Review
Reprinted from: *Healthcare* **2021**, *9*, 1339, doi:10.3390/healthcare9101339 93

Christina Malini Christopher, Bhuvan KC, Ali Blebil, Deepa Alex, Mohamed Izham Mohamed Ibrahim and Norhasimah Ismail et al.
Clinical and Humanistic Outcomes of Community Pharmacy-Based Healthcare Interventions Regarding Medication Use in Older Adults: A Systematic Review and Meta-Analysis
Reprinted from: *Healthcare* **2021**, *9*, 1577, doi:10.3390/healthcare9111577 101

Ahmed M. Alshehri, Lara A. Elsawaf, Shaikah F. Alzaid, Yasser S. Almogbel, Mohammed A. Alminggash and Ziyad S. Almalki et al.
Factors Affecting Pharmacy Students' Decision to Study in Pharmacy Colleges in Saudi Arabia: A Cross-Sectional Questionnaire-Based Analysis
Reprinted from: *Healthcare* **2021**, *9*, 1651, doi:10.3390/healthcare9121651 119

Agnieszka Zimmermann, Jakub Płaczek, Natalia Wrzosek and Artur Owczarek
Assessment of Pharmacists Prescribing Practices in Poland—A Descriptive Study
Reprinted from: *Healthcare* **2021**, *9*, 1505, doi:10.3390/healthcare9111505 129

Sultan Alghadeer and Mohammed N. Al-Arifi
Community Pharmacists' Practice, Awareness, and Beliefs about Drug Disposal in Saudi Arabia
Reprinted from: *Healthcare* **2021**, *9*, 823, doi:10.3390/healthcare9070823 141

Wei-Ho Chen, Pei-Chen Lee, Shu-Chiung Chiang, Yuh-Lih Chang, Tzeng-Ji Chen and Li-Fang Chou et al.
Pharmacist Workforce at Primary Care Clinics: A Nationwide Survey in Taiwan
Reprinted from: *Healthcare* **2021**, *9*, 863, doi:10.3390/healthcare9070863 149

Shigeo Yamamura, Tomoko Terajima, Javiera Navarrete, Christine A. Hughes, Nese Yuksel and Theresa J. Schindel et al.
Reproductive Health Services: Attitudes and Practice of Japanese Community Pharmacists
Reprinted from: *Healthcare* **2021**, *9*, 1336, doi:10.3390/healthcare9101336 161

Sultan M. Alshahrani, Khalid Orayj, Ali M. Alqahtani and Mubarak A. Algahtany
Community Pharmacists' Perceptions towards the Misuse and Abuse of Pregabalin: A Cross-Sectional Study from Aseer Region, Saudi Arabia
Reprinted from: *Healthcare* **2021**, *9*, 1281, doi:10.3390/healthcare9101281 175

Claire Brandish, Frances Garraghan, Bee Yean Ng, Kate Russell-Hobbs, Omotayo Olaoye and Diane Ashiru-Oredope
Assessing the Impact of a Global Health Fellowship on Pharmacists' Leadership Skills and Consideration of Benefits to the National Health Service (NHS) in the United Kingdom
Reprinted from: *Healthcare* **2021**, *9*, 890, doi:10.3390/healthcare9070890 187

Jill Pence, Shannon Ashe, Georges Adunlin and Jennifer Beall
A Comparison of Nursing and Pharmacy Students' Perceptions of an Acute Care Simulation
Reprinted from: *Healthcare* **2022**, *10*, 715, doi:10.3390/healthcare10040715 207

Saad Saeed Alqahtani
Community Pharmacists' Opinions towards Poor Prescription Writing in Jazan, Saudi Arabia
Reprinted from: *Healthcare* **2021**, *9*, 1077, doi:10.3390/healthcare9081077 215

Darrow Thomas, John A. Soldner, Cheryl D. Cropp and Jennifer Beall
Pharmacy Student Perceptions of a Virtual Pharmacogenomics Activity
Reprinted from: *Healthcare* **2022**, *10*, 286, doi:10.3390/healthcare10020286 225

Georges Adunlin and Kevin Pan
Pharmacy Students' Attitudes and Perceptions toward Financial Management Education
Reprinted from: *Healthcare* **2022**, *10*, 683, doi:10.3390/healthcare10040683 235

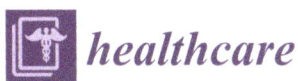

Article

Profile of Prescription Medication in an Internal Medicine Ward

Carla Perpétuo [1,2], Ana I. Plácido [2,3], Jorge Aperta [1,2], Maria Teresa Herdeiro [3] and Fátima Roque [1,4,*]

[1] Research Unit for Inland Development, Polytechnic Institute of Guarda (UDI-IPG), 6300-559 Guarda, Portugal; carladicarol@ipg.pt (C.P.); apertajorge@gmail.com (J.A.)
[2] Local Health Unit of Guarda, 6300-035 Guarda, Portugal; anaplacido@ipg.pt
[3] Institute of Biomedicine (iBiMED-UA), Department of Medical Sciences, University of Aveiro, 3810-193 Aveiro, Portugal; teresaherdeiro@ua.pt
[4] Health Science Research Center (CICS-UBI), University of Beira Interior, 6201-001 Covilhã, Portugal
* Correspondence: froque@ipg.pt

Abstract: Aging-related loss of resilience associated with the lack of evidence regarding the therapeutic efficacy of medicines can prompt a lack of efficacy of treatments and multiple prescriptions. This work aims to characterize the medication profile of Portuguese older adult inpatients and explore the relationship between hospitalization days and the consumption of medicines. A retrospective data analysis study in older patients who were admitted to a medical internal medicine ward during 2019. The median age of the 616 patients included was 85 years. During the hospitalized period, patients took on average 18.08 medicines. The most prescribed drugs belong to the subgroup of (a) anti-thrombotic agents (6.7%), with enoxaparin being the most prescribed, (b) other analgesics and antipyretics (6.6%), paracetamol being the most frequent, and (c) the Angiotensin Conversion Enzyme Inhibitor (ACE) (6.5%), captopril being the most frequent. The high number of prescriptions in older adults during their hospitalization suggests the need of changing therapeutics to achieve a better efficacy of treatment, which corroborates the hypothesis that the lack of scientific evidence concerning the risk/benefits of many medical therapies in older adults can make it difficult to achieve good clinical outcomes and promote the wastage of health resources.

Keywords: older adults; polypharmacy; internal medicine ward

1. Introduction

In the last century, the development of health technologies and the improvement in socio-economic conditions have enhanced health and improved life expectancy, which in association with the decrease in fertility has contributed to an aging population [1,2]. Aging is characterized by progressive alterations in psychological, biological (with drug pharmacodynamics and pharmacokinetics alterations), and even social functions and greater susceptibility to disease [3]. Such alterations can cause a decrease in the ability to recover from unhealthy conditions and consequently can increase the consumption of health resources, which includes medicines [4,5]. Recently, it was reported that about four out of 10 older adults consume five or more medicines (polypharmacy) [6]. Pharmacotherapy can improve quality of life, cure, prevent, or relieve symptoms, but in the older population, special care must be taken with the occurrence of adverse drug reactions (ADR) [7]. The increased prevalence of ADR in older adults is not only related to aging-related increases in susceptibility but also the lack of scientific evidence concerning the risk/benefits of many medical therapies of the older adults [8]. Across history, older adults have been systematically excluded from clinical trials [9], and even when they were included, they are younger than the mean age of older adults' population [8]. As a result, sometimes, prescription can occur without adequate clinical data, which can compromise clinical outcomes and the well-being of the patients [8,9].

For this reason, new approaches are needed to improve the therapeutic efficacy of older adults as well as their quality of life. In this context, the knowledge medication profile of older adults is preponderant. This work aims to characterize the medication consumption profile of inpatient older adults, as well as attempt to establish a correlation between the medication profile and the diseases and hospitalization days.

2. Materials and Methods

A retrospective study was performed to characterize the medication profile among older inpatients of a general internal medicine service of a first-level hospital located in the inner center region of Portugal. All older patients (aged $\geq$ 65) hospitalized in the internal medicine service for at least 4 days during 2019 were eligible to participate in the study. Older patients hospitalized for less than 4 days were excluded. For patients hospitalized more than once in the internal medicine service, the number of days hospitalized was obtained through the sum of the days of each hospitalization. Data were retrospectively collected from the hospital's electronic medical record and included patient age, patient gender (male/female), patient diagnoses, hospitalization days, and drugs prescribed. The list of all medication, extracted from the electronic records, was converted to the corresponding Anatomical Therapeutic Classification (ATC) code, using the WHO Collaborating Centre for Drug Statistics Methodology's web [10], and patient's diagnoses were classified according to the International Statistical Classification of Diseases and Related Health Problems, 10th Revision (ICD-10). Statistical and descriptive analysis was conducted using the IBM SPSS software version 25.0 and Microsoft Excel. Spearman's test was used to examine the relationship between age, gender, hospitalization days, the most prescribed pharmacological subgroups, and the number of simultaneous prescribed medicines. Numerical and ordinal data were analyzed using descriptive statistics and presented in frequency and percentage and using mean, median, and quartile values.

3. Results

A total of 616 participants were included in the study (median age = 85.0, Min 65, Max 100). Most of the participants were male (51.84%), and 90.2% had been hospitalized only one time (median of hospitalized days = 12). The most frequent diagnosis of the 616 inpatients in the study were as follows: (a) I00-I99-Diseases of the circulatory system (21.40%, N = 829), (b) E00-E89-Endocrine, nutritional, and metabolic diseases (N = 636, 16.40%), and (c) J00-J99-Diseases of the respiratory system (10.70%, N = 415) (Table 1). During the hospitalized period, patients took a median of 17.0 medicines (Min 5, Max 50), and the median of simultaneous medicines per day was 12 medicines (Min 3, Max 27) (Table 1).

Table 1. Study population characteristics.

Study Population Characteristics	N = 616
Age (years)	
Median (Q1–Q3)	85.0 (78.0–89.0)
65–74	98 (15.9%)
75–84	206 (33.4%)
$\geq$85	312 (50.7%)
Gender	
Female	298 (48.4%)
Male	318 (51.6%)

Table 1. Cont.

Study Population Characteristics	N = 616
Hospitalization days	
Median (Q1–Q3)	12 (8–20)
Range (minimum and maximum)	4–90
No. of hospitalizations	
1 hospitalization	556 (90.2%)
2 hospitalizations	54 (8.8%)
3 hospitalizations	6 (1.0%)
No. of prescribed medicines	
Median (Q1–Q3)	17 (13–22)
Range (minimum and maximum)	4–50
No. of simultaneous medicines prescribed per day	
Median (Q1–Q3)	12 (10–14)
Range (minimum and maximum)	3–27
ICD-10 diagnostics	N = 3873
A00-B99—Certain infectious and parasitic diseases	96 (2.50%)
C00-D49—Neoplasms	79 (2.00%)
D50-D89—Diseases of the blood and blood-forming organs and certain disorders involving the immune mechanism	220 (5.70%)
E00-E89—Endocrine, nutritional and metabolic diseases	636 (16.40%)
F0-F99—Mental, Behavioral, and Neurodevelopmental disorders	140 (3.60%)
G00-G99—Diseases of the nervous system	82 (2.10%)
H00-H59—Diseases of the eye and adnexa	11 (0.30%)
H60-H95—Diseases of the ear and mastoid process	14 (0.40%)
I00-I99—Diseases of the circulatory system	829 (21.40%)
J00-J99—Diseases of the respiratory system	415 (10.70%)
K00-K95—Diseases of the digestive system	125 (3.20%)
L00-L99—Diseases of the skin and subcutaneous tissue	50 (1.30%)
M00-M99—Diseases of the musculoskeletal system and connective tissue	80 (2.10%)
N00-N99—Diseases of the genitourinary system	396 (10.20%)
Q00-Q99—Congenital malformations, deformations, and chromosomal abnormalities	1 (0.00%)
R00-R99—Symptoms, signs, and abnormal clinical and laboratory findings, not elsewhere classified	278 (7.20%)
S00-T88—Injury, poisoning, and certain other consequences of external causes	53 (1.40%)
V00-Y99—External causes of morbidity	32 (0.80%)
Z00-Z99—Factors influencing health status and contact with health services	336 (8.70%)

Within the 11,159 prescribed medications, 285 were different medicines, 137 were dietary supplements, and 28 were enteral or parenteral nutrition. The most prescribed medicines belong to the ATC groups blood and blood-forming organs (23.4%), cardiovascular system (20.5%), nervous system (17.1%), and tract alimentary and metabolism (17.0%) (Appendix A, Table A1). The most prescribed drugs belong to the subgroup of (a) anti-thrombotic agents (6.7%), with enoxaparin being the most prescribed, (b) other analgesics and antipyretics (6.6%), paracetamol being the most frequent, (c) the Angiotensin Conversion Enzyme Inhibitor (ACE) (6.5%), captopril being the most frequent, and (e) irrigation solutions (6.3%), with sodium chloride solutions being the most used (Table 2).

Table 2. Most prescribed medicines, third level, pharmacological subgroup.

Most Prescribed Medicines (3rd Level, Pharmacological Subgroup)	Frequency	% N = 11,159
A02B—Drugs for Peptic Ulcer and Gastro-esophageal Reflux Disease (GORD)	489	4.4%
A06A—Drugs for Constipation	381	3.4%
A10A—Insulins and Analogues	489	4.4%
B01A—Antithrombotic Agents	746	6.7%
B05B—I.V. Solutions (I.V. solutions used in parenteral administration of fluids, electrolytes and nutrients)	385	3.5%
B05C—Irrigating Solutions (products used for bladder irrigation, surgical irrigation, incl. instruments)	707	6.3%
B05X—I.V. Solution Additives (I.V. solution additives are concentrated preparations containing substances used for correcting fluid and electrolyte balance and nutritional status)	377	3.4%
C03C—High-Ceiling Diuretics	437	3.9%
C07A—Beta Blocking Agents	334	3.0%
C09A—ACE Inhibitors	723	6.5%
J01C—Beta-Lactam Antibacterials, Penicillins	356	3.2%
N02B—Other Analgesics and Antipyretics	739	6.6%
N05A—Antipsychotics	320	2.9%
N05B—Anxiolytics	298	2.7%
R03A—Adrenergics, Inhalants	314	2.8%

We observed a positive correlation between the hospitalization days and the ICD-10 diagnosis: R00-R99—Symptoms, signs, and abnormal clinical and laboratory findings, not elsewhere classified ($R = 0.103$, $p = 0.010$) and S00-T88—Injury, poisoning, and certain other consequences of external causes ($R = 0.106$, $p = 0.009$) (Table 3).

Table 3. Spearman correlation between hospitalization days and ICD-10 diagnosis.

		Coefficient Value	p Value
Hospitalization days	R00-R99—Symptoms, signs, and abnormal clinical and laboratory findings, not elsewhere classified	0.103	0.010
	S00-T88—Injury, poisoning, and certain other consequences of external causes	0.106	0.009

A negative association between age and the medicines belonging to the subgroups A10A ($R = -0.111$, $p = 0.006$) and N05B ($R = -0.110$, $p = 0.006$). It was also observed a positive association between age and the medicines belonging to the subgroups B05C ($R = 0.165$, $p < 0.0001$), C03C ($R = 0.171$, $p < 0.0001$), J01C ($R = 0.119$, $p = 0.003$) and R03A ($R = 0.106$ and $p = 0.009$) (Table 4).

Table 4. Spearman correlation between age and medicines prescribed (third level, pharmacological subgroup).

		Coefficient Value	p Value
Age	A10A—Insulins and Analogues	−0.111	0.006
	N05B—Anxiolytics	−0.110	0.006
	B05C—Irrigating Solutions (products used for bladder irrigation, surgical irrigation, incl. instruments	0.165	<0.0001
	C03C—High-Ceiling Diuretics	0.171	<0.0001
	J01C—Beta-Lactam Antibacterials. Penicillins	0.119	0.003
	R03A—Adrenergics, Inhalants	0.106	0.009

We also observed a positive correlation between the number of hospitalization days and the number of simultaneous prescribed medicines per day (Table 5).

Table 5. Spearman correlation between the variables of hospitalization days and simultaneous medication per day.

		Coefficient Value	p Value
Hospitalization days	simultaneous medicines per day	0.089	0.045

4. Discussion

This study analyzed the medication profile of Portuguese inpatients at an internal medicine service and concluded that during hospitalization, the inpatients consumed a high number of medicines, suggesting that the high frailly of older adults associated with the lack of prescription guidelines for older adults made it difficult to achieve clinical outcomes and increased the time of hospitalization.

The high average age of the participants included in this study is not surprising, since according to Eurostat, Portuguese have an average life expectancy of 81.5, which is higher than the mean of 27 European Union countries (81.0). However, the increase in life expectancy is not accompanied by health quality; indeed, only 9% of Portuguese older adults are considered healthy, which is a lower number when compared with Austria (58.0%), Germany (38.0%), and France (37%) [11]. This unhealthy state and aging-related loss of resilience and pharmacokinetic and pharmacodynamics alterations that occur in older adults [12] can be a major contribution to the high average number of hospitalized days [13] as well as to the fact that almost 10% of the participants had more than one hospitalization during 2019.

On average, the participants consumed 18.08 medicines during their hospitalization, suggesting a high complexity of the therapeutic treatment that perhaps results from the multiple comorbidities presented by the participants. Similar results were observed by other studies in a long-term care hospitalization setting [14]. There is a lack of evidence for the use of certain medicines in older adults, which greatly limits knowledge about the effectiveness of medication [15] in this age group and leads to the need for a frequent change in medication. The drugs that act on the nervous system are one of the most frequently prescribed drugs among our patients [16]. Indeed, according to the literature, the consumption of these medicines is frequent not only in hospitalized patients but also in nursing home residents [17–19]. In our study, we observed a decrease in the consumed anxiolytics with aging, suggesting an attempt to deprescribe it with increasing ages [5,20,21].

Although the relevant information is provided, the data of this study are not representative of all populations, and they cannot be generalized to all hospitalized older adults; the information collected in this study reinforces the need for more scientific knowledge concerning the risk/benefits of polypharmacy in older adults.

5. Conclusions

The association between a high number of prescribed medicines and the number of hospitalization days observed suggests the need for more scientific evidence regarding therapeutic efficacy in older adults.

Author Contributions: All authors listed have made substantial, direct contributions to the work and approved it for publication. Conceptualization, F.R. and M.T.H.; methodology F.R. and M.T.H.; software, C.P. and A.I.P.; validation, F.R., M.T.H. and J.A.; formal analysis, C.P. and A.I.P.; investigation, C.P.; resources, C.P.; data curation, J.A., C.P. and A.I.P.; writing—A.I.P. and C.P.; writing—review and editing, J.A., F.R. and M.T.H.; visualization, F.R. and M.T.H.; supervision, F.R. and M.T.H.; project administration, F.R. and M.T.H.; funding acquisition F.R. and M.T.H. All authors have read and agreed to the published version of the manuscript.

Funding: This work was financially supported by the APIMedOlder project [PTDC/MED-FAR/31598 /2017], funded by the Operational Programme of Competitiveness and Internationalization (POCI), in its FEDER/FNR component POCI-01-0145-FEDER-031598, and the Foundation for Science and Technology (FCT).

Institutional Review Board Statement: This study obtained the ethical approval (01167) of the hospital on 7 of February 2020 and was carried out according to the European union (EU) general data protection regulation (GDPR).

Informed Consent Statement: Not applicable.

Data Availability Statement: Not applicable.

Conflicts of Interest: The authors declare that the research was conducted in the absence of any commercial or financial relationships that could be construed as a potential conflict of interest.

Appendix A

Table A1. Most prescribed medicines.

	Anatomical Main Group	Frequency	% N = 11,159
A	Alimentary Tract and Metabolism	1901	17%
B	Blood and Blood Forming Organs	2606	23.4%
C	Cardiovascular System	2283	20.5%
D	Dermatologicals	28	0.3%
G	Genito Urinary System and Sex Hormones	144	1.3%
H	Systemic Hormonal Preparations, excl. Sex Hormones and Insulins	220	2.0%
J	Anti-Infectives for Systemic Use	1043	9.3%
L	Antineoplastic and Immunomodulating Agents	17	0.2%
M	Musculo-Skeletal System	151	1.4%
N	Nervous System	1913	17.1%
P	Antiparasitic Products, Insecticides, and Repellents	2	0%
R	Respiratory System	800	7.2%
S	Sensory Organs	27	0.2%
V	Various	24	0.2%

References

1. United Nations. *World Population Ageing 2019 Highlights*; United Nations: New York, NY, USA, 2019.
2. Divo, M.J.; Martinez, C.H.; Mannino, D.M. Ageing and the epidemiology of multimorbidity. *Eur. Respir. J.* **2014**, *44*, 1055–1068. [CrossRef] [PubMed]
3. Grina, D.; Briedis, V. The use of potentially inappropriate medications among the Lithuanian elderly according to Beers and EU (7)-PIM list—A nationwide cross-sectional study on reimbursement claims data. *J. Clin. Pharm. Ther.* **2017**, *42*, 195–200. [CrossRef] [PubMed]
4. Stegemann, S.; Ecker, F.; Maio, M.; Kraahs, P.; Wohlfart, R.; Breitkreutz, J.; Zimmer, A.; Bar-Shalom, D.; Hettrich, P.; Broegmann, B. Geriatric drug therapy: Neglecting the inevitable majority. *Ageing Res. Rev.* **2010**, *9*, 384–398. [CrossRef]
5. Martins, I.D.S. Deprescribing no idoso. *Rev. Port. Clínica Geral* **2013**, *29*, 66–69. [CrossRef]
6. Lee, E.A.; Brettler, J.W.; Kanter, M.H.; Steinberg, S.G.; Khang, P.; Distasio, C.C.; Martin, J.; Dreskin, M.; Thompson, N.H.; Cotter, T.M.; et al. Refining the Definition of Polypharmacy and Its Link to Disability in Older Adults: Conceptualizing Necessary Polypharmacy, Unnecessary Polypharmacy, and Polypharmacy of Unclear Benefit. *Perm. J.* **2020**, *24*. [CrossRef]
7. Davies, E.A.; O'Mahony, M.S. Adverse drug reactions in special populations—The elderly. *Br. J. Clin. Pharm.* **2015**, *80*, 796–807. [CrossRef] [PubMed]
8. Gurwitz, J.H. Polypharmacy: A new paradigm for quality drug therapy in the elderly? *Arch. Intern. Med.* **2004**, *164*, 1957–1959. [CrossRef] [PubMed]
9. Thake, M.; Lowry, A. A systematic review of trends in the selective exclusion of older participant from randomised clinical trials. *Arch. Gerontol. Geriatr.* **2017**, *72*, 99–102. [CrossRef] [PubMed]
10. WHO Collaborating Centre for Drug Statistics Methodology—ATC/DDD. Available online: https://www.whocc.no/atc_ddd_index/ (accessed on 2 February 2021).
11. Chocano-Bedoya, P.O.; Bischoff-Ferrari, H.A. *DO-HEALTH: Vitamin D3-Omega-3-Home Exercise-Healthy Aging and Longevity Trial—Dietary Patterns in Five European Countries*; Springer: Cham, Switzerland, 2019.
12. Gutierrez Valencia, M.; Martinez Velilla, N.; Lacalle Fabo, E.; Beobide Telleria, I.; Larrayoz Sola, B.; Tosato, M. Interventions to optimize pharmacologic treatment in hospitalized older adults: A systematic review. *Rev. Clin. Esp.* **2016**, *216*, 205–221. [CrossRef] [PubMed]
13. Abegaz, T.M.; Birru, E.M.; Mekonnen, G.B. Potentially inappropriate prescribing in Ethiopian geriatric patients hospitalized with cardiovascular disorders using START/STOPP criteria. *PLoS ONE* **2018**, *13*, e0195949. [CrossRef] [PubMed]
14. Hernandez Martin, J.; Merino-sanjuán, V.; Peris-martí, J.; Correa-ballester, M.; Vial-escolano, R.; Merino-sanjuán, M. Applicability of the STOPP/START criteria to older polypathological patients in a long-term care hospital. *Eur. J. Hosp. Pharm.* **2018**, *25*, 310–316. [CrossRef] [PubMed]
15. Renom-Guiteras, A.; Meyer, G.; Thurmann, P.A. The EU(7)-PIM list: A list of potentially inappropriate medications for older people consented by experts from seven European countries. *Eur. J. Clin. Pharm.* **2015**, *71*, 861–875. [CrossRef]

16. Fahrni, M.L.; Azmy, M.T.; Usir, E.; Aziz, N.A.; Hassan, Y. Inappropriate prescribing defined by STOPP and START criteria and its association with adverse drug events among hospitalized older patients: A multicentre, prospective study. *PLoS ONE* **2019**, *14*, e0219898. [CrossRef] [PubMed]
17. O'Connor, M.N.; Gallagher, P.; Byrne, S.; O'Mahony, D. Adverse drug reactions in older patients during hospitalisation: Are they predictable? *Age Ageing* **2012**, *41*, 771–776. [CrossRef] [PubMed]
18. Blanc, A.L.; Spasojevic, S.; Leszek, A.; Théodoloz, M.; Bonnabry, P.; Fumeaux, T.; Schaad, N. A comparison of two tools to screen potentially inappropriate medication in internal medicine patients. *J. Clin. Pharm. Ther.* **2018**, *43*, 232–239. [CrossRef] [PubMed]
19. Ma, Z.; Zhang, C.; Cui, X.; Liu, L. Comparison of three criteria for potentially inappropriate medications in chinese older adults. *Clin. Interv. Aging* **2019**, *14*, 65–72. [CrossRef] [PubMed]
20. Roller-Wirnsberger, R.; Thurner, B.; Pucher, C.; Lindner, S.; Wirnsberger, G.H. The clinical and therapeutic challenge of treating older patients in clinical practice. *Br. J. Clin. Pharmacol.* **2020**, *86*, 1904–1911. [CrossRef] [PubMed]
21. Reeve, E.; Gnjidic, D.; Long, J.; Hilmer, S. A systematic review of the emerging definition of 'deprescribing' with network analysis: Implications for future research and clinical practice. *Br. J. Clin. Pharmacol.* **2015**, *80*, 1254–1268. [CrossRef] [PubMed]

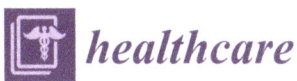

Article

Factors Facilitating and Hindering Development of a Medication Use Review Service in Eastern Europe and Iran-Cross-Sectional Exploratory Study

Anita Tuula [1,*], Daisy Volmer [1], Liisa Jõhvik [2], Ieva Rutkovska [3], Indre Trečiokienė [4], Piotr Merks [5], Magdalena Waszyk-Nowaczyk [6], Mariola Drozd [7], Alena Tatarević [8], Maja Radovanlija [9], Carmen Pacadi [10], Arijana Meštrović [11], Réka Viola [12], Gyöngyvér Soós [12], Cristina Rais [13], Adriana-Elena Táerel [13], Magdalena Kuzelova [14], Marziyeh Zare [15], Payam Peymani [16], Marje Oona [17] and Michael Scott [18]

1. Institute of Pharmacy, University of Tartu, 50411 Tartu, Estonia; daisy.volmer@ut.ee
2. Hospital Pharmacy, Tartu University Hospital, 50406 Tartu, Estonia; liisa.johvik@kliinikum.ee
3. Faculty of Pharmacy, Riga Stradins University, LV-1007 Riga, Latvia; ieva.rutkovska@gmail.com
4. Pharmacy Center, Faculty of Medicine, Vilnius University, 01513 Vilnius, Lithuania; indre.treciokiene@mf.vu.lt
5. Department of Pharmacology and Clinical Pharmacology, Faculty of Medicine, Collegium Medicum, Cardinal Stefan Wyszyński University in Warsaw, 01-938 Warsaw, Poland; p.merks@uksw.edu.pl
6. Department of Pharmaceutical Technology, Pharmacy Practice Division, Poznan University of Medical Sciences, 60-780 Poznan, Poland; mwaszyk@ump.edu.pl
7. Department of Humanities and Social Medicine, Medical University of Lublin, 20-093 Lublin, Poland; marioladrozd@umlub.pl
8. Istrian Pharmacies, 52100 Pula, Croatia; tatarevic.app@gmail.com
9. Pharmacy Rajić, 34000 Požega, Croatia; radovanlija.maja@gmail.com
10. Mandis Pharm Community Pharmacies, 10000 Zagreb, Croatia; carmenpacadi@gmail.com
11. Pharma Expert Consultancy and Education, 10040 Zagreb, Croatia; arijana.mestrovic@pharmaexpert.hr
12. Faculty of Pharmacy, University of Szeged, H-6720 Szeged, Hungary; tothne.viola.reka@szte.hu (R.V.); SoosGyongyver@szte.hu (G.S.)
13. Faculty of Pharmacy, Carol Davila University of Medicine and Pharmacy, 020956 Bucharest, Romania; cristina_rais@yahoo.com (C.R.); adriana.taerel@yahoo.com (A.-E.T.)
14. Department of Pharmacology and Toxicology, Faculty of Pharmacy, Comenius University in Bratislava, 83232 Bratislava, Slovakia; kuzelova@fpharm.uniba.sk
15. Health Policy Research Center, Institute of Health, Shiraz University of Medical Sciences, Shiraz 7134845794, Iran; marziyeh.zare70@gmail.com
16. Rady Faculty of Health Sciences, College of Pharmacy, University of Manitoba, Winnipeg, MB R3E 0T5, Canada; peymani.payam@gmail.com
17. Institute of Family Medicine and Public Health, University of Tartu, 50411 Tartu, Estonia; marje.oona@ut.ee
18. Medicines Optimisation Innovation Centre, Antrim BT41 2RL, UK; drmichael.scott@northerntrust.hscni.net
* Correspondence: anita.tuula@ut.ee; Tel.: +372-7375-286

Abstract: Polypharmacy is a common issue in patients with chronic diseases. Eastern-European countries and Iran are exploring possibilities for implementing the Medication Use Review (MUR) as a measure for optimizing medication use and ensuring medication safety in polypharmacy patients. The aim of this study was to gain insights into the development of the community pharmacy sector and map facilitators and barriers of MUR in Eastern Europe and Iran. The representatives of the framework countries received a questionnaire on community pharmacy sector indicators, current and future developments of pharmacies, and factors encouraging and hindering MUR. To answer the questionnaire, all representatives performed document analysis, literature review, and qualitative interviews with key stakeholders. The socio-ecological model was used for inductive thematic analysis of the identified factors. Current community pharmacist competencies in framework countries were more related to traditional pharmacy services. Main facilitators of MUR were increase in polypharmacy and pharmaceutical waste, and access to patients' electronic list of medications by pharmacists. Main barriers included the service being unfamiliar, lack of funding and private consultation areas. Pharmacists in the framework countries are well-placed to provide MUR, however, the service needs more introduction and barriers mostly on organizational and public policy levels must be addressed.

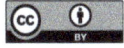

Keywords: MUR; medication review; barriers; pharmacist; community pharmacy

1. Introduction

In older patients with multiple chronic diseases, polypharmacy and drug-related problems are increasingly serious concerns. Polypharmacy patients have an increased risk of experiencing adverse drug reactions, geriatric syndromes, morbidity, and decreased medication adherence. Polypharmacy patients also receive inappropriate medications more frequently [1]. Although polypharmacy is often necessary, it is important to differentiate inappropriate polypharmacy, which occurs when the patient is receiving medication without an evidence-based indication, their medicines fail to achieve therapeutic goals, they experience or have a high risk of experiencing adverse drug reactions or they are not able to properly take their medications [2].

To support appropriate polypharmacy and ensure medication safety, many pharmacist-led services have been developed worldwide. Pharmacist-led medication review (MR) is a structured evaluation of a patient's medicines for detecting drug-related problems and recommending interventions with the aim of optimizing medicine use and improving health outcomes [3]. MR services have been shown to improve medication awareness including improved medication adherence and decreased drug-related problems [4–6]. The latter is particularly important, as adverse drug events are the 14th leading cause of patient morbidity and mortality globally with a substantial proportion of such medication-related harm being avoidable [2]. Although the effect of MR on mortality, hospitalizations, length of stay in hospital, emergency department visits, readmissions, physician visits, and healthcare utilization needs more evidence [4,7,8], the World Health Organization in their 2019 report has considered it to be one of the key steps for assuring medication safety in polypharmacy [2].

Different types of MR services such as medication therapy management, home medicines review and medicines use review have been offered by community pharmacists in United States of America, Australia, New Zealand, and United Kingdom for many years [9–12]. By 2017, 19 of 34 European countries were offering a MR service and it has been recognized as one of the most commonly provided advanced pharmacist-led cognitive service in Europe [13]. Eastern European countries have historically been more focused on traditional services as dispensing, compounding, and counselling regarding medication use. Existing extended services mainly include point-of-care tests (e.g., taking blood pressure) and are focused on complementing the traditional pharmacy service rather than expanding pharmacists' role in the broader healthcare system [14]. However, there have been some earlier attempts at applying an MR service in Bulgaria, Croatia, Czech Republic and Hungary [14,15].

One of the first Eastern-European countries to provide a nationally approved and funded MR service in community pharmacies was Slovenia in 2015 [13,16]. In relation to this service barriers to its provision were identified as lack of time in the pharmacy setting and recognition of the service by patients, physicians and health care payers. Positive patient feedback and extension of professional role were recognized as MR facilitators [16]. The main barriers to implementing MR identified in other studies have mostly been connected to pharmacy workflow, staffing issues, lack of access to patient's clinical information and cooperation with other healthcare specialists [9,17,18].

2. Aim

The aim of this study was to map and analyze healthcare and pharmacy sector indicators facilitating and hindering provision of the Medication Use Review (MUR) service in Eastern-European countries and Iran.

3. Materials and Methods

Background information: In September 2017, a working group of pharmacists, general practitioners, and key stakeholders from both healthcare and the pharmacy sector was established in Estonia with the aim of developing a standard for the MUR service and identify possibilities for the implementation of the above-mentioned service. In 2018 the Estonian MR standard was adapted and amended from the 2013 Pharmaceutical Care Network Europe statement for medication review [19]. The adapted standard includes three levels of MR:

1. Simple MUR conducted in a community pharmacy by a community pharmacist; the pharmacist receives information about the medication regimen and patient's diseases from the patient in a face-to-face interview and their general practitioner (GP); the service focuses on educating the patient on their diseases and medicines and detecting issues related to medication adherence and manifested drug related problems.
2. Comprehensive MR conducted in a community pharmacy by a community pharmacist who has passed an additional course in clinical pharmacy; additionally, requires information on the clinical test results from the GP as the pharmacist also evaluates the medication list for potential drug related problems.
3. MR service provided by a clinical pharmacist in the hospital setting; the clinical pharmacist additionally gets involved in establishing the treatment regimen for the patient [20].

In January 2019, the MUR pilot project started in Estonia and in March the international MUR network consisting of 11 countries (Estonia, Latvia, Lithuania, Poland, Croatia, Bosnia and Herzegovina, Hungary, Romania, Bulgaria, Slovakia and Iran) was launched to look further at the opportunities for advancing the MUR service on the first level according to the adapted standard, which can also be considered Type 2 MR according to Hatah et al. 2014 meta-analysis [21].

Study instrument: In September 2019, representatives of all 11 MUR framework countries received a study instrument compiled by researchers and practicing pharmacists from Estonia and consisting of the following questions:

- Country indicators: total population, gross national income per capita, life expectancy at birth male/female, quality life years male/female, total expenditure on health as percentage of gross domestic product—GDP (%), pharmaceutical spending as a percentage of health spending (%); share of population aged 65 and over (%), long term illness in elderly population (%).
- Pharmacy sector indicators: number of community pharmacies; number of community pharmacists; number of assistant pharmacists at community pharmacies.
- Current and future competencies and roles of community pharmacists; recent and future developments in community pharmacies.
- Factors which are facilitators and barriers to MUR.

To complete the questionnaire, the representatives of the MUR network were asked to use existing information and data sources specifically: literature review, document analysis and qualitative interviewing of key stakeholders (representatives of governmental institutions, professional organizations and higher education institutions providing pharmacy education). Interviews were conducted to answer the third and fourth question and were recorded by written notes. In May 2021, all representatives were asked for follow-up details on recent developments in the pharmacy sector and pharmacist's role. Ethics committee approval was not sought for this type of research, as the data collected for the study are not sensitive personal information, nor were any interventions conducted on the study participants. All participants were informed their answers will be used in the study and their anonymity will be guaranteed prior to the interviews.

Data analysis: the parameters of pharmacy sector and country indicators for Iran were different from the Eastern-European framework countries and thus were not included in equations for expenditure on health, share of elderly population and community pharmacy sector indicators.

The social ecological model (SEM) including individual, interpersonal, institutional/organizational, public policy, and social domains [22] was adapted and used for the inductive thematic analysis to identify which are the main factors currently affecting pharmacists in providing the service and on what level these factors need to be addressed. SEM analysis was used for all factors that were detected by at least two framework countries. The standards for reporting qualitative research (SRQR) were used for reporting the research results [23].

4. Results

Answers were collected in November 2019 from nine out of the eleven framework countries namely Croatia, Estonia, Latvia, Lithuania, Hungary, Poland, Iran, Slovakia and Romania.

4.1. Profile of Participant Countries

An overview of the country profiles is shown in Table 1. The average expenditure on health as a percentage of GDP in Eastern-Europe framework countries is 6.2%, being highest in Hungary (7.2%) and lowest in Poland (4.9%); Iran is slightly differing from others at 8.1% and has not been included in the equations. The share of elderly people in Eastern-European framework countries range between 15.5–23.5%, and roughly around 50–80% of them have at least one long-term illness (data of four network countries). The number of inhabitants per pharmacy ranges from 1822 to 4237 in Eastern-European countries, being on average 2880; Iran again differs with 7005 inhabitants per pharmacy. The average number of pharmacists per community pharmacy is 2.2 and the average number of assistant pharmacists per community pharmacy is 1.9 in Eastern-European framework countries.

Table 1. Profile of MUR framework countries.

	Croatia	Estonia	Hungary	Iran	Latvia	Lithuania	Poland	Romania	Slovakia
Population	4,130,000	1,326,000	9,685,000	82,914,000	1,908,000	2,760,000	37,888,000	19,365,000	5,457,000
GNI per capita (PPP $)	30,680	39,070	34,020	12,950	32,540	38,530	33,770	32,850	32,920
Life expectancy in years (m/f)	75/81	74/83	72/79	N/A	70/80	71/81	74/82	72/79	74/81
Quality life years (m/f)	N/A	54/59	59/60	N/A	50.6/52.2	56/60	N/A	59/59	56.4/57.0
Total expenditure on health, % of GDP	6.8	6.7	7.2	8.1	5.9	6.4	4.9	5	6.7
Pharmaceutical spending, % of health spending	23.3	18.2	22	N/A	27.4	29.1	N/A	20–22	26.4
Share of population aged over 65 (%)	19.6	19.4	23.5	6.1	20.0	19.6	18.2	19	15.5
Long term illness in elderly (%)	N/A	81.5 *	N/A	N/A	60 **	53.2 *	N/A	N/A	69.7 *
Number of community pharmacies	1181	495	2286	11,836	776	1515	12,286	9300	1716
Number of community pharmacists	2884 ***	894	5571	19,680	1591	2721	26,022	22,500	4183
Number of assistant pharmacists	2872 ****	774	7200	-	1284	1900	33,297	10,000	2304

* Data on patients aged 65 and above. ** Data on patients aged 60 and above. *** As number of MPharm working in health care system. **** As number of pharmacists technicians working in health care system. GNI—gross national income, PPP—purchasing power parity; m/f—male/female, N/A—not available.

4.2. Current Competencies of Community Pharmacists

Current competencies and roles of community pharmacists in all MUR framework countries include dispensing and counselling of prescription and over-the-counter medicines and compounding of extemporaneous medicines. Pharmacists also offer reporting or patient assistance in reporting adverse drug reactions, and patient education on disease prevention and maintenance of health in most framework countries. Usually, some point-of-care testing is provided (most common services named were blood pressure measurement, cholesterol, blood sugar and hemoglobin). In Lithuania, community pharmacists are offering an asthma management service and patient education on inhaler use techniques. In Croatia, pharmacists are improving patients' medication adherence by counselling service and sorting patients' medicines into weekly dispensers, and recently started dispensing biological therapies and counseling patients regarding their safe and proper use.

4.3. Future Competencies

Most often named future competencies of community pharmacists in framework countries were provision of extended services such as MR, influenza vaccination, diabetes screening, smoking cessation, international normalized ratio (INR) measurements, and new medicines service. Additionally, in Poland, performing simple diagnostic tests such as blood pressure monitoring, cholesterol and glucose measurements is expected to be a future competency.

4.4. Recent Developments and Future Plans

The primary recent development in the pharmacy sector for Estonia and Hungary was the ownership reform of community pharmacies and prohibition of vertical integration between wholesale and retail sale of medicines. Recent development for Romania includes an online pharmacy which dispenses over-the-counter medicines and parapharmaceuticals. For Poland, the recent development would be introduction of an E-Prescribing system.

Both Croatia and Estonia have been actively participating in the development of the electronic cross-border health services, which allows continuity of care for EU citizens while travelling abroad in EU. By 2021, both countries have implemented the electronic cross-border e-prescription system and are one of the first countries to do so.

Croatian working group also named several new regulations in pharmacy policies as a future development and by 2021, Croatian government has proposed the National Recovery and Resilience Plan for 2021–2026 which includes monitoring the outcomes of outpatient treatment and controlling and preventing medicine shortages in community pharmacies.

Future plans for Iran include an E-Prescribing system reaching everywhere in the country. In Lithuania, it was planned to introduce a state-run pharmacy network where state-owned hospital pharmacies would have outpatient departments to fulfil community pharmacy duties.

4.5. Factors Facilitating and Hindering MUR Development

In the project countries, the most often cited factors that were facilitating MUR were increase in polypharmacotherapy and pharmaceutical waste and access to an electronic list of medicines and medical records by pharmacists. The most often reported barriers were the service being unfamiliar to both physicians and pharmacists, the financing model of MUR, high workload in pharmacies and lack of private consultation rooms for MUR service in some community pharmacies. The SEM analysis detects which factors are currently facilitating or hindering the implementation of MUR in the practice of a community pharmacist. For the SEM analysis of facilitators and barriers, see Table 2.

Table 2. SEM for factors facilitating and hindering MUR service and the number of framework countries who detected the factor.

Domain	Barriers	Facilitators
First level individual	MUR service is not familiar to pharmacists (9) Lack of motivation in pharmacists (2)	Increased understanding about the importance and effectiveness of MUR service among pharmacists (3) Improved knowledge of pharmacists and physicians about the newest guidelines for pharmacotherapy and MUR service (2)
Second level intrapersonal	MUR service is not familiar to physicians (9) Insufficient collaboration between GPs and pharmacists (2)	Enhanced collaboration between healthcare professionals (3) Increased understanding about the importance and effectiveness of MUR service among physicians (3) Enhanced relations between pharmacists and patients (2) Development of the pharmacist role in the healthcare team (2)
Third level organizational/institutional	Lack of private rooms and electronic resources in community pharmacies (7) Service standard needs further development (7) High workload of pharmacists (6)	Developed MUR service tool (3)
Fourth level public policy	Financing model for the MUR service (8) Limited access to patient data for pharmacists (3) Pharmacists have no central system for documentation of patient data and pharmacist interventions (3)	Access to an electronic list of medicines and medical records or electronic prescriptions by pharmacists (5)
Fifth level society	MUR is unfamiliar to patients (3)	Increase in polypharmacotherapy and pharmaceutical waste (8) Increase in population ageing and number of patients with chronic illness (2) The results of MUR can support the development of new aspects in pharmacotherapy such as personalized medicines (2) MUR program can increase the adherence of patients to therapies as they can better understand the disease and medication (2)

5. Discussion

The development of the pharmacy sector in Eastern Europe and Iran could be considered similar. Pharmacist competencies mostly include providing traditional services such as dispensing, consulting and compounding, and there has been little development in pharmacist role regarding extended services so far. Thus, the barriers and facilitators of MUR service for the community pharmacist in these countries can be described jointly.

In framework countries, the initiative to introduce MUR has come from academics and active pharmacists, who understand that both polypharmacotherapy and pharmaceutical waste are serious concerns in the region, which have not been properly addressed by government institutions [24]. For comparison, the initiative to start providing Medicines Use Review in the United Kingdom as a nationally funded extended pharmacy service came from the National Health Service in 2005. The service was applied as a national approach to reduce health care costs, improve patients' management of their medicines and to introduced patient-centered services in community pharmacies [25,26]. The SEM analysis indicates that one of the most important barriers to the MUR service in Eastern Europe and Iran is the lack of support from policy makers. Key factors such as financing the service, creating a central system for documenting pharmacists' interventions, and allowing access to patient data necessary for providing MUR can only be solved on a national level.

Funding the service could prove to be difficult to overcome, as the average expenditure on healthcare in Eastern Europe and Iran is lower than the European Union average of 9.9% in all framework countries [27]. This might indicate that governments are less likely to fund healthcare as a sector and thus not support the provision of national remuneration for MUR. Currently there was no funding for the pilot project in Eastern Europe and Iran, which was considered one of the main barriers to the work by eight out of nine framework countries. The provision of MUR takes time and effort; hence the service could not be offered routinely without remuneration.

Access to digital records of the patient's medications is vital in order to be able to offer the MUR service and has been cited as a prime encouraging factor in previously published literature [28]. In some framework countries, these data are not available to the pharmacist. Although MUR could be provided by only accessing data that the GP and the patient have decided to share, it is not an ideal solution for providing the service long term, as the initiative for service must always come from the GP. A central documentation system for pharmacists' interventions would support the service, as effectively communicating MUR results to the patient's GP is important for achieving the best health outcomes.

The COVID-19 pandemic might have encouraged implementing pharmacist-led extended services on the public policy level in some countries. As an example, Polish community pharmacists can now independently prescribe medicines to themselves and their own family members [29].

One of the main barriers to MUR at the organizational level is the high workload of pharmacists. This issue could be solved by hiring more pharmacists, although the structure of the pharmacy sector in framework countries does not support this solution. In most framework countries, the number of patients per community pharmacy is rather low, while there are few pharmacists per community pharmacies. The large number of community pharmacies might hinder the development of MUR considering that it would therefore be difficult to find the additional workforce necessary for the extended services.

Other important organizational factors include lack of private rooms and electronic resources such as computers in community pharmacies. Community pharmacy owners might be more willing to invest in solving these organizational problems if the service received national remuneration. However, previous research has shown that lack of pharmacy staff, prioritization of other clinical activities and dissatisfaction with the consultation area seem to be persistent issues even in countries where MR has been funded [9,17,30].

Pharmacy chains have been known to promote implementing extended services such as MUR, especially with national funding. Promotion of MUR by pharmacy chains, however, contributes to the quality of the service being more questionable in the eyes of other healthcare professionals [9]. Some framework countries have recently applied restrictions to pharmacy ownership or are planning to establish a state-run pharmacy network. These changes could influence determining the national implementation but also the status of the service in the future.

Insufficient collaboration between general practitioners and pharmacists was reported as a barrier by only two framework countries. For the pilot in Eastern Europe and Iran, motivated and supportive physicians were included early on, which might have caused the misconception that opposition to the service by general practitioners would not be an issue. In previously published literature, lack of collaboration between healthcare professionals is often highlighted as one of the main barriers [9,17,30]. To address this potential issue, interprofessional education and collaborative practice between different healthcare workers, namely physicians, pharmacists, and nurses, could be developed much further in the framework countries, as earlier experience of working together can also support MR services [31].

MUR is still unfamiliar to many pharmacists and other health professionals, who could direct their patients to receive the service. More pharmacists need to provide MUR in order to normalize the service in the health sector. It is important for health workers to understand the potential benefits and have a positive experience with MUR to refer their patients to the service routinely. Thorough introduction is necessary for effective implementation of MUR in the framework countries.

According to the international vision and policy, the provision of professional services should be a priority for pharmacies and health systems. As with other health innovations, the implementation of professional pharmacy services is complex and represents an area in which pharmacy in the community has had limited experience [32]. Skills in areas such as leadership, task delegation, goal setting and teamwork seem equally important to pharmacists' clinical skills when it comes to integrating a new service into everyday practice. IT tools for data collection, legal support, training, and education, are just some of the drivers (or barriers) to change [33].

6. Conclusions

Key stakeholders in Eastern Europe and Iran are exploring the possibilities to apply extended pharmacy services such as MUR into practice. As an increase in polypharmacotherapy and pharmaceutical waste are increasing concerns in MUR framework countries, it is important to routinely assess patients' medication use. More health professionals need to be introduced to MUR and interprofessional practice which supports pharmacists working together with GPs. Pharmacists are in many ways well placed to provide MUR; however, it is necessary to gain government support and financing for the service in Eastern Europe and Iran. Several organizational barriers such as high workload and lack of private consultation rooms, as well of the lack of standards for the service need to be addressed for continuing with MUR.

Author Contributions: Conceptualization, D.V. and L.J.; methodology, D.V. and A.T. (Anita Tuula); data collection, D.V., L.J., I.R., I.T., P.M., M.W.-N., M.D., A.T. (Alena Tatarević), M.R., C.P., A.M., R.V., G.S., C.R., A.-E.T., M.K., M.Z. and P.P.; formal analysis, A.T. (Anita Tuula); data curation D.V., A.T. (Anita Tuula); writing—original draft preparation, A.T. (Anita Tuula), D.V., M.O., M.S.; writing— review and editing, all authors; visualization A.T. (Anita Tuula); supervision, D.V., M.O., M.S.; project administration, D.V. and A.T. (Anita Tuula); funding acquisition, D.V. All authors have read and agreed to the published version of the manuscript.

Funding: European Association of Faculties of Pharmacy PRD 2019 grant for the project "Development and Implementation of Medication Use Review Services at Community Pharmacy in Eastern European countries".

Institutional Review Board Statement: Ethical review and approval were waived for this study, due to the nature of the study. The current study did not include any interventions nor collection of personal data. All participants were aware their answers would be used anonymously for the study and were free to not participate.

Informed Consent Statement: Informed consent was obtained from all participants involved in the study.

Data Availability Statement: Data is contained within the article.

Acknowledgments: We acknowledge Elita Poplavska for initiating the project and contributing to data collection in Latvia.

Conflicts of Interest: The authors declare no conflict of interest.

References

1. Hajjar, E.R.; Cafiero, A.C.; Hanlon, J.T. Polypharmacy in elderly patients. *Am. J. Geriatr. Pharmacother.* **2007**, *5*, 345–351. [CrossRef]
2. World Health Organization. Medication Safety in Polypharmacy: Technical Report. 2019. Available online: https://www.who.int/publications/i/item/medication-safety-in-polypharmacy-technical-report (accessed on 7 February 2021).
3. Griese-Mammen, N.; Hersberger, K.E.; Messerli, M.; Leikola, S.; Horvat, N.; van Mil, J.W.F.; Kos, M. PCNE definition of medication review: Reaching agreement. *Int. J. Clin. Pharm.* **2018**, *40*, 1199–1208. [CrossRef]
4. Huiskes, V.J.; Burger, D.M.; van den Ende, C.H.; van den Bemt, B.J. Effectiveness of medication review: A systematic review and meta-analysis of randomized controlled trials. *BMC Fam. Pract.* **2017**, *18*, 5. [CrossRef]
5. Ali, P.S.; Mishra, A.; Palaksha, S.; Nataraj, B.R.; Kumar, M.B. Impact of Home Medication Review (HMR) Services on Medication Adherence in Elderly Population of Mysore. *Int. J. Ther.* **2018**, *1*, 39–43.
6. Hatah, E.; Tordoff, J.; Duffull, S.B.; Cameron, C.; Braund, R. Retrospective examination of selected outcomes of Medicines Use Review (MUR) services in New Zealand. *Int. J. Clin. Pharm.* **2014**, *36*, 503–512. [CrossRef]
7. Guisado-Gil, A.B.; Mejías-Trueba, M.; Alfaro-Lara, E.R.; Sánchez-Hidalgo, M.; Ramírez-Duque, N.; Santos-Rubio, M.D. Impact of medication reconciliation on health outcomes: An overview of systematic reviews. *Res. Soc. Adm. Pharm.* **2020**, *16*, 995–1002. [CrossRef]
8. Anderson, L.J.; Schnipper, J.L.; Nuckols, T.K.; Shane, R.; Sarkisian, C.; Le, M.M.; Pevnick, J.M. A systematic overview of systematic reviews evaluating interventions addressing polypharmacy. *Am. J. Health Syst. Pharm.* **2019**, *76*, 1777–1787. [CrossRef] [PubMed]
9. Bradley, F.; Wagner, A.C.; Elvey, R.; Noyce, P.R.; Ashcroft, D.M. Determinants of the uptake of medicines use reviews (MURs) by community pharmacies in England: A multi-method study. *Health Policy* **2008**, *88*, 258–268. [CrossRef] [PubMed]
10. Chen, T.F. Pharmacist-led home medicines review and residential medication management review: The Australian model. *Drugs Aging* **2016**, *33*, 199–204. [CrossRef] [PubMed]
11. Ramalho de Oliveira, D.; Brummel, A.R.; Miller, D.B. Medication Therapy Management: 10 Years of Experience in a Large Integrated Health Care System. *J. Manag. Care Pharm.* **2010**, *16*, 185–195. [CrossRef]
12. Lee, E.; Braund, R.; Tordoff, J. Examining the first year of Medicines Use Review services provided by pharmacists in New Zealand. *N. Z. Med. J.* **2009**, *122*, 1293.
13. Soares, I.B.; Imfeld-Isenegger, T.L.; Makovec, U.N.; Horvat, N.; Kos, M.; Arnet, I.; Hersberger, K.E.; Costa, F.A. A survey to assess the availability, implementation rate and remuneration of pharmacist-led cognitive services throughout Europe. *Res. Soc. Adm. Pharm.* **2020**, *16*, 41–47. [CrossRef] [PubMed]
14. European Expertise Centre for Pharmacy Education and Training. Country Profiles. Available online: https://eec-pet.eu/pharmacy-education/country-profiles/ (accessed on 16 December 2020).
15. Bulajeva, A.; Labberton, L.; Leikola, S.; Pohjanoksa-Mäntylä, M.; Geurts, M.M.E.; De Gier, J.J.; Airaksinen, M. Medication review practices in European countries. *Res. Soc. Adm. Pharm.* **2014**, *10*, 731–740. [CrossRef]
16. Nabergoj Makovec, U.; Kos, M.; Pisk, N. Community pharmacists' perspectives on implementation of Medicines Use Review in Slovenia. *Int. J. Clin. Pharm.* **2018**, *40*, 1180–1188. [CrossRef]
17. Cardwell, K.; Hughes, C.M.; Ryan, C. Community pharmacists' views of using a screening tool to structure medicines use reviews for older people: Findings from qualitative interviews. *Int. J. Clin. Pharm.* **2018**, *40*, 1086–1095. [CrossRef]
18. Dolovich, L.; Consiglio, G.; MacKeigan, L.; Abrahamyan, L.; Pechlivanoglou, P.; Rac, V.E.; Pojskic, N.; Bojarski, E.A.; Su, J.; Krahn, M.; et al. Uptake of the MedsCheck annual medication review service in Ontario community pharmacies between 2007 and 2013. *Can. Pharm. J. Rev. Des Pharm. Du Can.* **2016**, *149*, 293–302. [CrossRef]
19. PCNE Statement on Medication Review. 2013. Available online: https://www.pcne.org/upload/files/150_20160504_PCNE_MedRevtypes.pdf (accessed on 8 March 2019).
20. Volmer, D.; Randmäe, L. Mis on ravimite kasutamise hindamise teenus? *Apteek Täna* **2018**, *1*, 37–42.
21. Hatah, E.; Braund, R.; Tordoff, J.; Duffull, S.B. A systematic review and meta-analysis of pharmacist-led fee-for-services medication review. *Br. J. Clin. Pharmacol.* **2014**, *77*, 102–115. [CrossRef]
22. Kilanowski, J.F. Breadth of the socio-ecological model. *J. Agromed.* **2017**, *22*, 295–297. [CrossRef] [PubMed]
23. Standards for Reporting Qualitative Research. Available online: https://journals.lww.com/academicmedicine/fulltext/2014/09000/Standards_for_Reporting_Qualitative_Research___A.21.aspx (accessed on 21 May 2021).
24. Sepp, K.; Tuula, A.; Bobrova, V.; Volmer, D. Primary health care policy and vision for community pharmacy and pharmacists in Estonia. *Pharm Pract.* **2021**, *19*, 2404.

25. Bellingham, C. SEP 2004 TPJ. PJ Online. Contract 2005: What the new contract has in store. *Pharm. J.* **2004**, *273*, 385. Available online: https://www.pharmaceutical-journal.com/pj-online-contract-2005-what-the-new-contract-has-in-store/20012846.article (accessed on 22 December 2020).
26. Latif, A.; Pollock, K.; Boardman, H.F. The contribution of the Medicines Use Review (MUR) consultation to counseling practice in community pharmacies. *Patient Educ. Couns.* **2011**, *83*, 336–344. [CrossRef]
27. Healthcare Expenditure Statistics—Statistics Explained. Available online: https://ec.europa.eu/eurostat/statistics-explained/index.php/Healthcare_expenditure_statistics (accessed on 16 December 2020).
28. Uhl, M.C.; Muth, C.; Gerlach, F.M.; Schoch, G.-G.; Müller, B.S. Patient-perceived barriers and facilitators to the implementation of a medication review in primary care: A qualitative thematic analysis. *BMC Fam. Pract.* **2018**, *19*, 3. [CrossRef] [PubMed]
29. Merks, P.; Jakubowska, M.; Drelich, E.; Świeczkowski, D.; Bogusz, J.; Bilmin, K.; Sola, K.F.; May, A.; Majchrowska, A.; Koziol, M.; et al. The legal extension of the role of pharmacists in light of the COVID-19 global pandemic. *Res. Soc. Adm. Pharm.* **2021**, *17*, 1807–1812. [CrossRef] [PubMed]
30. Latif, A.; Pollock, K.; Boardman, H.F. Medicines use reviews: A potential resource or lost opportunity for general practice? *BMC Fam. Pract.* **2013**, *14*, 57. [CrossRef] [PubMed]
31. Chen, T.F.; de Almeida Neto, A.C. Exploring elements of interprofessional collaboration between pharmacists and physicians in medication review. *Pharm. World Sci.* **2007**, *29*, 574–576. [CrossRef]
32. Garcia-Cardenas, V.; Benrimoj, S.I.; Ocampo, C.C.; Goyenechea, E.; Martinez–Martinez, F.; Gastelurrutia, M.A. Evaluation of the implementation process and outcomes of a professional pharmacy service in a community pharmacy setting. A case report. *Res. Soc. Adm. Pharm.* **2017**, *13*, 614–627. [CrossRef]
33. Roberts, A.S.; Benrimoj, S.I.; Chen, T.F.; Williams, K.A.; Aslani, P. Practice change in community pharmacy: Quantification of facilitators. *Ann. Pharmacother.* **2008**, *42*, 861–868. [CrossRef]

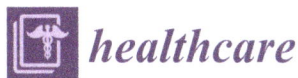

Article

Analysis of the Consumption of Non-Oncological Medicines: A Methodological Study on Patients of the Ada Cohort

Giulio Barigelletti [1,*], Giovanna Tagliabue [1], Sabrina Fabiano [1], Annalisa Trama [2], Alice Bernasconi [2], Claudio Tresoldi [1], Viviana Perotti [1], Andrea Tittarelli [1] and Ada Working Group [†]

[1] Cancer Registry Unit, Fondazione IRCCS Istituto Nazionale dei Tumori, Via Venezian 1, 20133 Milan, Italy; giovanna.tagliabue@istitutotumori.mi.it (G.T.); sabrina.fabiano@istitutotumori.mi.it (S.F.); claudio.tresoldi@istitutotumori.mi.it (C.T.); viviana.perotti@istitutotumori.mi.it (V.P.); andrea.tittarelli@istitutotumori.mi.it (A.T.)

[2] Evaluative Epidemiology Unit, Fondazione IRCCS Istituto Nazionale dei Tumori, Via Venezian 1, 20133 Milan, Italy; annalisa.trama@istitutotumori.mi.it (A.T.); alice.bernasconi@istitutotumori.mi.it (A.B.)

* Correspondence: giulio.barigelletti@istitutotumori.mi.it
† Ada Working Group is listed in Acknowledgments.

Abstract: Cancer patients are identified as fragile patients who are often immunodepressed and subject to secondary diseases. The Ada cohort comprises cancer survivors aged 15–39 years at diagnosis included in 34 Italian cancer registries. This study aimed to analyze the possible excess of non-cancer medicines use on the basis of the medicine database of the Ada cohort. Records of medicines present in the pharmaceutical flows collected by eight Lombardy cancer registries and used by patients with any type of cancer were extracted for the year 2012. Medicine consumption data were processed to assign a defined daily dose value and to evaluate the consumption of medicines belonging to different groups of the ATC (Anatomical Therapeutic Chemical) classification. The values were compared with values in the Lombardy population. Medicine consumption related to 8150 patients was analyzed, for a total of 632,675 records. ATC groups A and C for females and group N for both sexes showed significant increases. Group J for males and group M for females showed intermediate increases, and group H for both sexes showed smaller increases. This method allowed the identification of excess medicine use to reduce cancer therapy side effects and primary disease sequelae in this group of patients.

Keywords: medicine consumption; defined daily dose; adolescents and young adults; cancer patients; fragility; pain

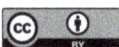

1. Introduction

The Ada project (Adolescent and Young Adult Cancer Survivors in Italy) [1], includes a database of patients who received a cancer diagnosis when aged between 15 and 39 years. In addition to information on the patients and their cancer types, the database lists the sources of the information, which are commonly collected by cancer registries (CRs). Among the most important sources are hospital discharge records, pathology laboratory data, outpatient data, and pharmaceutical prescription records.

The Ada database includes a total of 112,392 records of incident cancer cases between 1976 and 2015 related to 108,777 patients. The records were collected and sent to the database by 31 Italian population CRs and 3 Italian specialist CRs.

In recent years, there has been a significant decrease in the number of hospital discharge records (Figure 1), formerly the main source of epidemiological information. It is therefore useful to evaluate the potential of other sources of information, such as the source considered in the present study: medicine prescriptions.

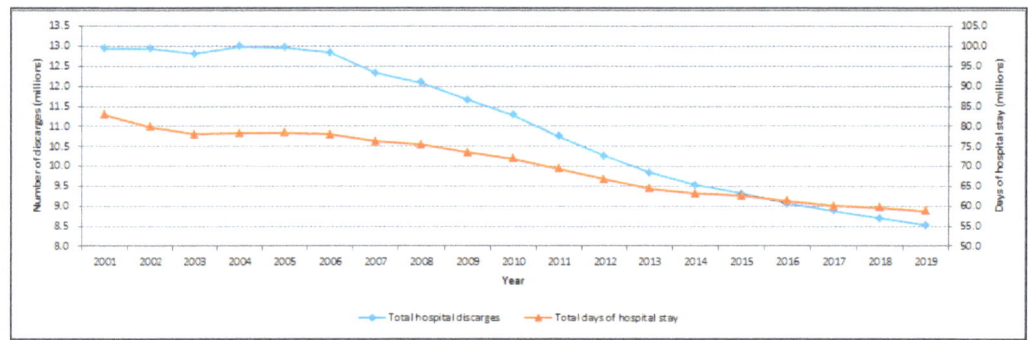

Figure 1. Italian trend of the overall volume of hospital discharges and days of hospital stay. Source: Italian Ministry of Health [2].

The pharmaceutical prescription records in the Ada database represent prescriptions issued according to the standards of the Italian National Health System (SSN). They may be subject to full or partial reimbursement according to the following prescription classes: A (life-saving medicines), C (non-essential medicines), and H (medicines for hospital use). Over-the-counter medicines and those prescribed without reimbursement by the SSN are not considered here since their prescription does not follow well-defined protocols, and they are not always reported.

The pharmaceutical prescription records are mainly composed of two data flows:

(1) The T flow is dispensed by community pharmacies, i.e., local pharmacies open to the public. This flow includes all medicines [3] distributed by the SSN upon payment of a co-payment or free of charge.
(2) The F flow is dispensed by hospital pharmacies or by the local services of the Public Health Agency (ATS, USL or AUSL in Italy). This flow comprises various types of medicines, which may vary from region to region and which in the Lombardy region include:

   a. Innovative hospital medicines;
   b. Outpatient medicines;
   c. Off-label medicines;
   d. Hyposensitizing therapies;
   e. Medicines issuable by specialist prescription only;
   f. Medicines administered to foreigners with an individual Temporarily Present Foreigner (STP) code;
   g. Medicines for rare diseases;
   h. Medicines delivered at hospital discharge for the first cycle of care;
   i. Medicines distributed by penitentiary institutions;
   j. Medicines distributed by Local Public Health Agencies;
   k. Medicines administered in hospital to patients with hemophilia;
   l. Medicines under risk-sharing agreements;
   m. Some blood components;
   n. New antiviral medicines for HCV treatment;
   o. Others.

Objectives

The hypothesis underlying the study was that there might be an excess consumption of non-cancer medicines in adolescent and young adult cancer patients. A consequent objective was to analyze and possibly justify the reasons for this consumption. As far as we know, there have been no previous studies analyzing the non-cancer medicine consumption in this specific group of fragile patients [4].

2. Materials and Methods

2.1. Data Selection

Of the 34 CRs contributing data to the Ada database, 14 provided pharmaceutical dispensation data. A total of 2,328,057 records for the years 1980–2012 were available. Since the highest coverage in the database was for the years 2010 to 2012, we decided to evaluate medicine consumption in 2012, the more recent year. The database included 280,812 registrations for 2012, relative to 12 CRs. To obtain correct and complete terms of comparison despite the absence of an internal standard, we chose 8 CRs in the Lombardy region among these 12 CRs, as their data could be compared with data available on the web (Lombardy Open Data [5]). The data of eight Lombardy population CRs were used for comparison, covering a total of 8,370,359 inhabitants, 4,307,101 females, and 4,063,258 males.

Since the goal was to evaluate and compare the consumption of medicines by adolescent and young adult cancer patients and since Lombardy Open Data allows to select data for the age group between 18 and 39 years, all patients of this age group with previous or recurrent cancer, incident according to the IARC (International Agency for Research on Cancer)-ENCR (European Network on Cancer Registries) criteria for all available years, who had taken medicines in 2012, were selected. For this group of patients, we extracted the medicine dispensation records in the pharmaceutical Ada database for flows T and F and prescription classes A (life-saving), C (non-essential), and H (hospital use).

2.2. Data Elaboration

All pharmaceutical records selected were subsequently processed in order to:

a. Calculate the punctual prescription units of medicines for 2012;
b. Group the records by pairing the patients with the marketing authorization numbers (AIC codes) of the medicines they had taken;
c. Add the NDP (number of defined daily doses (DDDs) in the package) to each patient + AIC pair;
d. Calculate the total number of DDDs for each patient + AIC pair.

The analysis involved the assignment for each type of dispensing (package with AIC) of an NDP, which is the result of multiplying the product of the DDDs by the total quantity of active ingredient present in the package.

Some problems were encountered at this point: some AICs lacked an NDP because the regulatory body had not assigned it due to technical impossibility, and several pharmaceutical records had wrong AICs or had been assigned an AIC-unrelated internal code.

After assignment of the NDP, the total DDD was calculated for each grouped record (patient + AIC pair). We then calculated the total DDD for each group of the Anatomical Therapeutic Chemical (ATC) classification system [6].

Since Lombardy Open Data provides only values as grouping by first ATC group (first letter of the ATC code) the values of the Ada data were grouped in the same way.

The DDD/1000 inhabitants/day (DDDid) was then calculated using formula (1) [7]:

$$\text{DDD}id = \frac{\text{NDP} \times \text{PP} \times 1000}{\text{POP} \times \text{RD}} \quad (1)$$

Or, in our case, using Formula (2):

$$\text{DDD}id = \frac{\text{DDD}tot \times 1000}{\text{POP} \times \text{RD}} \quad (2)$$

where NDP is the number of DDDs per package; PP is the number of packages prescribed; POP is the total population of the area, re-proportioned by age group 18–39 and sex; RD is the number of reference days, i.e., 365 (1 year); DDDtot is the number of total DDDs, obtained from the sum of the DDDs per ATC group of the grouped records.

The choice of the population in the denominator required special attention. In fact, the cohort whose medicine consumption we analyzed in this study was made up of an atypical set of cases, for which the use of the reference standard population for each age group could lead to misleading results. Therefore, we decided to select a population for the denominator that could best represent the whole, calculating it as a re-proportioning of the total population according to the scheme shown in Table 1. Thus, the population in the denominator was derived as a proportion of the total population covered by the CRs, multiplied by the ratio between the number of patients considered in the study and the total incident cases in one year in the coverage areas of the CRs for all ages.

Table 1. Re-proportioning of the reference population.

	M	F
Total cancer cases in the CR areas for all ages in 2012 (a)	30,671	27,322
Ada cohort patients aged 18–39 years in 2012, with medicine consumption in the same year (b)	3250	4900
Ratio between Ada cohort patients and total CR patients (b/a)	10.6%	17.9%
Total population in the CR coverage area	4,063,258	4,307,101
Reference re-proportioned population for calculation	430,556	772,447

CR = cancer registry.

3. Results

From the Ada database, 8150 patients with a cancer diagnosis between 1989 and 2012 and medicine consumption in 2012 were extracted. The group included 4900 females and 3250 males; distribution by life status was available at the most recent follow-up ($\leq$31 December 2017), as reported in Table 2. Most patients were diagnosed quite recently (from one to five years, as shown in Table 2), but there was also a sizeable group with a longer period of observation (up to 15 years).

Table 2. Distribution of cases selected for the analysis, by sex, time elapsed since diagnosis, and life status.

Years Since Diagnosis	0	1–5	6–15	16–25	Total	Alive	Dead	% Dead
Males	387	2092	745	26	3250	3008	242	7.4%
Females	637	3267	965	31	4900	4588	312	6.4%
Total	1024	5359	1710	57	8150	7596	554	6.8%

In Figures 2–5, the cases considered are presented by cancer type and sex according to the two main classifications in use: ICCC3 (International Classification of Childhood Cancer [8]) and ICD-10 (the WHO *International Classification of Diseases, 10th edition* [9]).

The processing of the pharmaceutical records selected for the analysis is summarized in Table 3.

Table 4 shows the set of values processed with the relative comparisons, where some excesses of consumption can be noted.

ATC group L, specific to cancer medicines, and groups G + V, which contain medicines used in cancer therapy, were excluded as they are outside the scope of this study.

ATC groups A (alimentary tract and metabolism) and C (cardiovascular system) for females, and ATC group N (nervous system) for both sexes showed significant increases.

ATC group J (anti-infectives for systemic use) for males and ATC group M (musculoskeletal system) for females showed intermediate increases, while group H (systemic hormonal preparations) for both sexes showed smaller increases.

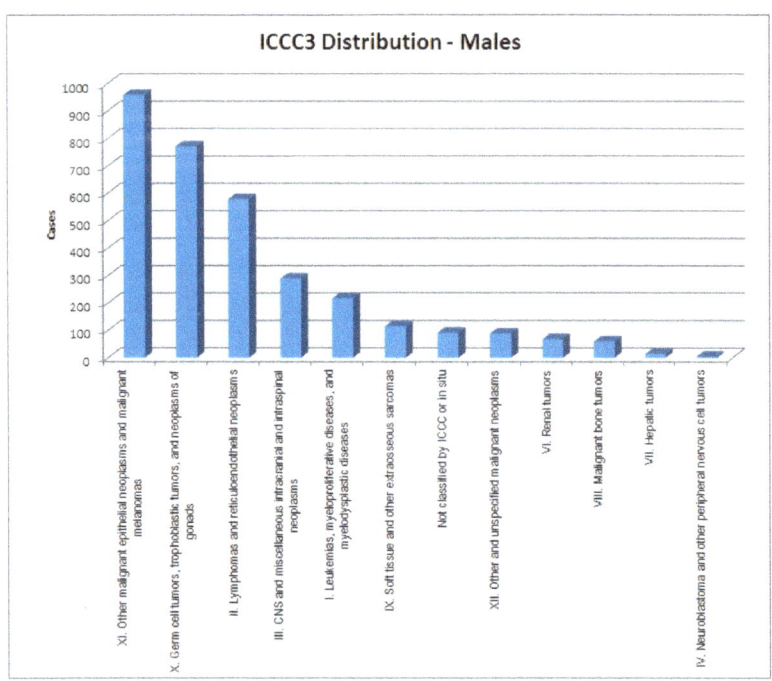

Figure 2. ICCC3 (standard) distribution of cases—males.

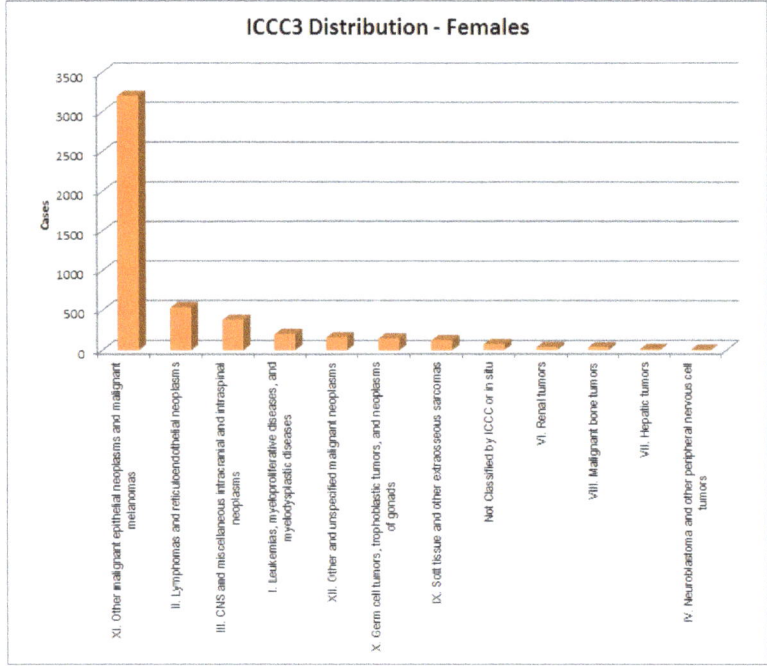

Figure 3. ICCC3 (standard) distribution of cases—females.

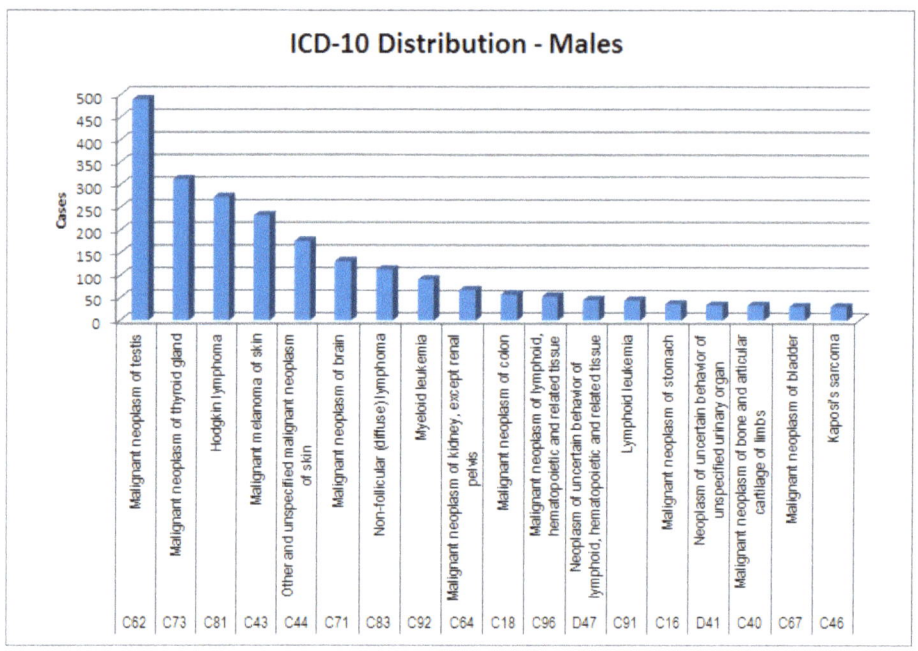

Figure 4. ICD-10 distribution of cases—males.

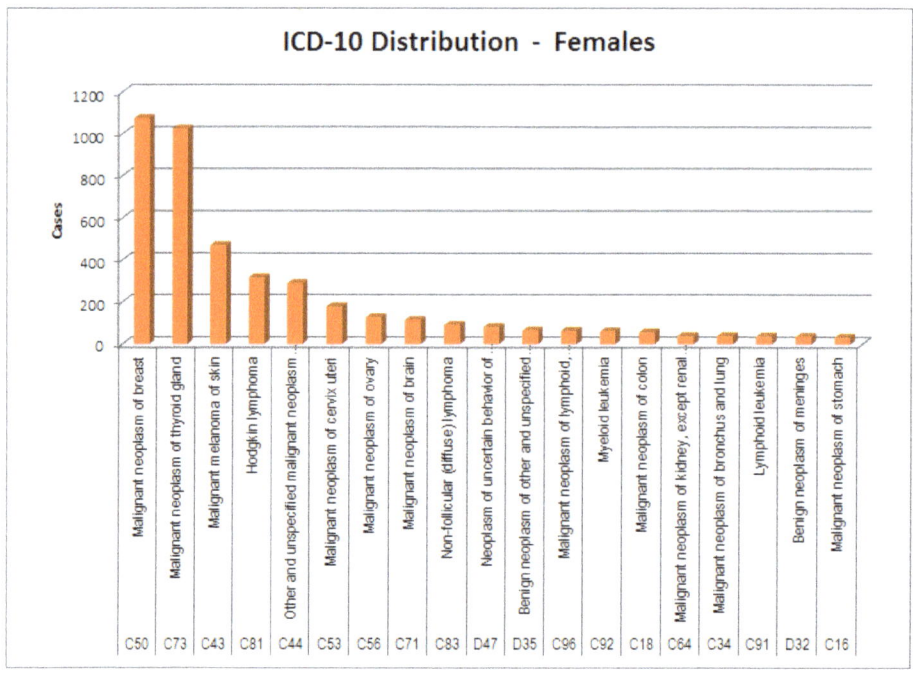

Figure 5. ICD-10 distribution of cases—females.

Table 3. Summary of elaborations on pharmaceutical records extracted from Ada database.

Description	Number of Records	Initial Year, Incident Cases	Final Year, Incident Cases	Notes
Patients with cancer and medicine consumption in 2012, aged between 18 and 39 years	8150	1989	2012	4900 females 3250 males
Records of medicines, 2012	632,675	2012	2012	
Records grouped by patient and AIC (a)	139,931	2012	2012	
Grouped records with invalid AIC	17,931			12.8% of total (a)
Grouped records not connectable to NDP or null NDP	1935			1.4% of total (a)
Total valid grouped records	120,065			

AIC = marketing authorization number; NDP = number of defined daily doses.

It should be noted that, for both sexes, ATC group R, relating to medicinal products for the respiratory system, presented a decrease in consumption.

The consumptions of ATC groups that showed significant increases was then analyzed by ATC subgroups (to the third and fourth digits). The results, shown in Figures 6–13, are expressed as the total number of DDDs prescribed for each group or subgroup and divided into three age groups.

The analysis of the relationship between cancer type, total DDDs of ATC group C, and age did not show significant associations, as shown in Table 5, in which an extract of this sub-analysis is presented. Normally, higher consumption is attributed to the older age group, although for lymphoid and ovarian diseases, the higher consumption is attributable to the intermediate age group (25–32 years).

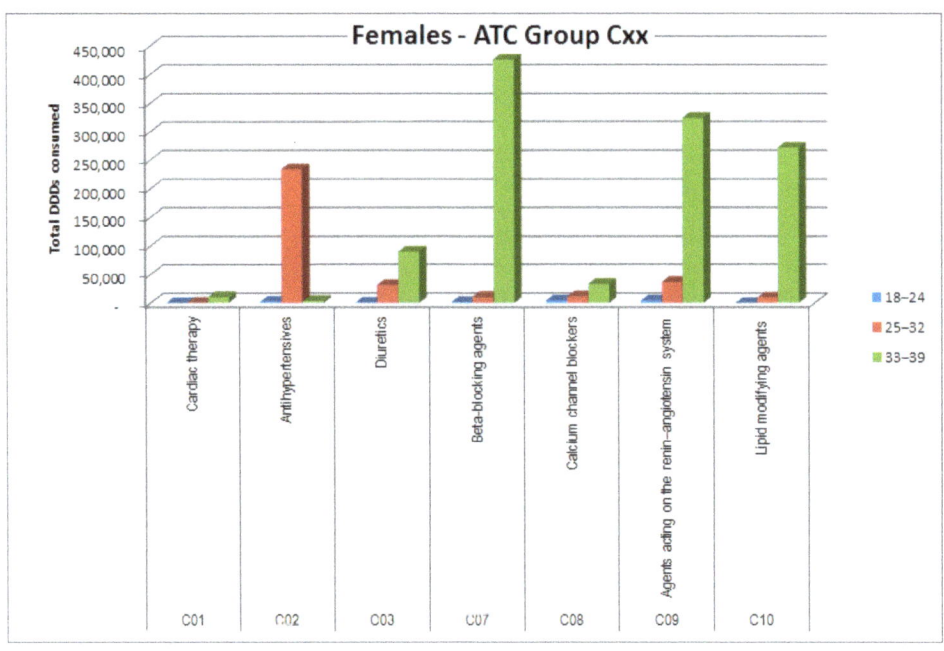

Figure 6. DDD consumption for females, ATC group Cxx.

Table 4. Comparisons between Ada cohort and Lombardy Open Data for ATC groups in 2012.

		↓Origin / ATC Group→	A Alimentary Tract and Metabolism	B Blood and Blood-Forming Organs	C Cardiovascular System	D Dermatologicals	G Genito-Urinary System and Sex Hormones	H Systemic Hormonal Preparations, Excluding Sex Hormones and Insulins	J Anti-Infectives for Systemic Use	L Antineoplastic and Immunomodulating Agents	M Musculoskeletal System	N Nervous System	P Antiparasitic Products, Insecticides and Repellents	R Respiratory System	S Sensory Organs	V Various
Year 2012 Males, age 18–39	1	Lombardy OPEN DATA 2012 M (DDD/1000 inhabitants/day)	20.18	4.99	23.92	2.63	0.86	6.28	12.6	1.00	3.5	24.86	0.15	22	1.07	0.14
	2	Consumption 2012, Ada DB M patients (DDD/1000 inhabitants/day)	20.04	8.33	12.19	0.32	0.59	17.58	88.40	3564.54	2.13	366.26	0.03	3.33	0.36	2.13
	3	Increase % (2 vs. 1)	−1%	67%	−49%	−88%	−31%	180%	601%	356,354%	−39%	1373%	−80%	−85%	−66%	1421%
Year 2012 Females, age 18–39	4	Lombardy OPEN DATA 2012 F (DDD/1000 inhabitants/day)	19.34	14.6	11.59	1.57	36.54	15.40	16.90	1.76	3.61	27.78	0.62	22	0.75	0.10
	5	Consumption 2012, Ada DB F patients (DDD/1000 inhabitants/day)	327.01	34.80	649.13	0.43	1275.91	51.64	23.08	2444.78	35.82	938.37	0.43	7.90	1.42	1.46
	6	Increase % (5 vs. 4)	1591%	138%	5501%	−73%	3392%	235%	37%	138,808%	892%	3278%	−31%	−64%	89%	1360%
		Excluded for use in cancer therapy														
		100–300%														
		300–1000%														
		>1000%														

DDD = defined daily dose; ATC = Anatomical Therapeutic Chemical classification; M = male; F = female.

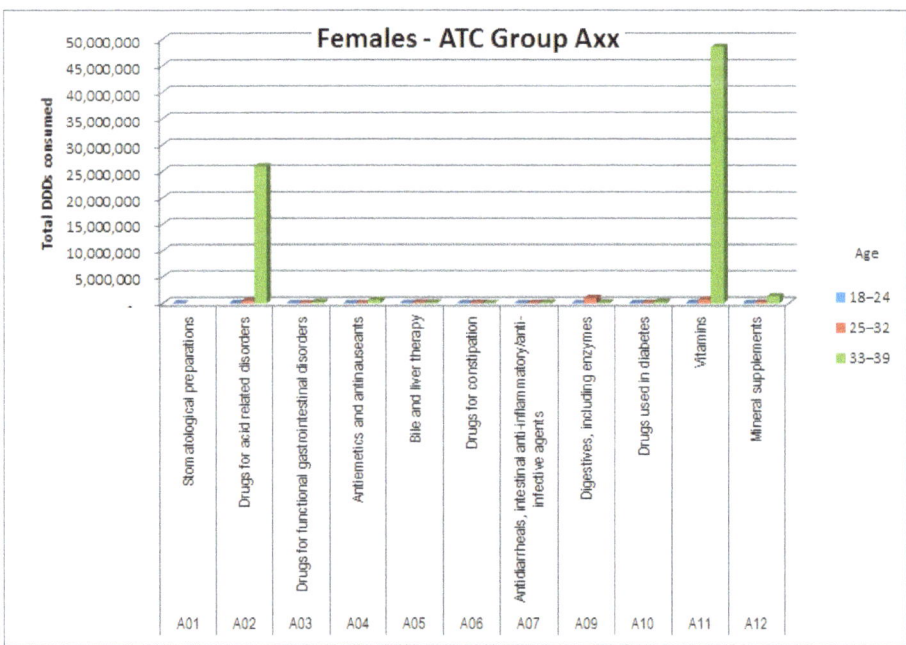

Figure 7. DDD consumption for females, ATC group Axx.

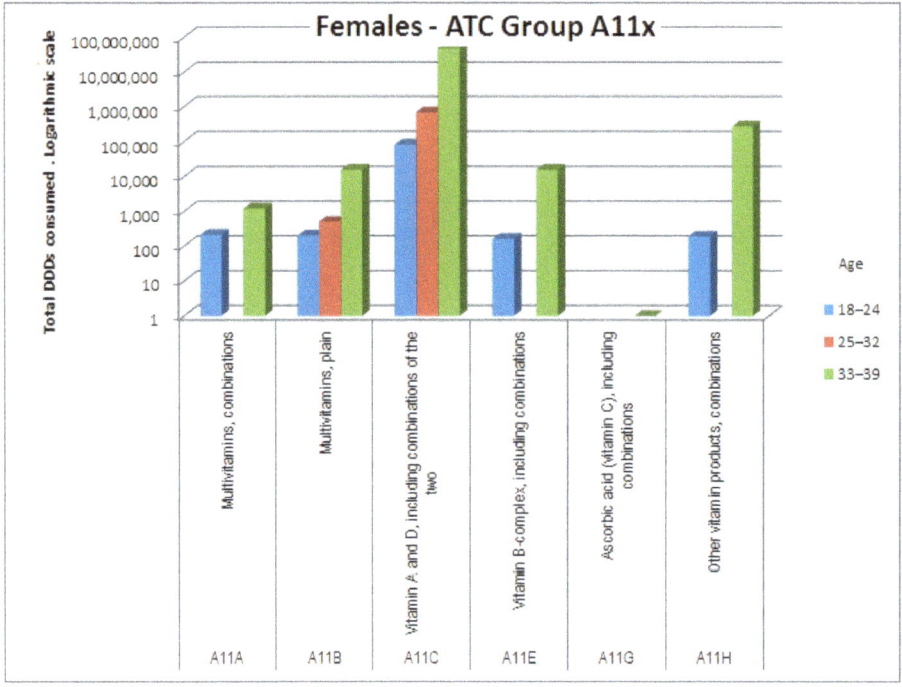

Figure 8. DDD consumption for females, ATC subgroup A11x (vitamins).

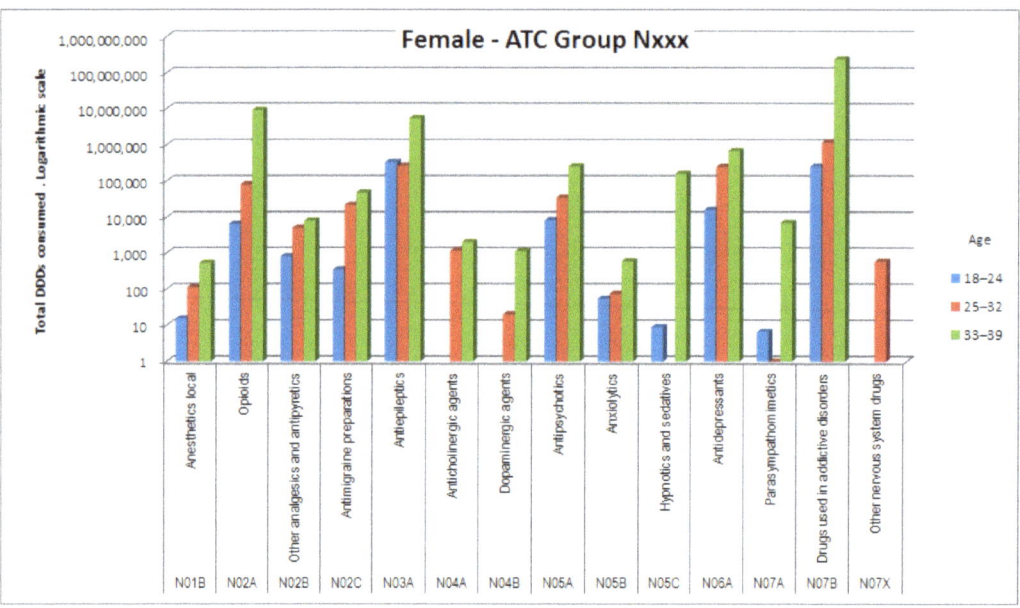

Figure 9. DDD consumption for females, ATC group Nxxx.

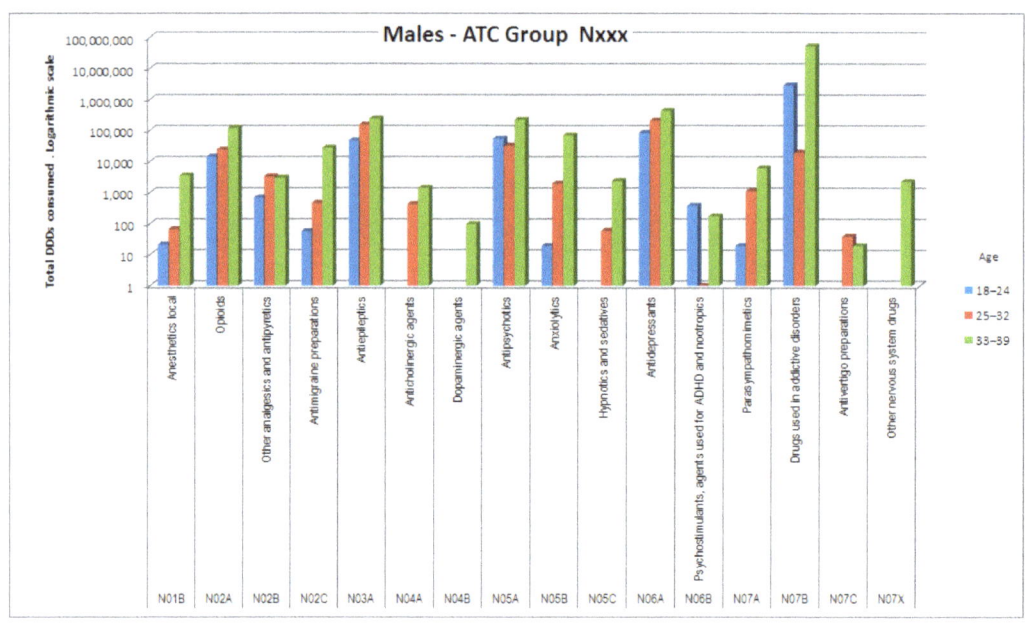

Figure 10. DDD consumption for males, ATC group Nxxx.

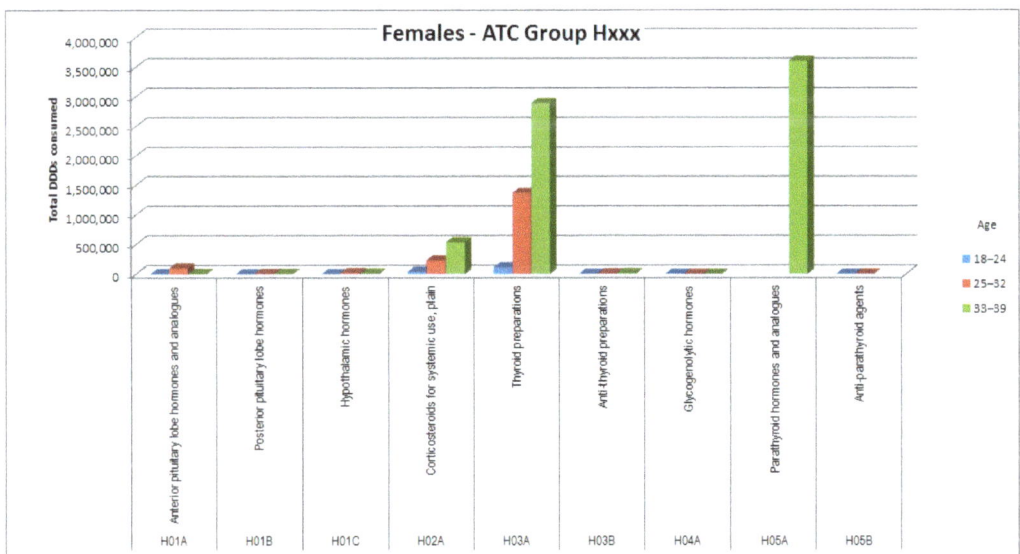

Figure 11. DDD consumption for females, ATC group Hxxx.

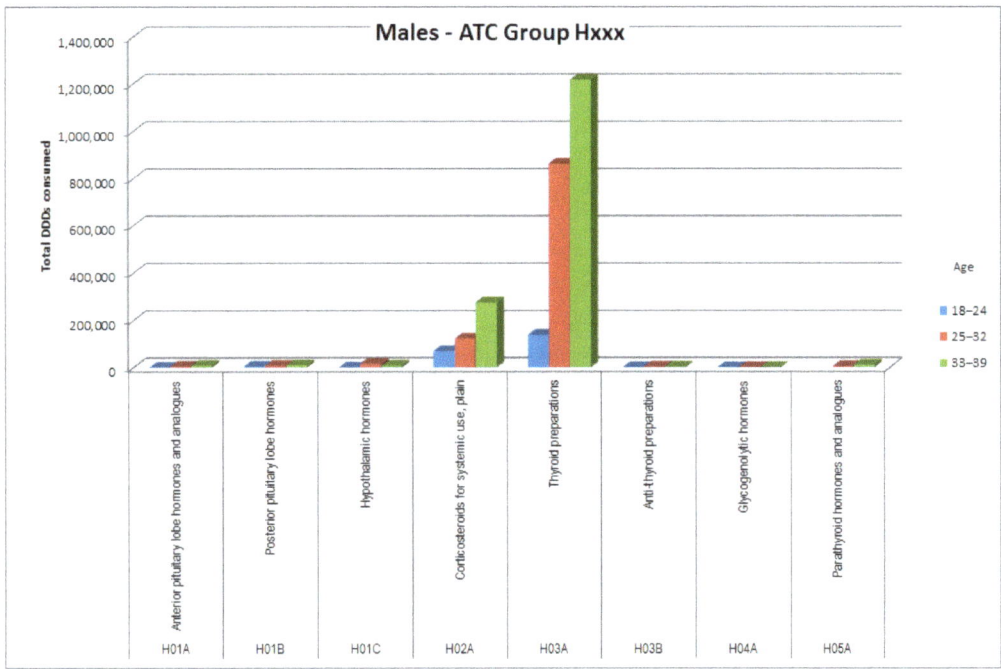

Figure 12. DDD consumption for males, ATC group Hxxx.

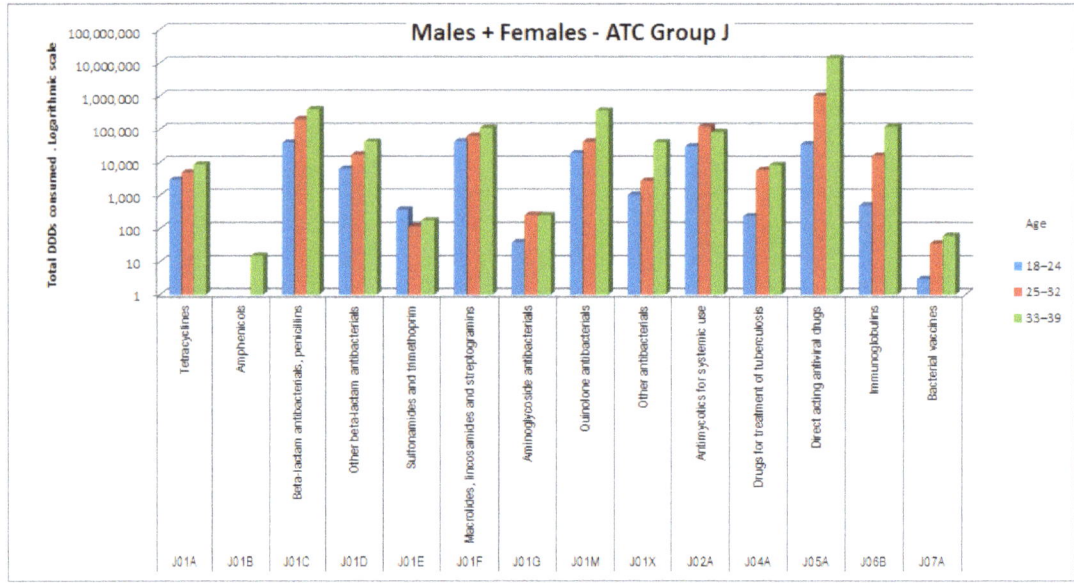

Figure 13. DDD consumption for males + females, ATC group Jxxx.

Table 5. Total DDDs for ATC group Cxx (females).

ICD-10	Description	Age	Total DDDs
C81	Hodgkin disease	33–39	306,236
C50	Malignant neoplasm of breast	33–39	256,674
C96	Malignant neoplasm of lymphoid, hematopoietic and related tissue	25–32	231,672
C73	Malignant neoplasm of thyroid gland	33–39	164,893
C83	Non-follicular lymphoma	33–39	126,998
C22	Malignant neoplasm of liver and intrahepatic bile ducts	33–39	100,059
C56	Malignant neoplasm of ovary	25–32	27,132
D46	Myelodysplastic syndrome	33–39	25,468
C49	Malignant neoplasm of connective and soft tissue	33–39	24.477
C44	Other and unspecified malignant neoplasm of skin	33–39	21,156
C53	Malignant neoplasm of cervix uteri	33–39	16,263

DDD = defined daily dose; ATC = Anatomical Therapeutic Chemical classification.

In Table 6, the consumption of H03A (thyroid preparations) and H05A (parathyroid hormones) medicines is analyzed, comparing patients with thyroid cancer (ICD-10 C73) and patients with other cancers (ICD-10 not C73), who showed substantial differences.

In Table 7, a detail of total DDD for subgroup N07B (medicines used in addictive disorders) is shown.

Table 6. Analysis of DDDs for thyroid preparations (H03A) and parathyroid hormones (H05A).

ICD10	ATC	TOTAL DDD
C73	H03A	5,617,183
All but not C73	H03A	984,064
C73	H05A	3,606,180
All but not C73	H05A	0

DDD = defined daily dose; ATC = Anatomical Therapeutic Chemical classification.

Table 7. Total DDDs for ATC subgroup N07B (males + females).

ATC Group	Description	Use	Total DDDs
N07BA02	Medicines used in smoke dependence	Medicines used in smoke dependence	30
N07BB	Medicines used in alcohol dependence	Medicines used in alcohol dependence	172,422
N07BC01	Betahistine	Medicines for nausea and vomiting	75,161
N07BC02	Methadone	Severe pain syndromes (dependence)	295,004,425
N07BC51	Buprenorphine, combinations	Buprenorphine, combinations	1,170,013

DDD = defined daily dose; ATC = Anatomical Therapeutic Chemical classification.

4. Discussion

Cancer patients have a need for more medicines of some of the ATC groups compared with a general patient population, as we found in our pilot study [10]. The cohort of cancer patients considered in this study, which was extrapolated from the Ada database, had particular characteristics, especially given the young age of the patients (18–39 years), but also given the specific peculiarity of the cancer types that most affect these patients [11]. This can greatly influence the consumption of medicines not directly involved in cancer treatment.

We performed analyses of some of the ATC groups that showed consumption increases, evaluating the ratios, gender differences, and clinical aspects of medicine prescriptions. The ATC groups L (antineoplastic), G (sex hormones), and V (miscellaneous) were excluded from the analysis because medicines belonging to these groups are normally used in cancer treatment.

ATC group C (cardiovascular system) showed excess consumption among female patients (Figure 6), to be attributed mainly to blood pressure and lipid regulators in the older age group (33–39 years). As shown in Table 5, this excess was not attributable to any particular cancer type, except as expected in the case of hormone replacement therapy in thyroidectomized patients.

Consumption of ATC group A medicines (alimentary tract and metabolism) was also higher in female patients (Figure 7). The increase was mainly related to subgroup A02 (antacids) and subgroup A11 (vitamins), with substantial consumption of vitamin D, as shown in Figure 8.

Both sexes, albeit with small differences between them, showed increased consumption of medicines belonging to ATC group N (nervous system), with the greatest increase observed for subgroup N07B (substances against abuse, listed in Table 6). In this group methadone (ATC N07BC02) was the agent with the greatest consumption, followed by opioids (N02A), antiepileptics (N03A), and antidepressants (N06A).

H03A (thyroid preparations) represented the subgroup with the highest consumption for ATC group H (systemic hormonal preparations); among female patients there was also a conspicuous peak for the H05A subgroup (parathyroid hormones). Comparative analysis of consumption in these two ATC subgroups between patients with thyroid cancer (ICD-10 C73) and patients with other cancers (ICD-10 not C73) revealed substantial differences, as shown in Table 6.

Additionally, ATC group J (anti-infectives for systemic use) showed a significant increase in consumption, due essentially to antibiotic and antiviral medicines.

4.1. Outline of Clinical Pharmacology

In ATC group A (alimentary tract and metabolism), the significantly higher prescription rate among women, almost exclusively in the older age group, was mainly attributable to the A11 subgroup (vitamins) and to a lesser extent to the A02 subgroup (antacids and analogues). Further sub-analysis of A11, also by age group, showed that vitamins are often prescribed in combination, and most prescriptions focus on vitamin A, E, and D combinations, probably because of their antioxidant (E) and anti-osteoporosis (D) effects, and on those of the B complex, probably for their effects on nerve fibers; these three aspects may be useful in counteracting some frequent side effects of cancer chemotherapy. The benefits of vitamin supplementation in cancer patients when not undergoing chemotherapy cycles are less clear and still debated [12,13]. Furthermore, although the increased use of vitamin D in the older age group of females appears consistent with the risk of osteoporosis, especially if they use corticosteroids, it is not clear how gender medicine can justify the other differences. It could be hypothesized that these medicines are used as placebo, and the appropriateness of prescribing them needs evaluation [14].

For ATC group C (cardiovascular system), the gender difference was even more pronounced. Males have a basal consumption in the reference population that is about double that of females, but in the observed cohort, their consumption halved (−49%), while for females a 55-fold increase in consumption was observed. As shown in Figure 6, these are mainly beta-blocking agents (C07) but also real antihypertensives (C02, C09) and anti-dyslipidemics (C10). Additionally, for this ATC group, gender medicine can provide some explanation, given that the hormone blockade in some oncology protocols can have opposite effects in the two sexes as regards the cardiovascular system, but the difference between the sexes was so high that this consideration appears insufficient, and again, the question of prescription appropriateness arises.

In ATC group H (systemic hormonal preparations), females tend to have a 2.5 times higher basal consumption than males, but in the patients of the Ada cohort, consumption almost tripled in both sexes. Disaggregating by ATC subgroup, we observed that females, in whom thyroid neoplasms have a double incidence compared with males (Figures 4 and 5), showed a prescription value of thyroid replacement therapy that was quadruple compared with males. It should be considered that in females there is a higher incidence of autoimmune thyroiditis; however, females have a specificity: unlike males, they also take replacement therapy for iatrogenic hypoparathyroidism, probably in consideration of the fact that they are at greater risk of osteoporosis than males, even before menopause [15].

Additionally, in ATC group J (anti-infectives for systemic use), there was an increase in consumption, modest in females but very marked in males. This increase was attributable to antibacterial medicines (bactericides more than bacteriostatics), antifungals, and antivirals, which are widely used in these patients who are often immunosuppressed as a result of the demanding cancer treatments [16].

In ATC group N (nervous system), females showed an overall triple consumption compared with males, indicating their greater propensity for medicine consumption in general [17–19]. The most commonly used medicines by both males and females in our cohort were those classified in the subgroup for substance abuse cessation, but which in these patients are used to treat chronic pain (methadone in 99.5% of cases, buprenorphine in 0.4%). Second in use were other subgroups of specific medicines for the treatment of painful symptoms, which appear relevant and diversified in pathogenesis [20]. These include substances with different mechanisms of action, such as N01B, N02A, N02B, and N02C, but also N06A and sometimes N03A. Last in this category were medicines used, together with non-medicinal techniques, to treat the psychological distress of these patients [21], which in addition to being frequent can in some cases reduce adherence to therapy [22] and sometimes lead to overt mental health issues (N05A, N05B, N05C, and again N06A) [23].

4.2. Observations and Limitations

(1) For a more effective analysis it would be preferable to use an internal standard, in the event that records of all prescriptions were available, as the references used (OsMed [24], Open Data, etc.) often have non-compliant characteristics or can limit the calculation needs.

(2) It is necessary to have a sufficiently large cohort to avoid a small number of individuals with diseases related to specific ATC groups or subgroups from skewing the results. With a sufficient number of data (not available in this study), the method could make it possible to stratify the excess consumption of medicines based on the time from diagnosis. In this way, possible differences between patients with the most recent diagnoses and other subgroups of patients could be detected, which would allow us to ascertain whether to associate the observed results with the side effects of specific therapies or with the distant outcomes of therapeutic interventions.

(3) The groupings of greater detail than the first ATC grouping (first character) are distorting because, although they belong to the same ATC subgroup, the medicines have different characteristics and therefore very different weights in DDD. Evaluating differences in DDD / 1000 inhabitants / day among these medicine subgroups makes no sense. Based on our experience, we have indicated the absolute value of DDD prescribed for some subgroups in order to identify the medicines that most influenced the changes in consumption within the primary group. The evaluation of consumption differences in the ATC subgroups can be performed by comparing the individual subgroups between cohorts with different characteristics, or between a cohort and a reference standard (as expressed in point 1).

(4) It is important to carry out appropriate quality control of the pharmaceutical sources, particularly regarding the correct attribution of AIC and ATC codes, which can be problematic when internal codes not corresponding to the official nomenclature are used.

5. Conclusions

The analysis of medicine consumption using DDD allows interesting observations to be made on consumption in specific patient populations. Fragile populations, such as the one considered for this study, consisting of cancer patients of the Ada database, show increases in consumption of specific ATC groups and significant differences between the sexes.

These findings can be used for better patient care, and they could be preparatory to actions to prevent and reduce the side effects of therapies and the sequelae of the primary disease, often present in this group of patients.

This technique can be implemented, with appropriate adaptations, for similar analyses in different patient groups. Moreover, if used in the context of the population and in comparison with exposure to environmental agents or adverse events, it can be employed as a sentinel event for monitoring situations of discomfort or suffering.

Author Contributions: G.B. contributed to study conception, designed the study, managed the Ada database to extract the data, performed the analyses, and wrote the first draft of the paper; G.T. contributed to study conception and writing the paper; S.F., A.B. and V.P. performed statistical controls; A.T. (Annalisa Trama) contributed to writing the paper; C.T. contributed to the clinical pharmacology analysis and to writing the paper; A.T. (Andrea Tittarelli) helped in managing the Ada database and in writing the paper. All authors read and approved the final manuscript.

Funding: This research received no external funding.

Institutional Review Board Statement: The study was conducted according to the guidelines of the Declaration of Helsinki, and approved by the Institutional Review Board (or Ethics Committee) of Fondazione IRCCS Istituto Nazionale Tumori (protocol code INT 134/17, date of approval 20 July 2017).

Informed Consent Statement: The data contained in the Ada database were collected with the approval of the related cancer registries. Each registry provided patient data in an anonymous format. Data collection was approved by the competent ethics committee. All data used in this study were processed and treated anonymously. The authors state that no informed consent nor further ethical approval was needed for the study.

Data Availability Statement: The data will be provided upon request.

Acknowledgments: The authors thank Marije de Jager for proofreading and correcting the English. Ada Working Group: Veneto Cancer Registry (CR) (Massimo Rugge), Milano CR (Maria Teresa Greco), Tuscany CR (Gianfranco Manneschi), Romagna CR (Stefania Giorgetti), Catania-Messina-Enna CR (Salvatore Sciacca), Liguria CR (Rosa Angela Filiberti), Brescia CR (Cinzia Gasparotti), Modena CR (Giuliano Carrozzi), Palermo CR (Walter Mazzucco), Reggio-Emilia CR (Lucia Mangone), Latina CR (Silvia Iacovacci), Napoli 3 Sud CR (Mario Fusco), Umbria CR (Fabrizio Stracci), Trento CR (Roberto Vito Rizzello), Ragusa CR (Giuseppe Cascone), Taranto CR (Sante Minerba), Bergamo CR (Giuseppe Sampietro), Lecce CR (Anna Melcarne), Mantova CR (Paolo Ricci, Luciana Gatti), Pavia CR (Lorenza Boschetti), Como CR (Maria Letizia Gambino), Monza-Brianza CR (Elisabetta Merlo), Barletta-Andria-Trani CR (Rossella Bruni), Caserta CR (Alessandra Sessa), Napoli 2 Nord CR (Giancarlo D'Orsi), Sondrio CR (Anna Clara Fanetti), Brindisi CR (Emma Cozzi), Trapani CR (Tiziana Scuderi), Campania Childhood CR (Francesco Vetrano), Marche CR (Iolanda Grappasonni), Valle D'Aosta CR (Salvatore Bongiorno), Emilia-Romagna Mesothelioma CR (Antonio Romanelli).

Conflicts of Interest: The authors declare no potential conflicts of interest with respect to the research, authorship, and/or publication of this article.

References

1. Bernasconi, A.; Barigelletti, G.; Tittarelli, A.; Botta, L.; Gatta, G.; Tagliabue, G.; Contiero, P.; Guzzinati, S.; Andreano, A.; Manneschi, G.; et al. Adolescent and Young Adult Cancer Survivors: Design and Characteristics of the First Nationwide Population-Based Cohort in Italy. *J. Adolesc. Young-Adult Oncol.* **2020**, *9*, 586–593. [CrossRef] [PubMed]
2. Italian Ministry of Health—The National Database of Hospital Admissions. Available online: http://www.salute.gov.it/portale/temi/p2_6.jsp?id=1236&area=ricoveriOspedalieri&menu=vuoto (accessed on 12 May 2021).
3. European Parlament—Medicines and Medical Devices Definition. Available online: https://www.europarl.europa.eu/factsheets/en/sheet/50/medicines-and-medical-devices (accessed on 12 May 2021).
4. Ethun, C.G.; Bilen, M.A.; Jani, A.B.; Maithel, S.K.; Ogan, K.; Master, V.A. Frailty and cancer: Implications for oncology surgery, medical oncology, and radiation oncology. *CA Cancer J. Clin.* **2017**, *67*, 362–377. [CrossRef] [PubMed]
5. Lombardy Region-Open Data. Available online: https://www.dati.lombardia.it (accessed on 12 May 2021).
6. WHO—Collaborating Center for Drug StatisticMethodologie. Available online: https://www.whocc.no/atc_ddd_index (accessed on 12 May 2021).
7. Eandi, M. Unita di consumo dei farmaci e valutazioni farmacoeconomiche: Uso e misuso di DDD e PDD. *Farmeconomia. Health Econ. Ther. Pathw.* **2002**, *3*, 209–222. [CrossRef]
8. Steliarova-Foucher, E.; Stiller, C.; Lacour, B.; Kaatsch, P. International Classification of Childhood Cancer, third edition. *Cancer* **2005**, *103*, 1457–1467. [CrossRef] [PubMed]
9. WHO-International Statistical Classification of Diseases and Related Health Problems 10th Revision. Available online: https://icd.who.int/browse10/2010/en (accessed on 12 May 2021).
10. Barigelletti, G. Pilot Study on the Comparison of Consumption of Medicines between Population and Fragile Cohorts, through the Use of DDDs (Defined Daily Dose). Available online: https://www.researchgate.net/publication/352211603_Pilot_study_on_the_comparison_of_consumption_of_medicines_between_population_and_fragile_cohorts_through_the_use_of_DDDs_Defined_Daily_Dose?channel=doi&linkId=60bf262e458515218f9f4233&showFulltext=true (accessed on 8 June 2021). [CrossRef]
11. Shaw, P.H.; Reed, D.; Yeager, N.; Zebrack, B.; Castellino, S.M.; Bleyer, A. Adolescent and Young Adult (AYA) Oncology in the United States: A specialty in its late adolescence. *J. Pediatr. Hematol.* **2015**, *37*, 161–169. [CrossRef] [PubMed]
12. Gibson, T.M.; Ferrucci, L.M.; Tangrea, J.A.; Schatzkin, A. Epidemiological and Clinical Studies of Nutrition. *Semin. Oncol.* **2010**, *37*, 282–296. [CrossRef] [PubMed]
13. Vernieri, C.; Nichetti, F.; Raimondi, A.; Pusceddu, S.; Platania, M.; Berrino, F.; de Braud, F. Diet and supplements in cancer prevention and treatment: Clinical evidences and future perspectives. *Crit. Rev. Oncol.* **2018**, *123*, 57–73. [CrossRef] [PubMed]
14. Bosetti, C.; Santucci, C.; Pasina, L.; Fortino, I.; Merlino, L.; Corli, O.; Nobili, A. Use of preventive drugs during the last year of life in older adults with cancer or chronic progressive diseases. *Pharmacoepidemiol. Drug Saf.* **2021**, *30*, 1057–1065. [CrossRef] [PubMed]
15. Kennedy, C.C.; Ioannidis, G.; Rockwood, K.; Thabane, L.; Adachi, J.D.; Kirkland, S.; Pickard, L.E.; Papaioannou, A. A Frailty Index predicts 10-year fracture risk in adults age 25 years and older: Results from the Canadian Multicentre Osteoporosis Study (CaMos). *Osteoporos. Int.* **2014**, *25*, 2825–2832. [CrossRef] [PubMed]

16. Anderson, C.; Lund, J.L.; Weaver, M.A.; Wood, W.A.; Olshan, A.F.; Nichols, H.B. Noncancer mortality among adolescents and young adults with cancer. *Cancer* **2019**, *125*, 2107–2114. [CrossRef] [PubMed]
17. Smelt, H.J.; Pouwels, S.; Smulders, J.F.; Hazebroek, E.J. Patient adherence to multivitamin supplementation after bariatric surgery: A narrative review. *J. Nutr. Sci.* **2020**, *9*, 46. [CrossRef] [PubMed]
18. AIFA—Italian Agency for Medicine—Le Differenze di Genere nel Consumo di Medicinali. Available online: https://www.aifa.gov.it/-/le-differenze-di-genere-nel-consumo-di-medicinali (accessed on 12 May 2021).
19. AIFA—Italian Agency for Medicine—I Dati OsMed. Available online: https://www.aifa.gov.it/-/prevalenza-d-uso-dei-farmaci-in-funzione-del-genere-e-dell-eta-ed-effetti-sulla-spesa-i-dati-osmed (accessed on 12 May 2021).
20. Urch, C.E.; Suzuki, R. Pathophysiology of somatic, visceral, and neuropathic cancer pain. In *Clinical Pain Management: Cancer Pain*, 2nd ed.; Sykes, N., Bennett, M.I., Yuan, C.S., Eds.; Hodder Arnold: London, UK, 2008; pp. 3–12.
21. Zebrack, B.J. Psychological, social, and behavioral issues for young adults with cancer. *Cancer* **2011**, *117*, 2289–2294. [CrossRef] [PubMed]
22. Trevino, K.M.; Fasciano, K.; Prigerson, H.G. Patient-Oncologist Alliance, Psychosocial Well-Being, and Treatment Adherence among Young Adults with Advanced Cancer. *J. Clin. Oncol.* **2013**, *31*, 1683–1689. [CrossRef] [PubMed]
23. Trevino, K.M.; Ba, C.H.A.; Fisch, M.J.; Friedlander, R.J.; Duberstein, P.R.; Prigerson, H.G. Patient-oncologist alliance as protection against suicidal ideation in young adults with advanced cancer. *Cancer* **2014**, *120*, 2272–2281. [CrossRef] [PubMed]
24. AIFA-OsMed Reports. Available online: https://www.aifa.gov.it/rapporti-osmed (accessed on 12 May 2021).

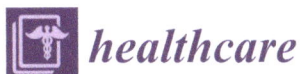

Article

Population-Based Study on the All-Cause and Cause-Specific Risks of Mortality among Long-Term Opioid Analgesics Users without Cancer in Taiwan

Po-Feng Lee [1,2,†], Chung-Yi Li [1,3], Yen-Chin Liu [4,5], Chang-Ta Chiu [6,†] and Wen-Hsuan Hou [7,8,9,*]

1. Department of Public Health, College of Medicine, National Cheng Kung University, Tainan 704, Taiwan; adusk0910@gmail.com (P.-F.L.); cyli99@mail.ncku.edu.tw (C.-Y.L.)
2. Jianan Psychiatric Center, Ministry of Health and Welfare, Tainan 717, Taiwan
3. Department of Public Health, College of Public Health, China Medical University, Taichung 406, Taiwan
4. Department of Anesthesiology, School of Post-Baccalaureate, College of Medicine, Kaohsiung Medical University, Kaohsiung 807, Taiwan; anesliu@kmu.edu.tw
5. Department of Anesthesiology, College of Medicine, National Cheng Kung University, Tainan 704, Taiwan
6. Department of Dentistry, An Nan Hospital, China Medical University, Tainan 709, Taiwan; chiouchangta@yahoo.com.tw
7. Department of Physical Medicine and Rehabilitation, Taipei Medical University Hospital, Taipei 110, Taiwan
8. School of Gerontology Health Management & Master Program in Long-Term Care, College of Nursing, Taipei Medical University, Taipei 110, Taiwan
9. Graduate Institute of Clinical Medicine, College of Medicine, Taipei Medical University, Taipei 110, Taiwan
* Correspondence: houwh@tmu.edu.tw
† Po-Feng Lee and Chang-Ta Chiu contributed equally to this article.

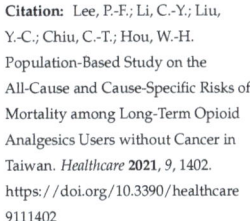

Citation: Lee, P.-F.; Li, C.-Y.; Liu, Y.-C.; Chiu, C.-T.; Hou, W.-H. Population-Based Study on the All-Cause and Cause-Specific Risks of Mortality among Long-Term Opioid Analgesics Users without Cancer in Taiwan. *Healthcare* 2021, 9, 1402. https://doi.org/10.3390/healthcare9111402

Academic Editors: Paolo Cotogni and Georges Adunlin

Received: 9 September 2021
Accepted: 14 October 2021
Published: 20 October 2021

Publisher's Note: MDPI stays neutral with regard to jurisdictional claims in published maps and institutional affiliations.

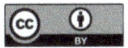

Copyright: © 2021 by the authors. Licensee MDPI, Basel, Switzerland. This article is an open access article distributed under the terms and conditions of the Creative Commons Attribution (CC BY) license (https://creativecommons.org/licenses/by/4.0/).

Abstract: (1) Background: The prevalence of opioid use in Taiwan increased by 41% between 2002 and 2014. However, little is known regarding the risk of mortality among long-term opioid analgesics users who do not have cancer. This study investigated this mortality risk with an emphasis on the calendar year and patients' age and sex. (2) Methods: This retrospective cohort study included 12,990 adult individuals without cancer who were long-term users of opioid analgesics and were randomly selected from the data set of Taiwan's National Health Insurance program from 2000 to 2012. They were then followed up through 2013. Information on the underlying causes of death was retrieved from the Taiwan Death Registry. Age, sex, and calendar year-standardized mortality ratios (SMRs) of all-cause and cause-specific mortality were calculated with reference to those of the general population. (3) Results: With up to 14 years of follow-up, 558 individuals had all-cause mortality in 48,020 person-years (cumulative mortality: 4.3%, mortality rate: 11.62 per 1000 person-years). Compared with the general population, the all-cause SMR of 4.30 (95% confidence interval (95% CI): 3.95–4.66) was significantly higher: it was higher in men than in women, declined with calendar year and age, and was significantly higher for both natural (4.15, 95% CI: 3.78–4.53) and unnatural (5.04, 95% CI: 3.88–6.45) causes. (4) Conclusions: Long-term opioid analgesics use among individuals without cancer in Taiwan was associated with a significantly increased risk of mortality. The notably increased mortality in younger adults warrants attention. Strategies to reduce long-term opioid analgesics use, especially their overuse or misuse, are in an urgent need.

Keywords: prescription opioids; mortality; standardized mortality ratio; underlying cause of death

1. Introduction

Over the past 20 years, the consumption of opioid analgesics has significantly increased in many North American and European countries. Overwhelming international concern has arisen regarding the increase in opioid analgesics addiction and black marketing as well as in opioid intoxication and mortality. Taiwan is no exception. From 2002 to 2007, opioid consumption in Taiwan increased by 55% from 362 to 560 defined daily doses per million inhabitants per day; Taiwan thus ranked 56th out of 181 countries and regions worldwide in opioid consumption, according to the 2005–2007 data set of the International Narcotics Control Board [1]. This trend continued to rise despite the Taiwanese government implementing strict guidelines on the prescription of opioid analgesics. For example, opioid consumption still increased by 41% between 2002 and 2014 [2]. The potential adverse health impacts of the long-term use of opioid analgesics are of both clinical and public health importance due to the increase in opioid consumption.

Both the prevalence and health risks associated with opioid analgesics use have been well documented in the literature. Several studies have compared different countries' trends in consuming opioid analgesics [3–5]. Furthermore, some studies have investigated the mortality risks associated with the use of different opioid analgesics in different populations [6–9]. However, the trends of all-cause and cause-specific mortality have revealed substantial heterogeneity among nations, calendar years, target populations, and types of opioid analgesics consumed [10–12]. A recent meta-analysis of 10 cohorts reported a pooled all-cause crude mortality rate of 28.8 per 1000 person-years (95% confidence interval (95% CI): 17.9–46.4) with substantial heterogeneity ($I^2 = 99.9\%$) [13]. However, another recent meta-analysis of 16 cohorts estimated a pooled all-cause crude mortality rate of 1.24 per 100 person-years (95% CI: 0.86–1.78) for people with regular or problematic cocaine use; the study also revealed considerable heterogeneity ($I^2 = 98.8\%$). [14] Moreover, researchers have rarely used age and sex as stratifications when investigating the effects of long-term opioid analgesics use on mortality [13,14].

The potentially increased risk of mortality among the increasing number of individuals without cancer who are long-term users of opioid analgesics in Taiwan has not received adequate attention. Additionally, information regarding the mortality risk associated with consuming opioid analgesics largely originates from Western societies, and little is known of this relationship in Asian populations. This study therefore investigated the all-cause and cause-specific risks of mortality associated with long-term opioid analgesics consumption among individuals without cancer in Taiwan. The risk of all-cause mortality was further stratified according to calendar year, age, and sex.

2. Materials and Methods

This study was approved by the Institutional Review Board of Jianan Psychiatric Center, Taiwan Ministry of Health and Welfare (No. 16-007). The requirement of written informed consent was waived due to the deidentification of all data. Data management and all analyses were performed onsite at the Health and Welfare Data Science Center of the Taiwan Ministry of Health and Welfare.

The authors assert that all procedures contributing to this work comply with the ethical standards of the relevant national and institutional committees on human experimentation and with the Helsinki Declaration of 1975, as revised in 2008.

2.1. Data Sources

The data analyzed in this study were retrieved from data sets of the National Health Insurance (NHI) program and the Taiwan Death Registry (TDR) from 2000 to 2013. The NHI data sets contain the records of all of Taiwan's inpatient/outpatient medical claims and the drugs prescribed for treatment, and the National Health Insurance Administration performs a quarterly expert review of a random sample of medical claims to ensure the claims' accuracy [15]. Additionally, the TDR is considered to be accurate and complete because all deceased residents of Taiwan must be registered, and physicians must provide all patient information on the death certificate, including the patient's demographic characteristics, underlying cause of death (UCOD), place of death, and marital status [16].

This study used a randomly selected sample of 2 million beneficiaries who were registered in the NHI in 2000. NHI claims and TDR information of this sample between 2000 and 2013 were retrieved and analyzed. This random sample was verified by the Department of Statistics of Taiwan's Ministry of Health and Welfare for its preventiveness of all Taiwanese residents with respect to age, sex, and geographical distribution of residence [15].

2.2. Study Cohort and End Points

The NHI claims revealed that between 2001 and 2012, 92,615 adults received opioid analgesics (i.e., oral morphine, oral fentanyl, oral codeine, oral tramadol, transdermal morphine, or transdermal fentanyl) as either a single prescription for >14 days or a cumulative prescription for >28 days in a 90-day period. We excluded the following users of opioid analgesics: (1) 62,731 users who had cancer-related diagnoses (International Classification of Diseases, Ninth Revision, Clinical Modification (ICD-9-CM)codes: 140–239) in 2000–2013; (2) 16,783 users who were aged <18 or >65 years when they were first prescribed the drugs; (3) 68 users who either had been prescribed opioid analgesics or had received opioid-related diagnoses (ICD-9-CM codes: 292, 305.51–305.53, 304.0, 304.7, 304.9, 965.0, E935.0, E850.1, E950.0, E980.0, and E935.1-935.2) before 2001; and (4) 43 users who had been prescribed two types of opioid analgesics at the same time. The remaining 12,990 adults comprised the study cohort.

2.3. Study Design

The study cohort was linked to the TDR according to the patients' unique personal identification numbers to identify those who had died by the end of 2013. All patients received at least 1 year of follow-up. The UCODs were classified according to ICD-9-CM (for calendar years 2000–2007) or International Classification of Diseases, Tenth Revision, Clinical Modification (for calendar years 2008–2013) codes. During the 14 years of interest, 558 of the included individuals died, namely 362 men and 196 women.

2.4. Statistical Analysis

The person-years observed for each person accumulated from the date of cohort enrollment to either date of death or the last day of 2013. Ages at cohort enrollment were categorized as follows: 18–24, 25–34, 35–44, 45–54, and 55–64 years. The person-years were then categorized according to calendar year, sex, and patient age during follow-up. The study cohort contributed a total of 48,020 person-years during the follow-up period (mean ± standard deviation: 2.81 ± 2.14 years).

We compared opioid analgesics users' risks for all-cause and cause-specific mortality with those of the general population with comparable sex and age during specific calendar years. The UCODs analyzed in this study included various natural causes of death (i.e., infection, neoplasms, metabolic diseases, hematologic diseases, mental disorders, neurological disorders, circulatory diseases, respiratory diseases, digestive diseases, genitourinary diseases, pregnancy, childbirth or complications during the puerperium, skin or subcutaneous diseases, musculoskeletal diseases, perinatal conditions, congenital malformations or deformities, or symptoms/signs not classified elsewhere), unnatural causes of death (i.e., accidents or violence, suicide, or homicide), and unspecified causes of death. Supplementary Table S1 lists the ICD codes for the UCODs analyzed in this study.

To calculate the expected number of deaths among long-term opioid analgesics users, the annual mortality rates were stratified according to age and sex, with those of the general population of Taiwan serving as a reference. The annual age- and sex-specific population sizes during the study period were derived from the national annual household registration statistics published by Ministry of the Interior of Taiwan (https://pop-proj.ndc.gov.tw/main_en/dataSearch.aspx?uid=78&pid=78, accessed on 31 May 2020). The annual average size of the general population during the study period (i.e., 2001–2013) was 22,881,081. Moreover, we calculated the all-cause and cause-specific standardized mortality ratios (SMRs). The all-cause SMR was further stratified according to the calendar year of cohort enrollment, patient age at cohort enrollment, and patient's sex. The 95% CI for the SMRs was estimated according to the exact estimation [17]. The UCOD distributions were compared between men and women and between patients of different ages at cohort enrollment. The analysis was performed with SAS (version 9.4; SAS Institute, Cary, NC, USA), and the level of significance was set to $\alpha = 0.05$.

3. Results

Table 1 lists the characteristics of the study cohort (60.25% men vs. 39.75% women). Although most patients were enrolled at the age of 45 years or older (67.09%), 15.19% of patients became long-term opioid analgesics users during young adulthood (<35 years). Codeine was the most commonly used opioid analgesics in patients who enrolled in 2001–2003 (57.7%), but the prevalence decreased thereafter to 5.2% between 2010 and 2012. Tramadol, however, gained prevalence over time, accounting for 88.9% (11,553/12,990) of all opioid analgesics that patients initially used (Supplementary Table S2). By the end of 2013, 558 patients had all-cause mortality over 48,020 person-years, representing a cumulative mortality and mortality rate of 4.3% and 11.62 per 1000 person-years. respectively. The calendar year, age, or sex-specific mortality rates are presented in Table 2 and Supplementary Figure S1.

Table 1. Characteristics of the study cohort.

Characteristics	n	%
Total	12,990	100.00
Calendar year of enrollment [a]		
2001–2003	360	2.77
2004–2006	789	6.07
2007–2009	3798	29.24
2010–2012	7843	60.38
Age at cohort enrollment (years)		
18–24	474	3.65
25–34	1499	11.54
35–44	2302	17.72
45–54	3682	28.34
55–64	5033	38.75
Mean ± SD	48.52 ± 11.63	
Sex		
Male	7826	60.25
Female	5164	39.75
Years of follow-up		
<2	5445	41.92
2–3	3878	29.85
4–5	2301	17.71
6–7	713	5.49
8–9	300	2.31
10–14	353	2.72
Mean ± SD	2.81 ± 2.14	
Survival status at the end of 2013		
Survivors	12,432	71.42
Nonsurvivors	558	28.58

[a] Based on the date of the first inpatient/outpatient visit with opioid analgesics usage between 2000 and 2013. Abbreviation: SD, standard deviation.

The study cohort had a significantly higher risk of all-cause mortality than the general population, with an age–sex–calendar SMR of 4.30 (95% CI: 3.95–4.66). Both men and women had significantly increased SMRs (4.56 and 3.89, respectively). Patients of all age stratifications also had significantly increased SMRs. Notably, the youngest group (patients aged 18–24 years) had an even higher SMR (13.17, 95% CI: 8.68–18.58). The age-specific SMRs gradually decreased with increases in age. Enrollment in an earlier calendar year was also significantly associated with a greater SMR; the highest (11.73) and lowest (3.13) SMRs were observed for patients enrolled between 2001 and 2003 and between 2010 and 2012, respectively (Table 2).

Table 2. All-cause standardized mortality ratios among individuals without cancer who were long-term users of opioid analgesics.

All-Cause Mortality	Obs.	Mortality Rate (per 10^3 Person-Years)	Exp.	Standardized Mortality Ratio [a]		
				Estimate	95% CI	
Overall	558	11.62	129.77	4.30	3.95	4.66
By calendar year of enrollment						
2001–2003	23	16.74	1.96	11.73	7.44	17.61
2004–2006	67	14.31	8.17	8.20	6.36	10.41
2007–2009	132	9.84	23.54	5.61	4.69	6.65
2010–2012	336	10.90	96.10	3.50	3.13	3.89
By age at cohort enrollment (years)						
18–24	27	1.77	2.05	13.17	8.68	18.58
25–34	94	6.16	14.33	6.56	5.30	7.95
35–44	93	8.31	18.36	5.07	4.09	6.15
45–54	144	11.56	31.07	4.63	3.91	5.42
55–64	200	15.92	63.96	3.13	2.71	3.57
By sex						
Men	362	13.40	79.85	4.56	4.10	5.04
Women	196	9.14	49.92	3.89	3.36	4.45

[a] Standardized for sex, age, and calendar year. Abbreviations: Obs., observed number; Exp., expected number; CI, confidence interval.

Despite the differences in sex-specific and age-specific all-cause SMRs, the UCOD distributions were not significantly different between deceased men and women or across all deceased patients. The deaths of the 85.1% of men and 88.3% of women were attributable to various natural causes (Supplementary Table S3). The leading natural causes of death in men were circulatory disease ($n = 91$), digestive disease ($n = 75$), and metabolic disease ($n = 37$), whereas the leading natural causes of women's deaths were mainly attributable to metabolic disease ($n = 42$), circulatory disease ($n = 36$), and genitourinary disease ($n = 19$) (not listed in the tables). Unnatural causes of death accounted for 11.6% and 10.7% of the total deaths of men and women, respectively. The discrepancy in UCOD distribution between men and women was not statistically significant ($p = 0.234$).

Supplementary Table S4 presents the age-specific number and proportion of various causes of death. The proportion of natural causes of death (74.1% of patients aged 18–24 years and 89.5% of those aged 55–64 years) tended to be higher among individuals who were older at cohort enrollment. Furthermore, unnatural causes of death and unspecified causes of death were more prevalent in younger adults. Nonetheless, these age-related discrepancies in UCOD distribution had no statistical significance ($p = 0.519$).

Cause-specific analyses revealed that the study cohort had a significantly increased risk of mortality from both natural (SMR = 4.15, 95% CI: 3.78–4.53) and unnatural causes (SMR = 5.04, 95% CI: 3.88–6.45). While the cause of death with the greatest increase in SMR was congenital anomalies (SMR = 58.15, 95% CI: 11.69–139.97), it was based on only three deaths. Such an increased SMR is unreliable and should be interpreted with caution because of a very wide confidence interval. Musculoskeletal and connective tissue diseases (20.88), infections and parasitic diseases (12.93), diseases of the nervous system or sensory organs (11.93), and hematological diseases (10.26) were all associated with greater long-term use of opioid analgesics, with an SMR that was 10 times higher than that of the controls. By contrast, the SMR for cancer was significantly lower among long-term users of opioid analgesics (SMR = 0.29, 95% CI: 0.16–0.47). For unnatural causes, significantly more deaths due to accidents/violence (SMR = 4.52, 95% CI: 3.15–6.14) or suicide (SMR = 5.88, 95% CI: 3.91–8.25) were observed in people without cancer who were long-term users of opioid analgesics (Table 3).

Table 3. Cause-specific standardized mortality ratios in individuals without cancer who were long-term users of opioid analgesics.

Underlying Cause of Death	Obs.	Mortality Rate (10³ Person-Years)	Exp.	Standardized Mortality Ratio [a]	
				Estimate	95% CI
Natural causes of death	481	10.02	116.30	4.15	3.78 4.53
Infection and parasitic diseases	29	0.60	2.24	12.93	8.66 18.05
Neoplasms [b]	13	0.27	44.27	0.29	0.16 0.47
Metabolic and immunity diseases	79	1.65	10.27	7.69	6.09 9.48
Hematological diseases	3	0.06	0.29	10.26	2.06 24.70
Mental disorders	2	0.04	0.64	3.14	0.35 8.74
Diseases of the nervous system and sensory organs	16	0.33	1.34	11.93	6.81 18.45
Circulatory diseases	127	2.65	26.62	4.77	3.98 5.64
Respiratory disease	42	0.87	9.52	4.41	3.18 5.84
Digestive diseases	88	1.83	10.67	8.25	6.61 10.06
Genitourinary disease	47	0.98	5.98	7.85	5.77 10.25
Complications of pregnancy, childbirth, and the puerperium	0	0.00	0.00	NA	
Skin and subcutaneous disease	3	0.06	0.67	4.45	0.89 10.71
Musculoskeletal and connective tissue diseases	13	0.27	0.62	20.88	11.11 33.68
Congenital anomalies	3	0.06	0.05	58.15	11.69 139.97
Conditions originating in the perinatal period	0	0.00	0.00	NA	
Symptoms/signs not classified elsewhere	16	0.33	3.12	5.12	2.93 7.92
Unnatural causes of death	63	1.31	12.49	5.04	3.88 6.45
Accidents and violence	35	0.73	7.73	4.52	3.15 6.14
Suicide	28	0.58	4.76	5.88	3.91 8.25
Homicide	0	0.00	0.18	NA	
Unspecified causes of death	14	0.29	0.77	18.25	9.97 28.99

Abbreviations: Obs., observed number; Exp., expected number; CI, confidence interval; NA, not applicable due to limited number of deaths. [a] Standardized for sex, age, and calendar year. [b] These deceased cancer patients were not present in NHI claims during the follow-up period.

4. Discussion

This study identified a relatively high all-cause SMR in 12,990 individuals without cancer who were long-term users of opioid analgesics in Taiwan, both among individuals with all-cause mortality across different calendar year, age, and sex stratifications as well as among individuals who died of natural and unnatural causes. To the best of our knowledge, this study is the first of its kind with an Asian cohort, and the results are comparable to the findings presented in studies with Western cohorts. Global opioid consumption increased substantially after the year 2000, disproportionately so in high-income countries, with severe consequences for mortality and morbidity. Codeine remains the most commonly used opioid analgesic, but stronger opioids, such as oxycodone, are becoming more common [18]. In contrast to international statistics on tramadol use, tramadol has been the most common opioid analgesic used long term by individuals without cancer in Taiwan.

Based on 10 cohorts, Larney et al. estimated a pooled all-cause crude mortality rate of 28.8 per 1000 person-years for people who were prescribed opioids, but their estimations exhibited substantial heterogeneity not only between countries, but also within countries [13]. The lowest and highest all-cause crude mortality rates were reported by Foster et al. in the United States (8.95 per 1000 person-years) [19] and Du et al. in Germany (57.70 per 1000 person-years), respectively [20]. More recently, Peacock et al. reviewed 16 cohort studies and reported a pooled all-cause crude mortality rate of 12.4 per 1000 person-years among people with regular or problematic cocaine use [14]. Similar to the findings of Larney et al. [13], Peacock et al. also indicated considerable geographic variations in all-cause crude mortality rate, with the highest figure being noted for studies conducted in tropical Latin America (22.8 per 1000 person-years), followed by studies from high-income North American countries (15.6 per 1000 person-years) and Western European countries (9.3 per 1000 person-years) [14]. Based on 92 papers with 101 cohorts ($n = 101 \sim 229,274$) that measured all-cause mortality and opioid overdose-specific mortality in North America, Australia, several Eastern and Western European countries, and Asia, Bahji et al. found the overall all-cause mortality rate was 18.7 per 1000 PY (95% CI: 17.1–20.3). The overall overdose-specific mortality rate was 7.0 per 1000 PY (95% CI: 6.1–8.0). All-cause and overdose-specific mortality were substantially higher in low/middle-income countries, among those with HIV, and among people who use injection drugs [21]. Over 48,020 person-years, 558 all-cause deaths were observed our study cohort (the mortality rate, representing an all-cause mortality of 11.62 per 1000 person-years, is comparable to international figures).

By using 16 cohorts and analyzing a total of 69,932 people with regular or problematic cocaine use, Peacock et al. obtained a pooled all-cause SMR of 6.13, with apparent sex (men/women: 3.42/4.59, respectively), age (<30 years/30 years: 7.75/3.09, respectively), and regional heterogeneity (tropical Latin American/Western European/high-income North American countries: 14.75/6.01/5.13, respectively) differences [14]. Based on 43 cohorts, Larney et al. estimated all-cause and cause-specific mortality among people using extra-medical opioids and found a pooled all-cause SMR of 10.0 (95% CI: 7.6–13.2). Excess mortality was observed across a range of causes, including overdose, injuries, and infectious and noncommunicable diseases [22]. Although our study obtained similar results, we also noted a decline in SMR over time, which was likely due to a shorter follow-up period for patients who were enrolled in relatively recent years. In fact, there are no data available suggesting a period most relevant to address the association of opioids with mortality. Among the 13 cohort studies included in the systematic review and meta-analysis of all-cause and overdose mortality risk among people prescribed opioids [13], only 2 studies followed study participants for at least 1 year, 1 study set a follow-up period of at least 5 years, and the others did not set any minimum time period required for follow-up. Moreover, Dart et al. described trends in the diversion and abuse of prescription opioid analgesics in the US between 2002 and 2013 and found that prescriptions for opioid analgesics increased substantially from 2002 through 2010 in the US but then decreased slightly from 2011 through 2013. The rate of opioid-related deaths rose and fell in a similar pattern, suggesting no obvious lag between opioid use and mortality [23].

Nonetheless, researchers should proceed with caution when interpreting the relatively increased SMRs because of the potential of confounding by indication, wherein the underlying medical conditions of users of opioids may also influence mortality. To address this potential methodological problem, Tölle et al. included four studies with seven study arms and 120,186 patients, and they calculated a pooled covariate adjusted hazard ratio (aHR) of 1.69 (95% CI: 1.47–1.95) for all-cause mortality [24]. When they confined mortality risk to out-of-hospital deaths, they obtained a pooled aHR of 2.12 (95% CI: 1.46–3.09) [24]. Moreover, the use of opioid analgesics is typically accompanied by the use of other pain relievers, such as nonsteroidal anti-inflammatory drugs, which makes the specific association of opioid analgesics with mortality difficult to evaluate. Although comparisons of SMRs across studies have potential problems [25], our study results were generally comparable to the findings of other research studies.

In the aforementioned studies by Peacock et al. and Tölle et al., congenital anomalies and hematological diseases exhibited a more than tenfold increase in SMR; however, both studies were based on a relatively small number of deaths. The increase in mortality from natural causes was associated with musculoskeletal and connective tissue diseases, infection and parasitic diseases, and diseases of the nervous system and sensory organs. Musculoskeletal pain is pain that affects bones, joints, ligaments, muscles, and tendons and is prevalent in both middle-aged and older adults. Chronic pain resulting from musculoskeletal and connective tissue diseases is one of the leading causes of disability [26], which might in turn increase the risk of mortality. The increased SMR for neurological diseases may be attributable to certain neuroplastic events within the mesocorticolimbic system that emerge due to chronic exposure to opioids. It may have a determinative influence on behavioral symptoms associated with opioid use disorder, which is a chronic relapsing clinical condition with remarkably high morbidity and mortality [27]. The remarkably low SMR for neoplasm in the present is due to the study cohort being restricted to people without cancer.

In our study, suicide was an unnatural cause of death that had one of the most elevated SMRs, which aligns with previous findings that patients with chronic pain are at an increased risk of suicide [28,29]. Many factors promote the initiation and persistence of opioid use, but the pathways toward vulnerability to overdose and suicide are related to biological, medical, and social factors [30]. A recent meta-analysis also reported increased SMRs for suicide (SMR: 7.93, 95% CI: 5.69–11.04), unintentional injury (SMR: 6.85, 95% CI: 4.41–10.64), and violence (SMR: 9.75, 95% CI: 6.60–14.39) [22]. Although our study also observed increased SMRs (4.52) for accidents and violence, no deaths due to homicide were observed in our study cohort.

Opioid use disorders affect over 16 million people worldwide, including over 2.1 million in the United States, and over 120,000 deaths worldwide annually are attributed to opioid use [31]. Although the rates of misuse of prescription medicine, including opioids, have been reported to be lower in countries in the Asia–Pacific region than in many Western countries (such as the United States and United Kingdom), adolescents and young adults in Asia–Pacific and Western countries exhibit similar trends of misuse. The problems with misuse in the Asia–Pacific region could be overlooked because the association between drug misuse and health consequences, such as mortality, are not well documented by most countries in the region [32].

Chronic pain is one of the most common symptoms reported by patients in outpatient clinics. However, failure to manage chronic pain and opioid dependence associated with chronic pain can result in high rates of morbidity and mortality. Moreover, pain-related expenses are extremely high and represent a substantial burden [26]. Besides, interventions such as marijuana laws, harm-reduction interventions, health insurer policies, and patient/health care provider education, as well as simultaneous interventions on opioid-related outcomes, have also been used to reduce the inappropriate prescription of drugs [33]. Some patients with chronic pain are treated with opioid analgesics regularly for pain relief, and likely to become long-term opioid analgesics users. Awareness and health literacy regarding the potential adverse effect from opioid use should be enhanced by shared decision making, a process by which the clinician and the patient share all applicable information and negotiate a plan of pain treatment that is acceptable to both [34].

Although this study used a population-based approach with a large number of unselected study participants, which minimized the likelihood of selection bias and allowed for analyses of mortality from specific causes, several limitations should be noted. First, we were unable to differentiate between misuse/overuse and appropriate use of opioids. Second, medical claims do not cover the information of extra-medical opioid use, which could entail certain degrees of exposure misclassification and could likely underestimate the association between long-term opioid analgesics use and mortality. Third, despite that an elevated risk of mortality was found in long-term opioid analgesics users, we did not weigh the risks and benefits of long-term opioid analgesics use. After all, pain control by medications is essential in assuring the quality of life in patients with chronic pain.

5. Conclusions

In conclusion, long-term opioid analgesics use among individuals without cancer in Taiwan was associated with a significantly increased risk of mortality. The notably increased mortality in younger adults warrants attention. Strategies to reduce long-term opioid analgesics use, especially their overuse or misuse, are urgently needed.

Supplementary Materials: The following are available online at https://www.mdpi.com/article/10.3390/healthcare9111402/s1, Supplementary Table S1: International Classification of Diseases' codes for the diseases analyzed in this study; Supplementary Table S2: Comparison of opioid analgesics consumed by patients enrolled in different calendar years; Supplementary Table S3: Comparison of underlying causes of death between male and female users of long-term opioid analgesics; Supplementary Table S4: Comparison of underlying causes of death among long-term users of opioid analgesics with respect to their age at cohort enrollment; Supplementary Figure S1: Mortality rate according to calendar year of enrollment (upper), age (years) at cohort enrollment (middle), or sex (lower).

Author Contributions: Conceptualization, P.-F.L. and C.-Y.L.; methodology, P.-F.L. and C.-Y.L.; formal analysis, P.-F.L., C.-Y.L. and W.-H.H.; investigation, P.-F.L. and C.-Y.L.; resources, P.-F.L. and C.-Y.L.; data curation, P.-F.L., C.-Y.L. and W.-H.H.; writing—original draft preparation, P.-F.L., C.-Y.L. and W.-H.H.; writing—review and editing, C.-Y.L., Y.-C.L., C.-T.C. and W.-H.H. All authors have read and agreed to the published version of the manuscript.

Funding: This research was funded by Taiwan Ministry of Science and Technology, Grant number MOST 109-2629-B-006-001.

Institutional Review Board Statement: This study was approved by the Institutional Review Board of Jianan Psychiatric Center, Taiwan Ministry of Health and Welfare (No. 16-007). The requirement of written informed consent was waived due to the deidentification of all data. Data management and all analyses were performed onsite at the Health and Welfare Data Science Center of the Taiwan Ministry of Health and Welfare.

Informed Consent Statement: Patient consent was waived due to the deidentification of all data.

Data Availability Statement: Data management and all analyses were performed onsite at the Health and Welfare Data Science Center of the Taiwan Ministry of Health and Welfare. Data is not available to the public and data sharing is prohibited under the current government regulations.

Acknowledgments: We are grateful to Chih-Hui Hsu from the Biostatistics Consulting Center, National Cheng Kung University Hospital for providing statistical consultation services. The authors are also grateful to Health Data Science Center, National Cheng Kung University Hospital for providing administrative and technical support.

Conflicts of Interest: The funders had no role in the design of the study; in the collection, analyses, or interpretation of data; in the writing of the manuscript, or in the decision to publish the results.

References

1. Pan, H.H.; Ho, S.T.; Lu, C.C.; Wang, J.O.; Lin, T.C.; Wang, K.Y. Trends in the consumption of opioid analgesics in Taiwan from 2002 to 2007: A population-based study. *J. Pain Symptom Manag.* **2013**, *45*, 272–278. [CrossRef]
2. Kang, K.H.; Kuo, L.F.; Cheng, I.C.; Chang, C.S.; Tsay, W.I. Trends in major opioid analgesic consumption in Taiwan, 2002–2014. *J. Formos. Med. Assoc.* **2017**, *116*, 529–535. [CrossRef]
3. Garcia del Pozo, J.; Carvajal, A.; Viloria, J.M.; Velasco, A.; Garcia del Pozo, V. Trends in the consumption of opioid analgesics in Spain. Higher increases as fentanyl replaces morphine. *Eur. J. Clin. Pharmacol.* **2008**, *64*, 411–415. [CrossRef]
4. Hamunen, K.; Paakkari, P.; Kalso, E. Trends in opioid consumption in the Nordic countries 2002–2006. *Eur. J. Pain* **2009**, *13*, 954–962. [CrossRef]
5. Roxburgh, A.; Hall, W.D.; Dobbins, T.; Gisev, N.; Burns, L.; Pearson, S.; Degenhardt, L. Trends in heroin and pharmaceutical opioid overdose deaths in Australia. *Drug Alcohol Depend.* **2017**, *179*, 291–298. [CrossRef]
6. Ekholm, O.; Kurita, G.P.; Hojsted, J.; Juel, K.; Sjogren, P. Chronic pain, opioid prescriptions, and mortality in Denmark: A population-based cohort study. *Pain* **2014**, *155*, 2486–2490. [CrossRef]
7. Kiang, M.V.; Basu, S.; Chen, J.; Alexander, M.J. Assessment of changes in the geographical distribution of opioid-related mortality across the United States by opioid type, 1999–2016. *JAMA Netw. Open* **2019**, *2*, e190040. [CrossRef]
8. Rose, A.J.; Bernson, D.; Chui, K.K.H.; Land, T.; Walley, A.Y.; LaRochelle, M.R.; Stein, B.D.; Stopka, T.J. Potentially inappropriate opioid prescribing, overdose, and mortality in Massachusetts, 2011–2015. *J. Gen. Intern. Med.* **2018**, *33*, 1512–1519. [CrossRef]
9. Ruhm, C.J. Corrected US opioid-involved drug poisoning deaths and mortality rates, 1999–2015. *Addiction* **2018**, *113*, 1339–1344. [CrossRef]
10. Bahji, A.; Cheng, B.; Gray, S.; Stuart, H. Reduction in mortality risk with opioid agonist therapy: A systematic review and meta-analysis. *Acta Psychiatr. Scand.* **2019**, *140*, 313–339. [CrossRef]
11. Degenhardt, L.; Bucello, C.; Mathers, B.; Briegleb, C.; Ali, H.; Hickman, M.; McLaren, J. Mortality among regular or dependent users of heroin and other opioids: A systematic review and meta-analysis of cohort studies. *Addiction* **2011**, *106*, 32–51. [CrossRef]
12. Ma, J.; Bao, Y.-P.; Wang, R.-J.; Su, M.-F.; Liu, M.-X.; Li, J.-Q.; Degenhardt, L.; Farrell, M.; Blow, F.C.; Ilgen, M.; et al. Effects of medication-assisted treatment on mortality among opioids users: A systematic review and meta-analysis. *Mol. Psychiatry* **2019**, *24*, 1868–1883. [CrossRef]
13. Larney, S.; Peacock, A.; Tran, L.T.; Stockings, E.; Santomauro, D.; Santo, T.; Degenhardt, L. All-cause and overdose mortality risk among people prescribed opioids: A systematic review and meta-analysis. *Pain Med.* **2020**, *21*, 3700–3711. [CrossRef]
14. Peacock, A.; Tran, L.T.; Larney, S.; Stockings, E.; Santo, T., Jr.; Jones, H.; Santomauro, D.; Degenhardt, L. All-cause and cause-specific mortality among people with regular or problematic cocaine use: A systematic review and meta-analysis. *Addiction* **2021**, *116*, 725–742. [CrossRef]
15. Chen, H.F.; Ho, C.A.; Li, C.Y. Risk of heart failure in a population with type 2 diabetes versus a population without diabetes with and without coronary heart disease. *Diabetes Obes. Metab.* **2019**, *21*, 112–119. [CrossRef]

16. Lu, T.H.; Lee, M.C.; Chou, M.C. Accuracy of cause-of-death coding in Taiwan: Types of miscoding and effects on mortality statistics. *Int. J. Epidemiol.* **2000**, *29*, 336–343. [CrossRef]
17. Dobson, A.J.; Kuulasmaa, K.; Eberle, E.; Scherer, J. Confidence intervals for weighted sums of Poisson parameters. *Stat. Med.* **1991**, *10*, 457–462. [CrossRef]
18. Maia, L.O.; Daldegan-Bueno, D.; Fischer, B. Opioid use, regulation, and harms in Brazil: A comprehensive narrative overview of available data and indicators. *Subst. Abuse Treat. Prev. Policy* **2021**, *16*, 12. [CrossRef]
19. Foster, D.; Udayachalerm, S.; Wang, J.; Murray, M. Characterization of opioid use and adverse outcomes using longitudinal data from a statewide health information exchange. *Pharmacotherapy* **2017**, *37*, e189.
20. Du, Y.; Wolf, I.K.; Busch, M.A.; Knopf, H. Associations between the use of specific psychotropic drugs and all-cause mortality among older adults in Germany: Results of the mortality follow-up of the German National Health Interview and Examination Survey 1998. *PLoS ONE* **2019**, *14*, e0210695. [CrossRef]
21. Bahji, A.; Cheng, B.; Gray, S.; Stuart, H. Mortality among people with opioid use disorder: A systematic review and meta-analysis. *J. Addict. Med.* **2020**, *14*, e118–e132. [CrossRef]
22. Larney, S.; Tran, L.T.; Leung, J.; Santo, T., Jr.; Santomauro, D.; Hickman, M.; Peacock, A.; Stockings, E.; Degenhardt, L. All-cause and cause-specific mortality among people using extramedical opioids: A systematic review and meta-analysis. *JAMA Psychiatry* **2020**, *77*, 493–502. [CrossRef]
23. Dart, R.C.; Surratt, H.L.; Cicero, T.J.; Parrino, M.W.; Severtson, S.G.; Bucher-Bartelson, B.; Green, J.L. Trends in opioid analgesic abuse and mortality in the United States. *N. Engl. J. Med.* **2015**, *372*, 241–248. [CrossRef]
24. Tölle, T.; Fitzcharles, M.A.; Häuser, W. Is opioid therapy for chronic non-cancer pain associated with a greater risk of all-cause mortality compared to non-opioid analgesics? A systematic review of propensity score matched observational studies. *Eur. J. Pain* **2021**, *25*, 1195–1208. [CrossRef]
25. Armstrong, B.G. Comparing standardized mortality ratios. *Ann. Epidemiol.* **1995**, *5*, 60–64. [CrossRef]
26. Dydyk, A.M.; Yarrarapu, S.N.S.; Conermann, T. Chronic Pain. In *StatPearls*; StatPearls Publishing: Treasure Island, FL, USA, 2021.
27. Thompson, B.L.; Oscar-Berman, M.; Kaplan, G.B. Opioid-induced structural and functional plasticity of medium-spiny neurons in the nucleus accumbens. *Neurosci. Biobehav. Rev.* **2021**, *120*, 417–430. [CrossRef]
28. Gill, H.; Perez, C.D.; Gill, B.; El-Halabi, S.; Lee, Y.; Lipsitz, O.; Park, C.; Mansur, R.B.; Rodrigues, N.B.; McIntyre, R.S.; et al. The Prevalence of suicidal behaviour in fibromyalgia patients. *Prog. Neuropsychopharmacol. Biol. Psychiatry* **2021**, *108*, 110078. [CrossRef]
29. Kirtley, O.J.; Rodham, K.; Crane, C. Understanding suicidal ideation and behaviour in individuals with chronic pain: A review of the role of novel transdiagnostic psychological factors. *Lancet Psychiatry* **2020**, *7*, 282–290. [CrossRef]
30. Bohnert, A.S.B.; Ilgen, M.A. Understanding links among opioid use, overdose, and suicide. *N. Engl. J. Med.* **2019**, *380*, 71–79. [CrossRef]
31. Dydyk, A.M.; Jain, N.K.; Gupta, M. Opioid Use Disorder. In *StatPearls*; StatPearls Publishing: Treasure Island, FL, USA, 2021.
32. Chan, W.L.; Wood, D.M.; Dargan, P.I. Prescription medicine misuse in the Asia-Pacific region: An evolving issue? *Br. J. Clin. Pharmacol.* **2021**, *87*, 1660–1667. [CrossRef]
33. Ansari, B.; Tote, K.M.; Rosenberg, E.S.; Martin, E.G. A rapid review of the impact of systems-level policies and interventions on population-level outcomes related to the opioid epidemic, United States and Canada, 2014–2018. *Public Health Rep.* **2020**, *135*, 100S–127S. [CrossRef] [PubMed]
34. Lewiecki, E.M. Risk communication and shared decision making in the care of patients with osteoporosis. *J. Clin. Densitom.* **2010**, *13*, 335–345. [CrossRef] [PubMed]

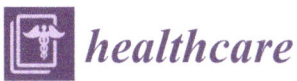

Article

Evaluating the Impact of Medication Risk Mitigation Services in Medically Complex Older Adults

Hubert Jin [1], Sue Yang [1], David Bankes [2], Stephanie Finnel [1], Jacques Turgeon [3] and Alan Stein [1,*]

[1] Office of Healthcare Analytics, Tabula Rasa HealthCare, Moorestown, NJ 08057, USA; hjin@trhc.com (H.J.); syang@trhc.com (S.Y.); sfinnel@trhc.com (S.F.)
[2] Office of Translational Research and Residency Programs, Tabula Rasa HealthCare, Moorestown, NJ 08057, USA; dbankes@trhc.com
[3] Precision Pharmacotherapy Research and Development Institute, 13485 Veteran's Way, Suite 410, Lake Nona, Orlando, FL 32827, USA; jturgeon@trhc.com
* Correspondence: astein@trhc.com; Tel.: +1-856-242-2595

Abstract: Adverse drug events (ADEs) represent an expensive societal burden that disproportionally affects older adults. Therefore, value-based organizations that provide care to older adults—such as the Program of All-Inclusive Care for the Elderly (PACE)—should be highly motivated to identify actual or potential ADEs to mitigate risks and avoid downstream costs. We sought to determine whether PACE participants receiving medication risk mitigation (MRM) services exhibit improvements in total healthcare costs and other outcomes compared to participants not receiving structured MRM. Data from 2545 PACE participants from 19 centers were obtained for the years 2018 and 2019. We compared the year-over-year changes in outcomes between patients not receiving (control) or receiving structured MRM services. Data were adjusted based on participant multimorbidity and geographic location. Our analyses demonstrate that costs in the MRM cohort exhibited a significantly smaller year-to-year increase compared to the control (MRM: USD 4386/participant/year [95% CI, USD 3040–5732] vs. no MRM: USD 9410/participant/year [95% CI, USD 7737–11,084]). Therefore, receipt of structured MRM services reduced total healthcare costs ($p < 0.001$) by USD 5024 per participant from 2018 to 2019. The large majority (75.8%) of the reduction involved facility-related expenditures (e.g., hospital admission, emergency department visits, skilled nursing). In sum, our findings suggest that structured MRM services can curb growing year-over-year healthcare costs for PACE participants.

Keywords: Program of All-Inclusive Care for the Elderly; adverse drug events; medication-related problems; drug-related problems; pharmacists; medication safety; Medicare; Medicaid

1. Introduction

The Program of All-Inclusive Care for the Elderly (PACE) provides comprehensive, supportive services to individuals older than 55 who are certified by their state to require a "nursing home level of care" [1]. The average PACE participant is about 77 years old, has six chronic comorbidities, takes several prescription medications per month, and needs help with at least one activity of daily living [2]. A central objective of PACE is to avoid long-term institutionalization by supporting independent community living [1]. To meet these goals, PACE organizations receive capitated payments (i.e., fixed-rate dollar amount per participant) from the federal government and their state's Medicaid program [1]. Capitation permits clinicians to provide any service needed to achieve positive outcomes in the mid to long term. Conversely, capitation implies that clinicians must strive to avoid expensive, preventable problems (e.g., preventable emergency department (ED) or hospital utilization) and unnecessary services that are unlikely to achieve participant goals of care.

While meeting this goal requires a multidimensional approach [3], medication-related morbidity is a costly societal burden that is relevant to PACE. The value-based, capitated

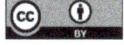

payment model means that PACE organizations are 100% at-risk for negative outcomes; thus, negative sequelae resulting from poor medication-related outcomes would have a direct negative impact on the economics of PACE organizations. For instance, a 2018 cost-of-illness model suggested that it costs about USD 2500, on average, to treat an individual who experiences treatment failure or a new medical problem after initial prescription use [4]. Medically-complex older adults—such as PACE participants—are particularly high risk of negative economic and clinical outcomes associated with drug-related harm [1,5,6]. For instance, one study found that for every dollar spent on medications, USD 1.33 is spent to treat associated medication-related problems (MRPs) in nursing home patients [7]. Another meta-analysis found that the odds of being hospitalized for an adverse-drug event (ADE) are four times greater in older adults compared to their younger counterparts [8]. Moreover, estimates suggest that 10–30% of hospitalizations are caused by ADEs in older adults [5].

Fortunately, the literature suggests that drug-related harm can often be avoided [9]. In particular, medication risk mitigation (MRM) services could enable PACE organizations to avoid some of the costly, negative outcomes associated with medication-related morbidity. MRM encompasses a suite of clinical pharmacy services and technological solutions that aim to optimize medication use in vulnerable older adults. Specifically, MRM services and solutions include ADE risk stratification [10]; clinical decision support software (CDSS) that aids pharmacists in the optimization of medication regimens [11]; pharmacogenomic (PGx) assessments [12]; provision of expert drug information to PACE prescribers [13]; and comprehensive medication adherence support. Until now, no controlled study has evaluated the impact of MRM services on economic outcomes in PACE. Therefore, the objective of this study is to evaluate whether PACE participants receiving MRM solutions exhibit improvements in healthcare costs and other pertinent healthcare outcomes compared to similar participants who do not receive MRM.

2. Materials and Methods

2.1. Study Design, Data Source, and Approvals

This was a retrospective, naturalistic, quasi-experimental study of 2018 and 2019 administrative medical claims data. This study was granted a waiver of informed consent from an independent institutional review board.

2.2. Intervention Description: TRHC's MRM Services

For prescription needs, many PACE programs partner with one pharmacy. CareKinesis, a Tabula Rasa HealthCare (TRHC) subsidiary, is a national PACE pharmacy that provides a suite of MRM solutions to 15 K participants from more than 60 PACE organizations across the US. CareKinesis provides these MRM services to complement the physical provision of prescribed medications. A detailed summary of the specific MRM solutions is provided in Table 1.

Table 1. Summary of TRHC's key medication risk mitigation (MRM) components in PACE.

MRM Component	Detailed Description
MedWise risk score (MRS)	• Risk assessment tool that helps identify PACE participants at high risk of ADEs and in need of risk-mitigating interventions. • Constructed from 5 modifiable risk factors derived from a drug regimen's PK and PD characteristics [14,15]. Scored from 0 to 53; ≥ 20 is considered high risk [14]. Among PACE participants served by CareKinesis, mean MRS is 18.5 [10]. • In PACE, each point rise in MRS is associated with: 8.6% increase in odds of ADEs; USD 1037 in annual medical spending; 3.2 and 2.1 additional ED visits and hospitalizations, respectively, per 100 participants per year [10]. • Results confirmed in other settings, demonstrating additional associations with mortality and falls [16,17].

Table 1. Cont.

MRM Component	Detailed Description
MedWise	<ul><li>This is an advanced CDSS used by TRHC pharmacists to assist clinical interventions [18].</li><li>It presents visualizations of a medication regimen within context of MRS risk factors and allows for identification of simultaneous multidrug interactions [11].</li><li>By working in tandem with the MRS, pharmacists can identify MRPs that contribute to ADEs.</li><li>Visuals of Medwise abound in the literature [19–23].</li></ul>
Pharmacogenomics services (PGx)	<ul><li>CareKinesis PACE Pharmacy offers PGx testing with clinical interpretation/intervention for PACE programs choosing to further personalize their participants' medication regimens [12].</li><li>CDSS ingests PGx results to help pharmacists identify drug-induced phenoconversion [24]. Thus, pharmacists can interpret consensus guidelines (e.g., CPIC) in the context of the entire drug regimen [25].</li><li>PGx services identify 2.5–3.0 gene-based interactions per PACE participant [26].</li></ul>
Drug information support	<ul><li>Clinical pharmacists provide expert advice to prescribers needing drug information prior to making a clinical decision [13].</li><li>PACE prescribers ask TRHC pharmacists a heterogeneous array of questions related to medication management. Prescribers implement about 80% of answers within drug regimens [13].</li></ul>
Comprehensive adherence support	<ul><li>TRHC's dispensary can provide participant medications in customized adherence packaging.</li><li>Refills for chronic medications are synchronized and dispensed automatically on a regular cycle basis.</li></ul>
Staff competency	<ul><li>As a condition of employment:<ul><li>Pharmacists must be (or become) board-certified in geriatric pharmacotherapy (i.e., BCGP) [27] and certified to use the proprietary CDSS (i.e., Certified MedWise Advisor™ pharmacists).</li></ul></li><li>Pharmacy technicians must have (or obtain) the Certified Pharmacy Technician Credential (i.e., CPhT) [28].</li></ul>
Medication safety review (MSR)	<ul><li>A service performed by pharmacists. By applying MRM components, pharmacists identify MRPs and provide recommendations to resolve them. Involves consultations with prescribers.</li><li>Pharmacists utilize prospective and retrospective review methods in PACE:<ul><li>Prospective MSRs address MRPs at prescribing-dispensing interface (prior to drug ingestion).</li><li>Retrospective MSRs address MRPs found in a pre-existing regimen (after drug ingestion).</li></ul></li><li>MSRs can be delivered telephonically or electronically (e.g., e-mail, instant message, or fax).</li><li>In MSRs, pharmacists identify about 2 MRPs per PACE participant. About 80% of all MRPs in PACE involve DDIs (36%), ADRs (18%), high doses (14%), and unindicated medications (13%). MRPs are often resolved through deprescribing (25%), changing drugs (25%), or changing doses (20%). Prescribers accept nearly 80% of recommendations [11].</li></ul>

Abbreviations: ADE = adverse drug event; ADR = adverse drug reaction; CDSS = clinical decision support software; CPIC = Clinical Pharmacogenetics Implementation Consortium; DDI = drug interaction; ED = emergency department; MRP = medication-related problem; PACE = Programs of All-inclusive Care for the Elderly; PD = pharmacodynamic; PK = pharmacokinetic; TRHC = Tabula Rasa HealthCare.

When MRM solutions are deployed into PACE pharmacy practice, pharmacists are enabled to identify MRPs and to issue recommendations to resolve them [11]. Pharmacist-provided "Medication Safety Reviews" (MSRs) are the conduit through which such interventions are delivered to PACE providers. As a formal definition, "MSRs apply the principals of pharmacodynamics, pharmacokinetics, pharmacogenomics, and chronopharmacology to enhance medication safety and prevent ADEs. Additionally, MSRs address simultaneous multidrug interactions in the context of the entire drug regimen" using the aforementioned CDSS [11].

In PACE, MSRs can vary substantially in their timing, intensity, and delivery. Regarding timing, MSRs can be retrospective or prospective. A retrospective MSR involves clinical interventions that aim to resolve MRPs for medications that have already been prescribed, dispensed, or ingested. A prospective MSR issues interventions that aim to prevent MRPs for medications that have not been ingested or dispensed yet. Regarding intensity, MSRs can aim to resolve one or more MRPs per patient. Regarding delivery, MSRs can be delivered telephonically or electronically. Telephonic delivery might involve an ad hoc call with the prescriber or a formal conference call with the PACE team to review multiple MRPs for multiple patients (operationally defined as a "polypharmacy call"). Electronic delivery could involve instant messaging through the prescription management system (EireneRx®, CareKinesis, Inc. and TabulaRasa HealthCare, Inc., Moorestown, NJ, USA), encrypted e-mails, or formal faxed reports.

Figure 1 summarizes the MRM solutions in a workflow diagram:

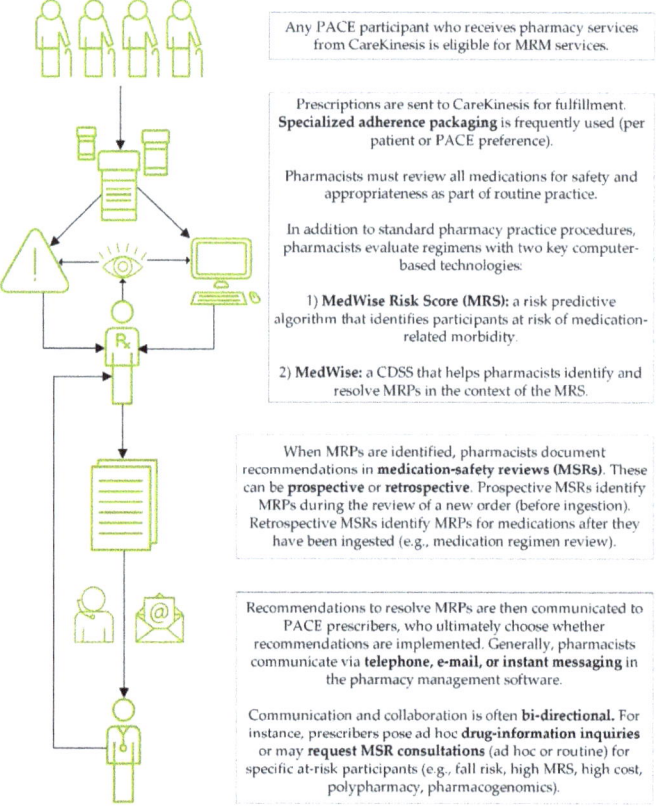

Figure 1. MRM workflow. Abbreviations: CDSS = clinical decision support software; MRM = medication risk mitigation, MRP = medication-related problem; PACE = The Program of All-Inclusive Care for the Elderly.

2.3. Subjects and Outcomes

In addition to the PACE pharmacy subsidiary (CareKinesis), TRHC also has a subsidiary that acts as a third-party administrator for several PACE organizations (CareVention HealthCare™ Third Party Administration). Therefore, TRHC has full administrative medical claims data for two types of PACE programs: (1) PACE clients that receive pharmacy (i.e., MRM services) through CareKinesis (intervention group) and (2) PACE clients that choose to receive pharmacy services elsewhere (control group). Thus, our study sample was non-randomized; all members for whom we had administrative claims were initially eligible for inclusion. Moreover, cohort selection was naturalistic since PACE organizations self-selected CareKinesis (i.e., MRM) services.

Because our intention was to compare the 2018-to-2019 changes in outcomes for both cohorts, we first excluded any participant that was not continuously enrolled during 2018 and 2019. We identified 19 PACE organizations for which (a) administrative medical records were available for the entirety of calendar years 2018 and 2019 and (b) had data use agreements that permitted retrospective research. Of these 19 organizations, 12 organizations received pharmacy services through CareKinesis (MRM), and 7 did not (no MRM).

We compared the following outcomes between the two groups:

- Medical costs. We evaluated the total combined facility (e.g., hospital) and physician (e.g., outpatient services, office visit) expenditures as well as each type of expenditure individually (i.e., hospital, physician). Costs were defined as the total amount that was adjudicated each year (i.e., 2018 and 2019) in US dollars in the claims data. Facility and physician costs were defined from the claim details field in the data. Facility and physician charges were encoded as UB92 and HCFA, respectively. Thus, the total costs were the sum of UB92 and HCFA.
- Fraction of participants with ≥ 1 reported ADE. ADEs were defined as any A- or B-level International Classification of Diseases, Tenth Revision, Clinical Modification (ICD-10) code as defined previously by Hohl et al. [29].
- Fraction of participants with ≥ 1 fall. Falls were defined using the following W-group ICD-10 codes: 01, 03–11; 17–19 as well as R29.6.
- Number of ED visits and hospital admissions. Both were identified by line-item claims.

2.4. Analysis

PACE organizations are free to select their pharmacy provider. Organizations either select CareKinesis' MRM services or obtain pharmacy services elsewhere. Thus, differences across relevant confounding variables could bias results. Typically, propensity score matching is deployed in observational studies as a way to adjust for potentially influential covariates [30]. However, this approach appeared less relevant since our control group was smaller than our intervention group, which limited our capability to do appropriate matching of individuals. To ensure a fair comparison between our two groups, we decided to weight our analyses using participants' baseline hierarchical condition category (HCC) scores.

For context, HCC scores are—broadly—a marker of multimorbidity and patient acuity. The Centers for Medicare and Medicaid Services (CMS) use HCC scores to adjust annual capitation payments for individual PACE participants [31]. A summary HCC score is derived using (a) a participant's ICD-10 codes from the previous calendar year and (b) participant demographic data (age, sex, Medicaid status, disability status) [32]. We used each participant's December 2019 HCC score because this reflected all 2018 diagnoses. Some health services researchers have found that HCC scores can serve as a valid predictive tool for hospitalizations, ED visits, and costs in various cohorts [33,34].

We performed the risk adjustment through the following four steps:

1. Set HCC bins with a set of boundaries.
2. Calculate weight for each participant. Let x_i represent the number of participants in the i-th bin for the MRM cohort. Let y_i represent the number of participants in the

same bin for the control cohort. Therefore, x_i/y_i represents the weight to apply to all participants in the i-th bin to make the control cohort equivalent to the MRM cohort.
3. For each bin, add a padding parameter—0.001—to avoid bins with zero participants and provide a smoothing effect.
4. Add a normalization step to ensure that the sum of the control cohort weights equals the control cohort sample size.

The normalized weights were then used to adjust each clinical outcome for control participants at each bin. For cost-related outcomes, we made one modification to this adjustment. Geographic differences between groups could bias results because medical costs in the US can substantially differ regionally [35]. In PACE, CMS accounts for this variation by applying a county-level adjustment to the HCC score [36]. Therefore, we adjusted the cost-specific outcomes using the actual capitated rate paid by CMS for each participant.

This adjustment procedure carries two implications for exclusion criteria. First, we excluded anyone without a baseline HCC score. Second, patients with end-stage renal disease (ESRD) were excluded since they are scored using a completely different HCC model [17], making the adjustments described above impossible. Regardless of HCC, excluding ESRD is reasonable since such patients tend to consume a disproportionate amount of financial resources [37].

After making all exclusions and adjustments, we first calculated the 2018-to-2019 changes in outcomes (i.e., financial and clinical outcomes) for both cohorts. For continuous outcomes, we compared the two cohorts' year-over-year changes (i.e., weighted mean difference) using a 2-sample t-test, weighted using each participant's baseline CMS HCC score (for non-cost outcomes) or capitated payment amount (for cost outcomes). Since costs tend to have skewed distributions, we also performed the comparisons using the Wilcoxon test. For the categorical outcomes (i.e., participants with ≥ 1 ADE or fall), we used a chi-square test (weighted by HCC) for comparisons. This test was applied to a 3×2 contingency table such as that shown in Table 2. Table 2 applies to ADEs; we used a comparable table for falls.

Table 2. Example contingency table.

	MRM	Control [1]
≥ 1 ADE in 2018 but not in 2019	# participants	# participants
No year-over-year change in ADEs	# participants	# participants
No ADE in 2018 but ≥ 1 in 2019	# participants	# participants

Abbreviations: MRM = Medication risk mitigation; [1] proportions were risk-adjusted based on weights of HCC distribution.

We considered p values < 0.05 statistically significant. All standard errors, confidence intervals, and p-values were computed using techniques suitable for weighted data (e.g., Kish's effective sample size) [38]. All analyses were conducted in R version 3.5.

3. Results

3.1. Cohort Description

The entire study consisted of 2545 PACE participants across the 19 PACE organizations. The sample was predominantly female (67.2%) with an average age of 77.0 (95% CI: 76.6, 77.3) years. The MRM and control cohorts were well-balanced across age and sex. However, patients in the MRM group had a greater level of multimorbidity, as defined by HCC (mean HCC 2.68 vs. 2.58, p = 0.042). The two groups also differed according to geographic distribution (p < 0.001). Specifically, PACE participants in the MRM group were predominantly from the Western (48.6%) and Southern (28.9%) regions of the US, whereas participants in the control cohort were largely from the Northeast (70.8%). Full participant demographics can be viewed in Table 3.

Table 3. Baseline demographics.

	MRM + Control	MRM	Control	p-Value [1]
Participants, n (%)	2545 (100)	1582 (62.2)	963 (37.8)	N/A
Male, n (%)	834 (32.8)	537 (33.9)	297 (30.8)	0.11
Age, mean (95% CI)	77.0 (76.6, 77.3)	76.7 (76.2, 77.2)	77.4 (76.8, 78.1)	0.09
HCC score, mean (95% CI)	2.64 (2.59, 2.69)	2.68 (2.62, 2.74)	2.58 (2.50, 2.65)	0.042
Conditions, n (%)				
Hypertension (I10)	1460 (57.4)	973 (61.5)	487 (50.6)	<0.001
Diabetes, type II (E11)	1137 (44.7)	776 (49.1)	361 (37.5)	<0.001
Dyslipidemia (E78)	1046 (41.1)	659 (41.7)	387 (40.2)	0.23
Dementia (F03)	506 (19.9)	329 (20.8)	177 (18.4)	0.14
COPD (J44)	490 (19.3)	293 (18.5)	197 (20.5)	0.23
Major depressive disorder (F33)	436 (17.1)	300 (19.0)	136 (14.1)	0.002
Heart failure (I50)	144 (5.7)	81 (5.1)	63 (6.5)	0.13
Location of PACE, n (%)				
Northeast [2]	859 (33.8)	177 (11.2)	682 (70.8)	<0.001
South [3]	623 (24.5)	457 (28.9)	166 (17.2)	
Midwest [4]	294 (11.6)	179 (11.3)	115 (11.9)	
West [5]	769 (30.2)	769 (48.6)	0 (0.0)	

Abbreviations: COPD = Chronic obstructive pulmonary disease; HCC = Hierarchical condition category scores; MRM = Medication risk mitigation; [1] Nominal variables were compared with the chi-square test and continuous variables were compared with the independent *t*-test. [2] Massachusetts, New Jersey, and Pennsylvania. [3] Florida, North Carolina, and South Carolina. [4] Arkansas, Iowa, Michigan, and Oklahoma. [5] California and Colorado.

3.2. Outcomes

As shown in Table 4, the mean total medical costs (i.e., combined facility and physician) increased from 2018 to 2019 in both cohorts, but the increase was smaller for the MRM cohort. Specifically, the MRM group's costs increased by a mean of USD 4386 (95% CI, USD 3040–5732) per participant, whereas the control group's costs increased by USD 9410 (95% CI, USD 7737–11,084) per participant. This USD 5024 difference between each group's year-over-year change was significant ($p < 0.001$); therefore, PACE organizations using MRM consumed USD 5024 less per participant from 2018 to 2019 relative to control. As depicted in Figure 2, 75.7% (USD 3807/USD 5024) of this reduction was related to facility expenditures. As shown in Table 4, both facility and physician expenditures increased less in the MRM cohort ($p < 0.001$).

Table 4. Year-over-year changes in medical expenditures adjusted by the actual capitated rate [1].

Group	2018, Mean (95% CI)	2019, Mean (95% CI)	Year-over-Year Change [2] (95% CI)	% Change (95% CI)	Weighted Mean Difference [3], Absolute	p-Value [4]
Mean total medical expenditures per participant: combined facility and physician (US Dollars)						
MRM	USD 22,841 (USD 21,465, USD 24,218)	USD 27,228 (USD 25,664, USD 28,792)	USD 4386 (USD 3040, USD 5732)	19.2% (13.3%, 25.1%)	USD 5024	t: <0.001 W: <0.001
Control	USD 25,418 (USD 23,781, USD 27,055)	USD 34,829 (USD 32,873, USD 36,784)	USD 9410 (USD 7737, USD 11,084)	37.0% (30.4%, 43.6%)		
Mean physician expenditures per participant (US Dollars):						
MRM	USD 11,932 (USD 11,295, USD 12,570)	USD 13,800 (USD 13,064, USD 14,536)	USD 1868 (USD 1399, USD 2336)	15.7% (11.7%, 19.6%)	USD 1217	t: <0.001 W: <0.001
Control	USD 10,727 (USD 10,061, USD 11,394)	USD 13,811 (USD 13,003, USD 14,621)	USD 3085 (USD 2493, USD 3676)	28.8% (23.2%, 34.3%)		

Table 4. *Cont.*

Group	2018, Mean (95% CI)	2019, Mean (95% CI)	Year-over-Year Change [2] (95% CI)	% Change (95% CI)	Weighted Mean Difference [3], Absolute	p-Value [4]
			Mean facility expenditures per participant (US Dollars)			
MRM	USD 10,909 (USD 9791, USD 12,027)	USD 13,428 (USD 12,165, USD 14,691)	USD 2519 (USD 1386, USD 3651)	23.1% (12.7%, 33.5%)	USD 3807	t: <0.001 W: <0.001
Control	USD 14,691 (USD 13,195, USD 16,187)	USD 21,017 (USD 19,088, USD 22,945)	USD 6326 (USD 4757, USD 7894)	41.3% (32.4%, 53.7%)		

Abbreviations: MRM = Medication risk mitigation; t = p-value from weighted t-test; W = p-value from Wilcoxon test. [1] The cost outcomes for 2018 and 2019 reported were adjusted by the actual capitated rate for each participant. Adjustments were applied to the control group's 2018 and 2019 costs. This ensured that geographic differences between MRM and control did not bias outcomes. [2] 2019–2018 costs. [3] Year-over-year change for control–year-over-year change for MRM. [4] Comparison is between each group's mean year-over-year change (weighted t-test) or median year-over-year change (Wilcoxon).

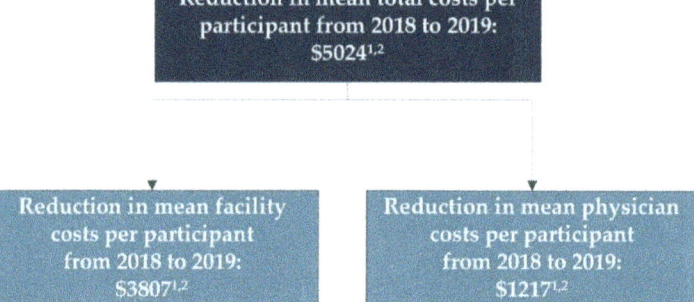

Figure 2. Breakdown in year-over-year cost reduction seen in MRM relative to control. [1] Cost reduction represents the difference between the intervention and control group's 2018-to-2019 change in medical costs. Adjustments were applied to the control group's 2018 and 2019 costs. Adjustments were based on the actual capitated rate. This ensured that geographic differences between MRM and control did not bias outcomes. [2] Denotes a statistically significant ($p < 0.05$) difference between MRM and control groups.

For the 2018-to-2019 changes in every other outcome (Table 5), the results directionally favored the MRM group; however, the difference between the groups was not statistically significant for any of the outcomes.

Table 5. Year-over-year changes in clinical outcomes adjusted by hierarchical condition category scores [1].

Group	2018 (95% CI)	2019 (95% CI) [1]	Year-over-Year Change, Absolute [2] (95% CI)	Year-over-Year Change, % (95% CI)	Weighted Difference [3], Absolute	p-Value [4]
		ADEs (fraction of participants with at least 1 ADE per year):				
MRM	0.068 (0.056, 0.081)	0.069 (0.056, 0.081)	0.001 (−0.015, 0.016)	0.9% (−21.4%, 23.2%)	0.023	χ^2: 0.17
Control	0.055 (0.040, 0.071)	0.079 (0.060, 0.097)	0.023 (0.003, 0.043)	42.2% (5.7%, 78.7%)		

Table 5. Cont.

Group	2018 (95% CI)	2019 (95% CI) [1]	Year-over-Year Change, Absolute [2] (95% CI)	Year-over-Year Change, % (95% CI)	Weighted Difference [3], Absolute	p-Value [4]
\multicolumn{7}{c}{Falls (fraction of participants with at least 1 fall per year)}						
MRM	0.11 (0.09, 0.12)	0.12 (0.10, 0.14)	0.013 (−0.007, 0.034)	12.4% (−6.8%, 31.9%)	0.016	χ^2: 0.65
Control	0.11 (0.09, 0.13)	0.14 (0.12, 0.16)	0.029 (0.000, 0.058)	25.9% (0.1%, 51.7%)		
\multicolumn{7}{c}{Emergency department visits (mean number of visits per participant per year)}						
MRM	1.5 (1.4, 1.7)	1.6 (1.4, 1.7)	0.04 (−0.12, 0.19)	2.4% (−7.9%, 12.6%)	0.14	t: 0.20 W: 0.27
Control	1.9 (1.7, 2.2)	2.1 (1.8, 2.4)	0.17 (−0.06, 0.47)	9.1% (−6.2%, 24.4%)		
\multicolumn{7}{c}{Hospital admissions (mean number of admissions per participant per year)}						
MRM	0.32 (0.28, 0.35)	0.36 (0.32, 0.40)	0.04 (−0.01, 0.09)	12.7% (−1.6%, 27.1%)	0.025	t: 0.26 W: 0.17
Control	0.33 (0.28, 0.38)	0.40 (0.34, 0.46)	0.07 (0.001, 0.13)	19.6% (0.2%, 39.0%)		

Abbreviations: ADE = Adverse drug events; MRM = Medication risk mitigation; t = p-value from weighted t-test; W = p-value from Wilcoxon test; χ^2 = p-value from chi-square test. [1] The outcomes reported were adjusted by hierarchical condition category scores. Adjustments were applied to the control group's 2018 and 2019 outcomes. This ensured that differences related to multimorbidity between MRM and control did not bias outcomes. [2] 2019–2018. [3] Year-over-year change for control–year over year change for MRM. [4] Comparison is between each group's change score.

4. Discussion

Healthcare economists have demonstrated that US healthcare expenditures are expected to rise through 2025 [39]. Reasons are multifactorial, but the upward cost trajectory is largely attributable to disease progression in an aging population [39]. Therefore, it is not surprising that we observed a year-over-year increase in total medical costs for more than 2500 medically complex older adults enrolled in 19 PACE programs dispersed across the US. However, PACE participants who received MRM services exhibited a significantly lower year-over-year increase in costs compared to participants who were not exposed to the same services, even after adjusting for the baseline capitated rate, which accounts for differences in multimorbidity and geographical location. Relative to control, the MRM group consumed USD 5024 less per participant year-over-year, where about 75% of the reduction came from facility-related expenditures. Though we did not demonstrate statistically significant differences in year-to-year changes for other outcomes, every result was directionally in favor of MRM and was clinically important, helping to explain the cost reduction. In sum, our findings suggest that MRM services can curb growing healthcare costs in PACE.

A recent study of MRM services in Medicare beneficiaries supports this idea. In an Enhanced Medication Therapy Management (EMTM) program [40], Stein et al. examined the impact of retrospective MSRs across nearly 11,500 Medicare beneficiaries [41]. The authors found that those who received MSRs consumed USD 958 less in Medicare costs (facility plus physician) year-over-year than those who did not. Similar to the study at hand, Stein et al. also found that the overwhelming majority (90%) of the savings were due to expenses incurred at facilities. The reproducibility of the financial outcomes in a more complex PACE cohort strongly suggests that the benefits of MRM services are consequential in different patient populations.

Reproducibility is logical considering how MSRs are deployed and executed in clinical practice. First, a novel risk assessment tool, the MedWise Risk Score (MRS), facilitates intervention deployment to those who are most at risk for ADEs [42]. High-MRS PACE participants have been shown to consume more medical resources (e.g., medical costs, hospitalizations, and ED visits) and suffer from more ADEs [10]. Since scores are derived from modifiable pharmacologic risk factors found within a drug regimen, pharmacists can act to mitigate risk factors contributing to negative outcomes. Though future studies need to evaluate whether PACE pharmacists' interventions can positively alter MRS-defined risk, the aforementioned evaluation of MSRs in EMTM indicates that this is possible as long as recommendations are implemented by prescribers [42].

Regarding clinical execution, Bankes et al. found that during MSRs, PACE pharmacists identify about two medication-related problems (MRPs) per participant, where four medication-safety related MRPs—drug interactions, adverse drug reactions, high doses, and unindicated medications—account for about 80% of all MRPs logged [11]. This distribution is highly comparable to what was seen when MSRs were deployed in the EMTM setting [42]. Others have found these types of medication-safety MRPs to be quite costly. For instance, a cost avoidance model suggested that resolving the aforementioned MRPs can avoid between USD 90–675 per occurrence [43]. Importantly, PACE prescribers accept about 80% of pharmacists' recommendations, which suggests that MRPs are indeed being resolved; thus, MRS-defined risk is being attenuated [11].

Unlike EMTM (where MSRs are performed retrospectively, after drugs have been prescribed and ingested), MRM in PACE offers pharmacists the ability to resolve such problems prospectively, at the point of prescribing. While this is likely the biggest contributor to the reduction in costs here than what was reported by Stein et al., other ancillary components of MRM that are unavailable in the EMTM setting could also help explain this difference. For example, adherence support services, pharmacogenomic consultations, and prescriber-initiated engagement of PACE pharmacists for drug information are all expected to optimize regimens and improve outcomes [13,44,45]. Future research must evaluate which MRM components are most impactful to economic and clinical outcomes. Moreover, prospectively designed research should determine whether our observed relative cost reduction represents cost savings, cost avoidance, or a blend of both.

It is expected that healthcare costs will continue to rise [39] amid Medicaid funding restrictions [46]. Our results suggest that comprehensive MRM provides a way for PACE to address this concern. This is important because PACE appears to be inattentive to medication-related morbidity from a regulatory standpoint. Specifically, current regulations do not require pharmacists to be part of the PACE interdisciplinary team [1]. This means that a PACE center may not have on-the-ground expertise in pharmacotherapeutics, pharmacology, and/or pharmacokinetics. For such centers, MRM appears to be valuable.

The primary limitation of this analysis is self-selection bias. We attempted to make the fairest comparison possible by adjusting for participant multimorbidity and geographic location. Yet, there could be some unmeasurable or unavailable variables that confounded the results. For instance, we were not able to consider the length of PACE enrollment. Next, generalizability may be limited for two reasons related to potential sampling bias. First, we only had access to administrative claims of 2500 participants from 19 PACE organizations. As of June 2021, this represents <5% of the entire PACE census and <14% of all programs [47]. Nevertheless, we had representation from various locations throughout the US, and our sample appeared similar across some demographics (e.g., age, sex) reported by the National PACE Association [2]. Second, with only seven centers in the control group, it is possible that we did not capture PACE organizations that have robust clinical pharmacy services. Still, those services would not be using the same clinical decision support systems. It is possible that the effect of MRM could be attenuated when compared against programs with robust clinical pharmacy service offerings [46,48–50]. Finally, we were unable to demonstrate statistically significant differences between groups for their year-over-year change in the proportion of patients with ADEs. Therefore, it is impossible to conclusively tie cost reduction to improvements in medication safety; medication safety is the main purpose of MRM. Our lack of significance is likely explained by our reliance on ICD-10 codes. Specifically, ADEs tend to be grossly underreported in administrative claims [51]. Therefore, our sample size was likely insufficient to detect significant differences for this outcome. Future studies should use a formal sample size calculation (which will necessitate a larger sample size) to draw more reliable conclusions about this important outcome.

5. Conclusions

In sum, PACE participants who received MRM services exhibited a smaller year-over-year increase in costs compared against risk-adjusted participants who were not exposed to MRM. Specifically, those who received MRM consumed USD 5024 less in total medical costs year-over-year than those who did not. Therefore, MRM appears to be effective at curbing rising healthcare costs in PACE.

Author Contributions: Conceptualization, A.S., H.J., S.Y. and S.F.; methodology, all authors; formal analysis, H.J., S.Y. and S.F.; investigation, H.J., S.Y. and S.F.; resources, A.S.; writing—original draft preparation, D.B.; writing—review and editing, all authors; visualization, H.J., S.Y., S.F. and D.B.; supervision, A.S.; project administration, A.S.; funding acquisition, J.T. All authors have read and agreed to the published version of the manuscript.

Funding: This research and the APC were funded by Tabula Rasa HealthCare, who was the employer of all authors at the time of initial writing.

Institutional Review Board Statement: The study was conducted according to the guidelines of the Declaration of Helsinki, and approved by the Institutional Review Board of The Biomedical Research Alliance of New York (protocol code 19-12-172-427, approved on 24 May 2019).

Informed Consent Statement: Patient consent was waived due to the low-risk, retrospective nature of this research.

Data Availability Statement: The data presented in this study are available on request from the corresponding author. The data are not publicly available due to privacy concerns.

Acknowledgments: The authors would like to thank Dana Fillippoli; Calvin Alt; Patty Bailey; Martha Blake; Jeffrey Knowlton; Lane Liles; and Richard Schamp.

Conflicts of Interest: All authors disclose that they are employees and stockholders of TRHC.

References

1. Bouwmeester, C. The PACE program: Home-based long-term care. *Consult. Pharm.* **2012**, *27*, 24–30. [CrossRef] [PubMed]
2. PACE by the Numbers. Available online: https://www.npaonline.org/sites/default/files/PDFs/5033_pace_infographic_update_july2021.pdf (accessed on 13 December 2021).
3. Sloane, P.D.; Oudenhoven, M.D.; Broyles, I.; McNabney, M. Challenges to cost-effective care of older adults with multiple chronic conditions: Perspectives of Program of All-Inclusive Care for the Elderly medical directors. *J. Am. Geriatr. Soc.* **2014**, *62*, 564–565. [CrossRef] [PubMed]
4. Watanabe, J.H.; McInnis, T.; Hirsch, J.D. Cost of prescription drug-related morbidity and mortality. *Ann. Pharm.* **2018**, *52*, 829–837. [CrossRef] [PubMed]
5. Parameswaran Nair, N.; Chalmers, L.; Peterson, G.M.; Bereznicki, B.J.; Castelino, R.L.; Bereznicki, L.R. Hospitalization in older patients due to adverse drug reactions -the need for a prediction tool. *Clin. Interv. Aging* **2016**, *11*, 497–505. [CrossRef] [PubMed]
6. Lavan, A.H.; Gallagher, P. Predicting risk of adverse drug reactions in older adults. *Ther. Adv. Drug Saf.* **2016**, *7*, 11–22. [CrossRef]
7. Bootman, J.L.; Harrison, D.L.; Cox, E. The health care cost of drug-related morbidity and mortality in nursing facilities. *Arch. Intern. Med.* **1997**, *157*, 2089–2096. [CrossRef]
8. Beijer, H.J.; de Blaey, C.J. Hospitalisations caused by adverse drug reactions (ADR): A meta-analysis of observational studies. *Pharm. World Sci.* **2002**, *24*, 46–54. [CrossRef] [PubMed]
9. Chan, M.; Nicklason, F.; Vial, J.H. Adverse drug events as a cause of hospital admission in the elderly. *Intern. Med. J.* **2001**, *31*, 199–205. [CrossRef]
10. Bankes, D.L.; Jin, H.; Finnel, S.; Michaud, V.; Knowlton, C.H.; Turgeon, J.; Stein, A. Association of a novel medication risk score with adverse drug events and other pertinent outcomes among participants of the Programs of All-Inclusive Care for the Elderly. *Pharmacy* **2020**, *8*, 87. [CrossRef] [PubMed]

11. Bankes, D.L.; Amin, N.S.; Bardolia, C.; Awadalla, M.S.; Knowlton, C.H.; Bain, K.T. Medication-related problems encountered in the Program of All-Inclusive Care for the Elderly: An observational study. *J. Am. Pharm. Assoc.* **2020**, *60*, 319–327. [CrossRef] [PubMed]
12. Bain, K.T.; Schwartz, E.J.; Knowlton, O.V.; Knowlton, C.H.; Turgeon, J. Implementation of a pharmacist-led pharmacogenomics service for the Program of All-Inclusive Care for the Elderly (PHARM-GENOME-PACE). *J. Am. Pharm Assoc.* **2018**, *58*, 281–289.e1. [CrossRef] [PubMed]
13. Bankes, D.L.; Schamp, R.O.; Knowlton, C.H.; Bain, K.T. Prescriber-initiated engagement of pharmacists for information and intervention in Programs of All-Inclusive Care for the Elderly. *Pharmacy* **2020**, *8*, 24. [CrossRef] [PubMed]
14. Cicali, B.; Michaud, V.; Knowlton, C.H.; Turgeon, J. Application of a novel medication-related risk stratification strategy to a self-funded employer population. *Benefits Q.* **2018**, *34*, 49–55.
15. Turgeon, J.; Michaud, V.; Cicali, B. Population-Based Medication Risk Stratification and Personalized Medication Risk Score. WO2019089725, 5 September 2019.
16. Ratigan, A.R.; Michaud, V.; Turgeon, J.; Bikmetov, R.; Gaona Villarreal, G.; Anderson, H.D.; Pulver, G.; Pace, W.D. Longitudinal association of a medication risk score with mortality among ambulatory patients acquired through electronic health record data. *J. Patient Saf.* **2020**, *17*, 249–255. [CrossRef] [PubMed]
17. Michaud, V.; Smith, M.K.; Bikmetov, R.; Dow, P.; Johnson, J.; Stein, A.; Finnel, S.; Jin, H.; Turgeon, J. Association of the MedWise Risk Score with health care outcomes. *Am. J. Manag Care* **2021**, *27* (Suppl. S16), S280–S291. [PubMed]
18. Knowlton, C.H. Medication risk mitigation matrix: A pharmaceutical care opportunity for precision medication. *J. Am. Pharm Assoc.* **2015**, *55*, 354–358. [CrossRef] [PubMed]
19. Tranchina, K.; Turgeon, J.; Bingham, J. Integrating a novel medication risk score and use of an advanced clinical decision support system into a pharmacist- and nurse-coordinated transition of care program to mitigate drug interactions. *Clin. Case Rep. J.* **2021**, *2*, 1–5.
20. Matos, A.; Bankes, D.L.; Bain, K.T.; Ballinghoff, T.; Turgeon, J. Opioids, polypharmacy, and drug interactions: A technological paradigm shift is needed to ameliorate the ongoing opioid epidemic. *Pharmacy* **2020**, *8*, 154. [CrossRef]
21. Bardolia, C.; Michaud, V.; Turgeon, J.; Amin, N.S. Deprescribing dual therapy in benign prostatic hyperplasia: A patient case. *Clin. Case Rep.* **2020**, *10*, 1–4.
22. Ballinghoff, T.; Bain, K.; Matos, A.; Bardolia, C.; Turgeon, J.; Amin, N.S. Opioid response in an individual with altered cytochrome P450 2D6 activity: Implications of a pharmacogenomics case. *Clin. Case Rep. J.* **2020**, *1*, 1–4.
23. Bain, K.T.; McGain, D.; Cicali, E.J.; Knowlton, C.H.; Michaud, V.; Turgeon, J. Precision medication: An illustrative case series guiding the clinical application of multi-drug interactions and pharmacogenomics. *Clin. Case Rep.* **2020**, *8*, 305–312. [CrossRef]
24. Shah, R.R.; Smith, R.L. Addressing phenoconversion: The Achilles' heel of personalized medicine. *Br. J. Clin. Pharmacol.* **2015**, *79*, 222–240. [CrossRef] [PubMed]
25. Deodhar, M.; Dow, P.; Al Rihani, S.B.; Turgeon, J.; Michaud, V. An illustrative case of phenoconversion due to multi-drug interactions. *Clin. Case Rep. J.* **2020**, *1*, 1–6.
26. Bain, K.T.; Matos, A.; Knowlton, C.H.; McGain, D. Genetic variants and interactions from a pharmacist-led pharmacogenomics service for PACE. *Pharmacogenomics* **2019**, *20*, 709–718. [CrossRef]
27. Board of Pharmacy Specialties: Geriatric Pharmacy. Available online: https://www.bpsweb.org/bps-specialties/geriatric-pharmacy/ (accessed on 26 August 2021).
28. Pharmacy Technician Certification Board. Available online: https://www.ptcb.org/ (accessed on 26 August 2021).
29. Hohl, C.M.; Karpov, A.; Reddekopp, L.; Stausberg, J. ICD-10 codes used to identify adverse drug events in administrative data: A systematic review. *J. Am. Med. Inform. Assoc.* **2013**, *21*, 547–557. [PubMed]
30. Kane, L.T.; Fang, T.; Galetta, M.S.; Goyal, D.K.C.; Nicholson, K.J.; Kepler, C.K.; Vaccaro, A.R.; Schroeder, G.D. Propensity score matching: A statistical method. *Clin. Spine Surg.* **2020**, *33*, 120–122. [CrossRef] [PubMed]
31. Kautter, J.; Ingber, M.; Pope, G.C. Medicare risk adjustment for the frail elderly. *Health Care Financ. Rev.* **2008**, *30*, 83–93.
32. Yeatts, J.P.; Sangvai, D. HCC coding, risk adjustment, and physician income: What you need to know. *Fam. Pract. Manag.* **2016**, *23*, 24–27.
33. Mosley, D.G.; Peterson, E.; Martin, D.C. Do hierarchical condition category model scores predict hospitalization risk in newly enrolled Medicare Advantage participants as well as probability of repeated admission scores? *J. Am. Geriatr. Soc.* **2009**, *57*, 2306–2310. [PubMed]
34. Haas, L.R.; Takahashi, P.Y.; Shah, N.D.; Stroebel, R.J.; Bernard, M.E.; Finnie, D.M.; Naessens, J.M. Risk-stratification methods for identifying patients for care coordination. *Am. J. Manag Care* **2013**, *19*, 725–732. [PubMed]
35. Committee on Geographic Variation in Health Care Spending and Promotion of High-Value Care; Board on Health Care Spending; Institute of Medicine. *Variation in Health Care Spending: Target. Decision Making, Not Geography*, 1st ed.; National Academy of Sciences: Washington, DC, USA, 2013.
36. Kautter, J.; Pope, G.C. CMS frailty adjustment model. *Health Care Financ. Rev.* **2004**, *26*, 1–19.
37. Foley, R.N.; Collins, A.J. End-stage renal disease in the United States: An update from the United States Renal Data System. *J. Am. Soc. Nephrol. JASN* **2007**, *18*, 2644–2648. [CrossRef]
38. Kish, L. *Survey Sampling*; John Wiley & Sons: New York, NY, USA, 1965.

39. Keehan, S.P.; Stone, D.A.; Poisal, J.A.; Cuckler, G.A.; Sisko, A.M.; Smith, S.D.; Madison, A.J.; Wolfe, C.J.; Lizonitz, J.M. National health expenditure projections, 2016–2025: Price increases, aging push sector to 20 percent of economy. *Health Aff.* **2017**, *36*, 553–563. [CrossRef] [PubMed]
40. Part D Enhanced Medication Therapy. Available online: https://innovation.cms.gov/initiatives/enhancedmtm/ (accessed on 13 December 2021).
41. Stein, A.; Finnel, S.; Bankes, D.; Jin, H.; Awadalla, M.S.; Johnson, J.; Turgeon, J. Health outcomes from an innovative enhanced medication therapy management model. *Am. J. Manag. Care* **2021**, *27* (Suppl. S16), S300–S308. [PubMed]
42. Bankes, D.; Pizzolato, K.; Finnel, S.; Awadalla, M.S.; Stein, A.; Johnson, J.; Turgeon, J. Medication-related problems identified by pharmacists in an enhanced medication therapy management model. *Am. J. Manag. Care* **2021**, *27* (Suppl. S16), S292–S299.
43. Hough, A.; Vartan, C.M.; Groppi, J.A.; Reyes, S.; Beckey, N.P. Evaluation of clinical pharmacy interventions in a Veterans Affairs medical center primary care clinic. *Am. J. Health Syst. Pharm.* **2013**, *70*, 1168–1172. [CrossRef] [PubMed]
44. Iuga, A.O.; McGuire, M.J. Adherence and health care costs. *Risk Manag. Healthc. Policy* **2014**, *7*, 35–44. [PubMed]
45. Bain, K.T.; Knowlton, C.H.; Matos, A. Cost avoidance related to a pharmacist-led pharmacogenomics service for the Program of All-inclusive Care for the Elderly. *Pharmacogenomics* **2020**, *21*, 651–661. [CrossRef]
46. McCarrell, J. PACE: An interdisciplinary community-based practice opportunity for pharmacists. *Sr. Care Pharm.* **2019**, *34*, 439–443. [CrossRef] [PubMed]
47. PACE in the States. Available online: https://www.npaonline.org/sites/default/files/PDFs/PACE%20in%20the%20States%20June%202021.pdf (accessed on 13 December 2021).
48. Vouri, S.M.; Tiemeier, A. The ins and outs of pharmacy services at a program of all-inclusive care for the elderly. *Consult. Pharm.* **2012**, *27*, 803–807. [CrossRef] [PubMed]
49. Bouwmeester, C.; Kraft, J.; Bungay, K.M. Optimizing inhaler use by pharmacist-provided education to community-dwelling elderly. *Respir. Med.* **2015**, *109*, 1363–1368. [CrossRef]
50. Covington, L.P.; McCarrell, J.; Hoerster, N.S. Prevalence of anticholinergic medication use in the Program of All-Inclusive Care for the Elderly. *Consult. Pharm.* **2016**, *31*, 168–174. [CrossRef] [PubMed]
51. Hazell, L.; Shakir, S.A. Under-reporting of adverse drug reactions: A systematic review. *Drug Saf.* **2006**, *29*, 385–396. [CrossRef] [PubMed]

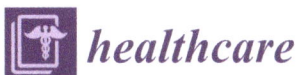

Study Protocol

A Nationwide Mystery Caller Evaluation of Oral Emergency Contraception Practices from German Community Pharmacies: An Observational Study Protocol

Christian Kunow, Moulika Aline Bello, Laura Diedrich, Laura Eutin, Yanneck Sonnenberg, Nele Wachtel and Bernhard Langer *

Department of Health, Nursing, Management, University of Applied Sciences Neubrandenburg, 17033 Neubrandenburg, Germany; christiankunow@googlemail.com (C.K.); gp20191@hs-nb.de (M.A.B.); gp20212@hs-nb.de (L.D.); gp20192@hs-nb.de (L.E.); gp20196@hs-nb.de (Y.S.); gp20213@hs-nb.de (N.W.)
* Correspondence: langer@hs-nb.de

Abstract: To prevent unwanted pregnancies, oral emergency contraception (EC) with the active ingredients levonorgestrel (LNG) and ulipristal acetate (UPA) is recommended by the guidelines of the German Federal Chamber of Pharmacists (BAK). In this respect, community pharmacies (CPs) in Germany have a major responsibility for information gathering, selecting the appropriate medicine, availability and pricing, among other things. Therefore, it would be appropriate to conduct a study with the aim of investigating information gathering, a possible recommendation as well as availability and pricing for oral EC in German CPs. A representative nationwide observational study based on the simulated patient methodology (SPM) in the form of covert mystery calls will be conducted in a random sample of German CPs stratified according to the 16 federal states. Each selected CP will be randomly called once successfully by one of six both female and male trained mystery callers (MCs). The MCs will simulate a product-based scenario using the request for oral EC. For quality assurance of the data collection, a second observer accompanying the MC is planned. After all mystery calls have been made, each CP will receive written, pharmacy-specific performance feedback. The only national SPM study on oral EC to date has identified deficits in the provision of self-medication consultations with the help of visits in the CPs studied. International studies suggest that UPA in particular is not always available. Significant price differences could be found analogous to another German study for a different indication.

Keywords: non-prescription medicines; emergency contraception; community pharmacies; information gathering; availability; pricing; mystery calls; ulipristal acetate; levonorgestrel; Germany

Citation: Kunow, C.; Bello, M.A.; Diedrich, L.; Eutin, L.; Sonnenberg, Y.; Wachtel, N.; Langer, B. A Nationwide Mystery Caller Evaluation of Oral Emergency Contraception Practices from German Community Pharmacies: An Observational Study Protocol. *Healthcare* **2021**, *9*, 945. https://doi.org/10.3390/healthcare9080945

Academic Editors: Georges Adunlin and Jonathan Tritter

Received: 25 April 2021
Accepted: 22 July 2021
Published: 26 July 2021

Publisher's Note: MDPI stays neutral with regard to jurisdictional claims in published maps and institutional affiliations.

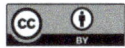

Copyright: © 2021 by the authors. Licensee MDPI, Basel, Switzerland. This article is an open access article distributed under the terms and conditions of the Creative Commons Attribution (CC BY) license (https://creativecommons.org/licenses/by/4.0/).

1. Introduction

To prevent unwanted pregnancies, the World Health Organization (WHO) recommends the use of emergency contraception (EC). The WHO distinguishes between the copper intrauterine device (Cu IUD) for insertion into the cavum uteri, the oral EC with the active ingredients levonorgestrel (LNG) and ulipristal acetate (UPA) and the combined oral contraceptives (COCs, Yuzpe method) [1], which are not recommended in Germany, as fewer adverse effects and higher clinical efficacy were associated with LNG and UPA [2–4]. In Germany, the Cu IUD is a prescription-only medicine (POM), whereas the oral EC—analogous to many other countries worldwide [5]—has been available since March 2015 as an over-the-counter (OTC) medicine without prescription [6,7]. In contrast, however, there are still a number of countries, such as South Korea, where oral EC is only available with prescription [5]. In this context, Poland plays a special role, as UPA was also available as an OTC medicine as of 2015, analogous to Germany, but was made subject to prescription again in 2017 despite controversial discussions and protests [8,9]. Oral EC may only be dispensed by community pharmacies (CPs) in Germany [10]. German CPs, therefore, have a great responsibility with regard to availability and pricing as important criteria for unhindered access [11,12]. With regard to the availability, this is particularly important in view of the fact that the effectiveness of oral EC is higher the faster it is taken [1]. With regard to the pricing, this is due to the fact that the German CPs are free to set the price of oral EC as an OTC medicine since the abolition of price maintenance in 2004 [13]. The actual prices for oral EC of the individual CPs are not available online, raising the question of what prices are actually charged by individual CPs. This lack of price transparency is one of the main reasons for price differences [14], especially as the prices are also usually only disclosed on-site at the CP at the end of the dispensing process [15].

German CPs dispensed 877,000 packs of oral EC in 2019, an increase of about 32% compared to the year of the OTC switch in 2015 (662,000 packs). Oral EC packs without prescription accounted for a share of about 71% of all oral EC packs in 2015 and even about 94% in 2019 [16]. Since more and more patients want to receive oral EC without a prior visit to their doctor, German CPs are also playing an increasingly important role in the provision of self-medication consultations. According to the guidelines of the German Federal Chamber of Pharmacists (BAK) on self-medication [17], the provision of self-medication consultations represents a multi-stage process from information gathering, selecting the appropriate medicine to giving advice in the context of dispensing. In principle, CPs in Germany have to ensure "adequate" provision of self-medication consultations. The provision of self-medication consultations must be carried out by a pharmacist, but can also be carried out by non-pharmacists (e.g., pharmacy technicians and pharmaceutical technical assistants) if the pharmacy manager has previously determined this in writing [18]. The BAK has issued corresponding guidelines for the provision of self-medication consultations for oral EC—first in 2015 [19] and last updated in 2020 [20]. In addition to giving advice, which should be applicable by the pharmacy staff in the respective conversation with the persons concerned, these guidelines also contain a checklist. This checklist should be available in CPs as a physical printed or digital version to ensure that the pharmacy staff asks the people concerned questions that are relevant for a possible recommendation of oral EC. In addition to the knowledge of the pharmacy staff, which is needed anyway, surveys have found knowledge deficits and incorrect knowledge about oral EC in adolescents [21–23], adults [24–27] and across populations [28,29] in Germany, especially with regard to the mechanism and period of time of action. This further underlines the importance of information gathering by the pharmacy staff including a possible recommendation of oral EC.

Unlike other countries such as the USA [11,12,30–47], the study situation for Germany for the provision of self-medication consultations, availability and pricing is rather poor so far. In nationwide interviews of 25 CPs conducted at the end of 2015, i.e., after the OTC switch in March 2015, 96% of the respondents reported using a checklist for the provision of self-medication consultations for oral EC. Of these, 52% said they worked with the checklist of the BAK. In addition, 96% of all interviewees stated that they had both LNG and UPA available [48]. In contrast to the dispensing recommendation of the BAK guidelines [20], a non-representative survey of 143 CPs in Hesse showed that oral EC is not always dispensed for women with the experience of sexual violence. Analogous results were found for women with poor German language skills [49], although this group is not explicitly mentioned in the BAK guidelines [20]. In a nationwide interview study, 12 female EC users interviewed wished, among other things, for more discretion and more patient-oriented information gathering [50]. In contrast, a non-representative online survey of 555 CPs concluded, among other things, that pharmacy staff refer women to gynaecologists in the case of safety concerns [51]. In contrast, however, no studies on pricing from German CPs to oral EC are known.

With regard to the methodology to be applied, however, the disadvantage of self-reported surveys and interviews—such as the previously presented studies on the practices of German CPs on oral EC—is that the validity of the study results could be limited due to social desirability bias, as the interviewed or surveyed pharmacy staff in particular tend to present their provision of self-medication consultations better than they actually provided them [52,53]. In the case of non-participant observations, the disadvantage is that pharmacy staff usually adjust their behaviour when they realise that they are being observed ("Hawthorne effect" [54]). To avoid the problems described above, the simulated patient methodology (SPM) is recommended [55,56] in the international literature as the "gold standard" [57]—also taking into account the relatively high administrative and financial effort as well as comparatively small sample sizes [57] and any intra- and inter-observer variabilities [58]—with which a lifelike conversational situation can be depicted [59]. However, only one SPM study on oral EC is known for Germany [60], which investigated the provision of self-medication consultations for oral EC, but neither availability nor pricing, and is also a representative analysis for only one federal state. Therefore, it would be appropriate to conduct a representative nationwide study with the following objectives:

- Primary objective: to investigate information gathering based on the BAK checklist, a possible recommendation as well as availability and pricing for oral EC.
- Secondary objective: to determine to what extent the study results differ with regard to possible influencing factors.

This study is planned on the basis of the present protocol. There is already a protocol on oral EC from Australian CPs, but it is based on interviews [61].

2. Materials and Methods

2.1. Study Design

The planned study is to be based on a cross-sectional design, conducted with the help of the SPM in the form of covert mystery calls and reported in accordance with the 'STROBE Statement—Checklist of items that should be included in reports of cross-sectional studies' [62]. Against the background of a nationwide study, calls are to be preferred to visits—which have already been used in German CPs [15,60,63,64], but only in relation to one city or one federal state—as the implementation of calls without the requirement of a physical presence in the CP is less costly and thus more feasible. Following the international literature [59,65–67], the SPM in the form of covert mystery calls is a covert participant observation

- by a person (**mystery caller (MC)**),
- who contacts a **CP**,
- with the help of a **call**,
- to simulate a lifelike conversation situation based on a predefined **scenario**.

This is followed by

- the **data collection** according to predefined criteria using an **assessment form** and
- the **data management and analysis**.

In addition,

- the CP contacted is given **performance feedback**, if applicable.

2.2. Mystery Caller

To conduct such a study, at least 1 person is needed as MC. In order to achieve generalisable and standardisable study results, more than 2 both female and male persons [65] should be recruited. However, since Watson et al. do not specify a precise upper limit [65], the use of 13 persons could be determined on average on the basis of a current SPM systematic review [66]. Although the guidelines of the BAK only refer to the provision of self-medication consultations for women [20]—in contrast to the Australian guidelines, for example [68]—the behaviour of the pharmacy staff should also be examined with men and thus with the help of a supposedly atypical selection for such a conversation situation. However, it is quite realistic to assess when a man calls for his wife or girlfriend and wants to take the call for her because she feels uncomfortable, ashamed or might even already be psychologically burdened [69–71]. In a German study, more than 82% of the CPs interviewed also considered it a problem that oral EC was not requested by the woman concerned, but by the respective man or a third person [51].

Since a former student (CK) had agreed to be a male MC before the research project was announced, female MCs in particular had to be acquired. In principle, this acquisition was promising, since previous research projects of the project leader (BL) usually involved more female students due to the health and care-related Master degree programmes. Finally, 1 male and 4 females could be acquired as student MCs, who with an age between 20 and 30 years are in the age range of average users of oral EC in Germany [25,72,73]. Thus, the now total of 6 acquired MCs—including the male non-student MC (age 38)—can contribute to the simulation of a lifelike conversation situation. The MCs participate in the project free of charge.

2.3. Setting and Participation

The planned study is to be carried out within the framework of a 3-semester research project of various Master degree programmes in the Faculty of Health, Nursing, Management of the University of Applied Sciences Neubrandenburg from the beginning of October 2020 until the end of February 2022. In order to be able to plan a representative nationwide study, a list of all CPs registered in Germany is first necessary to determine the basic population. The free pharmacy finder of the "Apotheken Umschau" [74] was used to create a list. Thus, information from the pharmacy finder with regard to name, postcode and location of all CPs in Germany has been extracted into an MS Excel file in December 2020. To check the accuracy, the total number of 18,777 CPs thus identified was compared with the latest available total number of 19,075 CPs provided annually by the Federal Union of German Associations of Pharmacists (ABDA) and most recently for the reference date 31 December 2019 [16]. Due to the slightly decreasing number of CPs in recent years [16], the population size determined should correspond to a fairly current status.

In Germany, there are no studies on availability and pricing of oral EC. Therefore, the degree of variability is unknown. The minimum necessary sample size (n) was determined for the corresponding population size (N) and an error margin (e) of 0.05 using the following formula based on a degree of variability of $p = 0.5$ and a 95% confidence interval [75]:

$$n = \frac{N}{1 + N(e)^2} = \frac{18,777}{1 + 18,777(0.05)^2} = \frac{18,777}{47.9425} = 391.66$$

The assumed degree of variability of $p = 0.5$ maximises the required sample size. The 18,777 CPs were stratified by location as an indicator for the respective German federal state and assigned a random number using the MS Excel random number generator. A simple random sample was then drawn in each stratum to the extent of that stratum's share of all CPs to select the required 392 CPs. To validate the selected CPs, a Google search was conducted and, if not already available, the telephone number was located. If, contrary to expectations, CPs are closed or cannot be found, it is planned to replace them by drawing more CPs in the corresponding stratum.

The distribution of the selected CPs to the MCs is to be done by means of the random principle, so that 65 to 66 CPs (392 CPs/6 MCs = 65.3 CPs) are assigned to each of the 6 MCs. Each of the selected CPs is to be called once successfully, so that in total there are also 392 calls (6 MCs × 65.3 CPs = 392 calls). The calls are to be made on different days of the week and at different times of the day. No costs are calculated for the execution of the calls, since all MCs have a telephone flat rate and the corresponding monthly basic fees for the MCs are incurred anyway.

In addition, 3 months before the start of the main study, 5 test calls (30 calls in total) will be made by each of the 6 MCs to CPs outside the random sample as part of a pilot study. This is to test the functionality of the SPM planned here in order to identify possible weaknesses. The MCs will conduct the test calls from home, but the project leader will be available at any time via a video conferencing system and the MCs are also required to discuss any problems that arise immediately together with the project leader in order to adjust the study protocol accordingly. These test calls also serve as practical training for the MCs, who have already familiarised themselves with the theoretical basics of the SPM and conducted a role play. After the role plays and the test calls, there will be a workshop to exchange experiences and inform each other about the special features of the scenario and the assessment form. If necessary, the scenario and the assessment form will be adapted accordingly.

2.4. Scenario

The conversation situation to be simulated, which should be as true to life as possible, should be based on a product-based scenario (Figure 1). The reason for planning a product-based rather than a symptom-based scenario is that the availability, pricing and provision of self-medication consultations for oral EC should be examined and the pharmacy staff should be specifically directed towards this. Basically, the scenario should only differ in the use of a female or male MC, i.e., in gender-specific answers or questions from the MCs.

The MCs should start the telephone conversation by saying that they probably need oral EC and then ask if the pharmacy staff can help. Thus, the person concerned should be disclosed at the beginning of the conversation. The disclosure of this rather little information at the beginning of the conversation can contribute to more comprehensive information gathering, since the pharmacy staff has to gather more information, e.g., about the reason for the call, by asking. In addition, the aim is to signal to the pharmacy staff with the word "probably" uncertainty about the need for oral EC and with the word pair "please help" a request for help for the immediate initiation of information gathering on the phone. From this point on, the pharmacy staff could want to end the conversation at any time and refer the supposedly affected person to a visit in the CP or a doctor's visit, for example. It is not necessary for MCs to ask for a pharmacist at the beginning of the conversation, as in Germany the provision of self-medication consultations is also possible through non-pharmacists.

If the pharmacy staff were to start information gathering, they could ask one or more questions from the BAK checklist [20]. The questions listed in Table 1 correspond completely to the questions of the BAK checklist relevant for everyday information gathering in Germany. Since one of our study objectives is to investigate the extent to which CPs ask questions from the BAK checklist, only these questions should be considered in the scenario. Therefore, further questions resulting from international guidelines (e.g., on weight) [76] should not be included in the scenario.

In connection with information gathering based on the checklist of the BAK [20], there should be corresponding answer guidelines for these questions for the MCs (Table 1), including that the girlfriend is 24 years old. Since it does not seem so realistic that the girlfriend has talked to the boyfriend about the strength, length and unusualness of the menstrual period (5th to 8th question) in the run-up to the call, the male MCs should answer "I don't know" if the pharmacy staff should ask about this. In principle, the answers of the MCs should be given in such a way that the conversation is quite easy for the MCs to simulate and the information gathering should be quite uncomplicated for the pharmacy staff. However, the pharmacy staff could also recommend only UPA, only LNG, UPA or LNG alternatively, the Cu IUD, oral EC without explicitly naming the active ingredient, or the need for no oral EC, regardless of whether information gathering is carried out appropriately. Otherwise, or in addition, the pharmacy staff could recommend a doctor's visit or a visit to the CP (sub-scenario 1).

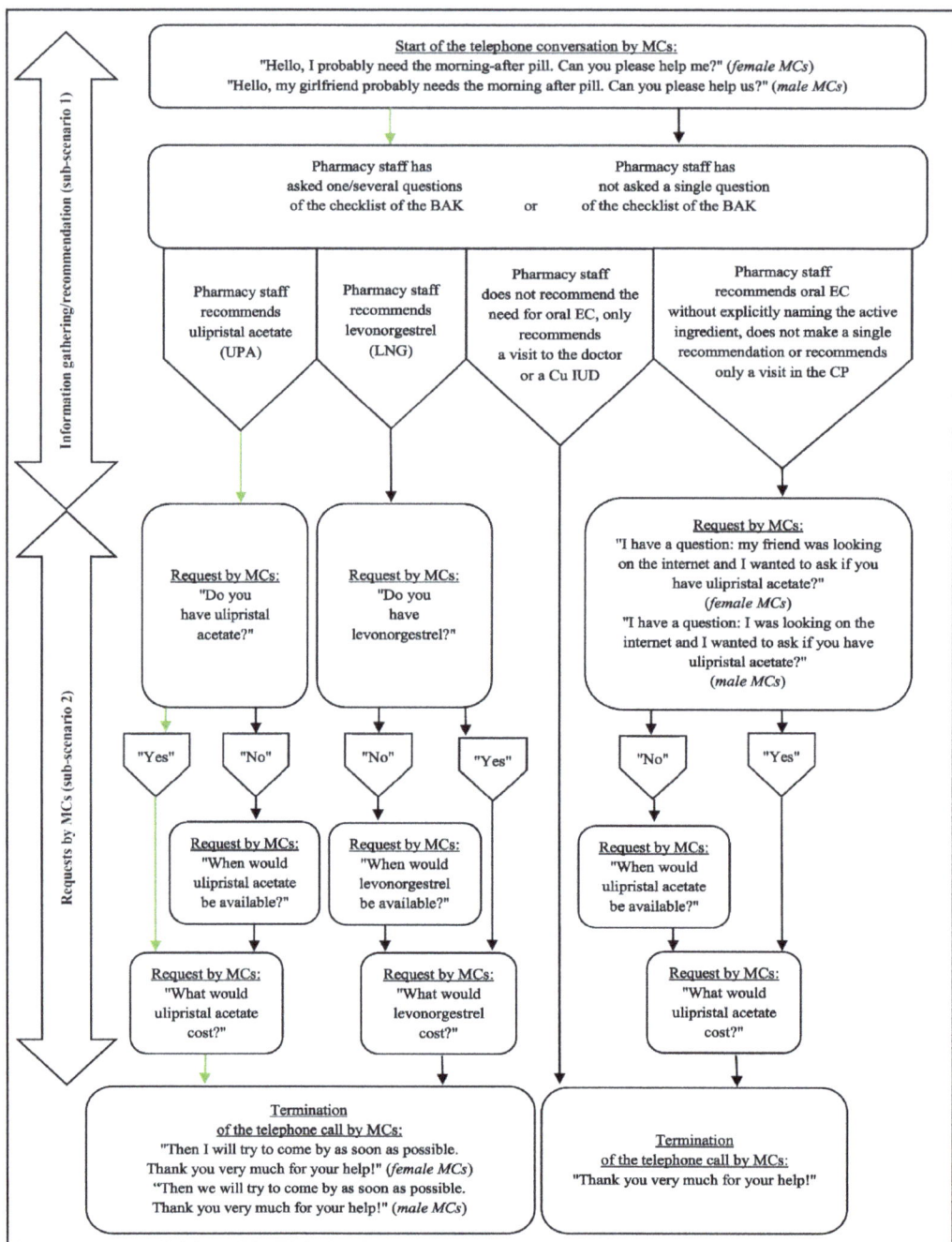

Figure 1. Scenario for female and male MCs using a flow chart. Note: The green arrows indicate the most optimal course of conversation.

Table 1. Sub-scenario 1 for female and male MCs (without the possible recommendation).

	Possible Questions by the Pharmacy Staff Based on the Questions of the BAK Checklist [20]	Response Specifications for MCs
1.	"How old are you?" "How old is your girlfriend?"	"I am 24." (female MCs) "She's 24." (male MCs)
2.	"Why do you need oral EC?"	"We had a condom failure."
3.	"When was the unprotected sexual intercourse?"	"4 days ago."
4.	"When was your last menstrual period?"	"11 days ago."
5.	"Is the date of the first day of the last menstrual period more than 28 days ago?"	
6.	"Was your last menstrual period weaker than usual?"	5th to 8th: "No." (female MCs)
7.	"Was the last menstrual period shorter than usual?"	5th to 8th: "I don't know." (male MCs)
8.	"Was the last menstrual period unusual in any other way?"	
9.	"Are you aware of any acute health problems or chronic illnesses?" "Is your friend aware of any acute health problems or chronic illnesses?"	"No." (female MCs) "No." (male MCs)
10.	"Are you currently breastfeeding?" "Is your girlfriend currently breastfeeding?"	"No." (female MCs) "No." (male MCs)
11.	"Are you currently taking any medication?" "Is your friend currently taking any medication?"	"No." (female MCs) "No." (male MCs)
12.	"Have you ever used oral EC before?" "Has your friend ever used oral EC?"	"No." (female MCs) "No." (male MCs)

After the possible information gathering activities and the recommendation of UPA or LNG, the MCs should ask follow-up questions: about availability and the costs of the recommended oral EC. If the pharmacy staff recommends the need for no oral EC, only a visit to the doctor or a Cu IUD, the MCs should not doubt the respective recommendation and end the conversation. If the pharmacy staff recommends oral EC without explicitly naming the active ingredient, does not make a single recommendation or only recommends a visit to the CP, the MCs should ask about the availability and the costs of UPA specifically, stating that their friend or they have informed themselves on the internet (sub-scenario 2).

Afterwards, the MCs are supposed to end the conversation—also according to the respective course—by thanking the pharmacy staff for the help and saying that they will try to come by as soon as possible. That the MCs should be given this statement is based on the fact that the use of the previously recommended oral EC is recommended as soon as possible after the unprotected sexual intercourse (UPSI) due to the greater effectiveness [20] and that the pharmacy staff might have given such a hint beforehand. If they have recommended the need for no oral EC, only a doctor's visit, a Cu IUD, oral EC without explicit mention of the active ingredient, only a visit in the CP or have not made a single recommendation, the MCs should only thank them for their help at the end.

2.5. Assessment

Analogous to the planned scenario, the items for the assessment should be based on the questions of the BAK checklist [20] and the possible recommendation (sub-scenario 1) as well as on the answers of the pharmacy staff on availability and pricing (sub-scenario 2). Since oral EC cannot be dispensed over the phone and the giving advice associated with dispensing usually takes place on-site at the CP, no items were collected for giving advice. Influencing factors obtained from the literature shall complete the assessment (Table 2). The planned items shall only be objective and mostly use dichotomous scales (closed yes/no questions).

Table 2. Assessment items for female and male MCs.

	Information Gathering Including a Possible Recommendation of Oral EC by Pharmacy Staff (Based on Sub-Scenario 1)		
1.	Did the pharmacy staff ask for the age?	Yes ☐	No ☐
2.	Did the pharmacy staff ask the reason for the request for oral EC?	Yes ☐	No ☐
3.	Did the pharmacy staff ask for the time of the UPSI?	Yes ☐	No ☐
4.	Did the pharmacy staff ask for the time of the last menstrual period?	Yes ☐	No ☐
	Did the pharmacy staff enquire whether ...		
5.	... the date of the first day of your last menstrual period was more than 28 days ago?	Yes ☐	No ☐
6.	... the last menstrual period was weaker than usual?	Yes ☐	No ☐
7.	... the last menstrual period was shorter than usual?	Yes ☐	No ☐
8.	... the last menstrual period was otherwise unusual?	Yes ☐	No ☐
9.	Did the pharmacy staff ask whether any acute health problems or chronic illnesses are known?	Yes ☐	No ☐
10.	Did the pharmacy staff ask if you are currently breastfeeding?	Yes ☐	No ☐
11.	Did the pharmacy staff ask whether any medicines are being taken?	Yes ☐	No ☐
12.	Did the pharmacy staff asked whether the morning-after pill has ever been used?	Yes ☐	No ☐
13.	Did the pharmacy staff recommend UPA?	Yes ☐	No ☐
14.	Did the pharmacy staff recommend LNG?	Yes ☐	No ☐
15.	Did the pharmacy staff recommend Cu IUD?	Yes ☐	No ☐
16.	Did the pharmacy staff recommend oral EC without naming the active substance?	Yes ☐	No ☐
17.	Did the pharmacy staff recommend not needing oral EC?	Yes ☐	No ☐
18.	What else did the pharmacy staff recommend?	Visit to the doctor ☐ Visit in CP ☐	
	Requests by MCs (Based on Sub-Scenario 2)		
19.	Did the CP have oral EC available?	Yes ☐ (UPA) Yes ☐ (LNG)	No ☐ (UPA) No ☐ (LNG)
19.a.	Did the pharmacy staff inform what CP might have the oral EC available?	Yes ☐ (UPA) Yes ☐ (LNG)	No ☐ (UPA) No ☐ (LNG)
20.a.	When would the CP have UPA available?	on the same day ☐ the next day ☐ later than the next day ☐ unknown ☐	
20.b.	When would the CP have LNG available?	on the same day ☐ the next day ☐ later than the next day ☐ unknown ☐	
21.	What is the (lowest) price quoted by the pharmacy staff for oral EC?	Price (UPA): ... Price (LNG): ...	
	Possible Influencing Factors		
22.	MC number?	...	
23.	What is the gender of the MC?	female ☐	male ☐
24.	What is the gender of the pharmacy staff?	female ☐	male ☐
25.	Does the CP have a quality certificate?	Yes ☐ No ☐ unknown ☐	
26.	How long did the telephone conversation last?	... , ... min.	
27.	Did the pharmacy staff ask questions or make statements that are not planned in the scenario? If "Yes", which ones?	Yes ☐	No ☐

Note: The possible influencing factors were taken from the specific literature sources cited in the manuscript.

In connection with the checklist and the guidelines of the BAK [20], the question of the age of the woman concerned (item 1) therefore plays a role, as the pharmacy staff should question the necessity of oral EC if the age is outside the childbearing age. In addition, dispensing oral EC to girls under 14 years of age without the consent of a legal guardian is not recommended [20]. The question about the reason for oral EC (item 2), on the other hand, is of central importance, since the pharmacy staff should only recommend oral EC if a UPSI has taken place [20]. The question of the timing of the UPSI (item 3) plays an even greater role here, since UPA and LNG are only effective in a certain period after UPSI [20].

In principle, UPA has the larger temporal window of effect, whereby UPA has also been shown to be more effective than LNG in terms of pregnancy rates in the first 24 or 72 h after the UPSI [77–79]. The guidelines of the BAK [20] advise the pharmacy staff, if the UPSI is no more than 72 h (3 days) ago, to recommend LNG or UPA to the person, if more than 72 h but no more than 120 h (5 days) ago, to recommend UPA exclusively. If, on the other hand, the UPSI occurred more than 120 h ago, a visit to a gynaecologist should be recommended instead of oral EC [20].

The questions about the last menstrual period (item 4–8) could give the pharmacy staff clues about an existing pregnancy, after which they should not recommend oral EC according to national guidelines [20], although it does not harm an existing pregnancy according to international guidelines [76]. The question about acute health problems or chronic diseases (item 9) is relevant because the pharmacy staff should recommend UPA in the case of an increased risk of thrombosis and the case of severe liver dysfunction a further visit to the doctor in addition to dispensing oral EC [20]. The question as to whether breastfeeding is taking place (item 10) is primarily aimed at information to be given by the pharmacy staff regarding a break from breastfeeding. For UPA, both national [20] and international guidelines [76] recommend a breastfeeding break of 1 week. In contrast, international guidelines [76] do not impose any restrictions for LNG, whereas national guidelines [20] recommend breastfeeding immediately after ingestion and a subsequent breastfeeding break of 8 h, as LNG passes into breast milk. The question about the use of medicines (item 11) is relevant because the pharmacy staff should point out that the effectiveness of UPA and LNG may be reduced if certain medicines are taken at the same time [20]. In addition, the question about the use of oral EC in the past (item 12) is relevant because, according to the national guidelines [20], repeated use of LNG within the same menstrual cycle should not be recommended by the pharmacy staff, whereas the international guidelines [76] do not make this restriction.

Based on the answers of the respective MC to the questions asked (item 1–12), the pharmacy staff should make a recommendation regarding EC (item 13–17) and recommend UPA ("appropriate outcome"). Since the MCs should not give any information in their answers about, for example, existing interactions or contraindications, the pharmacy staff could make this recommendation solely on the basis of the answer ("4 days ago.") to the question about the time of the UPSI (item 3). A recommendation for a visit to the doctor (item 18) would only make sense if a Cu IUD was recommended at the same time, which would not be effective in the planned scenario and would probably cost valuable time to prevent an unwanted pregnancy. A recommendation of a visit to the CP (item 18) would only make sense if UPA was recommended at the same time, since the person concerned would have to come to the CP to buy it anyway. In principle, the recommendation of a visit to the CP would be welcome, but only if it is clarified in the telephone consultation whether oral EC is necessary at all. Otherwise, an unnecessary journey would be imposed on the person concerned.

In addition, the (recommended) oral EC (item 19) should ideally be available immediately when asked about availability. If the oral EC is not available, it would be welcome from a service point of view if the pharmacy staff informs which CP could have it available (item 19a). In addition, if the time of availability is requested (item 20a), it should be available on the same day, since with a (stated) UPSI before 4 days, those affected would only have a few hours to receive the oral EC and then take it in order to be able to prevent an unwanted pregnancy. If LNG is recommended instead, its immediate availability (item 20b) would be welcomed in principle, but would not be helpful in this planned scenario, since according to the guidelines of the BAK [20], LNG should only be given up to 72 h (3 days) after UPSI. In connection with the assessment of the (lowest) indicated price of the (recommended) oral EC (item 21), it should be noted that in Germany—in contrast to LNG—there are currently significantly fewer preparations available on the market [80], so that there is less choice.

Influencing factors to be investigated include:
- the MC number (item 22) [81],
- the gender of the MC (item 23) [82],
- the gender of the pharmacy staff (item 24) [83], which is usually identifiable by the voice during the call,
- a possible quality certificate of the CP (item 25) [84], which should be determined by the MC on the same day of the call on the internet—if documented there—and which—if not yet determined—should be asked for on the basis of a further call after all calls have been completed
- as well as the length of the telephone call (item 26) [85] by using a clock accurate to the second.

In addition, questions or statements made by the pharmacy staff outside the planned scenario will be identified (item 27).

2.6. Data Collection

The assessment items will be transferred to an assessment form (Table 2) for data collection. In addition to the items, the call attempts are to be collected. In this regard, the MCs should try to reach the CP via their private mobile phone with a suppressed number a maximum of 3 times spread over a single possible day. If a CP could not be reached, the MCs shall mark the CP as unavailable, thus replacing it by drawing another CP in the corresponding stratum. If the call is held in a queue for at least 15 min, the MCs shall hang up and call again a little later on the same day. If an answering machine picks up the call, the MCs should hang up immediately and try calling again a little later on the same day. If the pharmacy staff inadvertently hangs up before the call is completed, the MCs should call back immediately. If the call is interrupted due to reception problems or if the MCs forget to ask questions before finishing the call, the MCs should also call back immediately. If the MCs suspect or are certain that their call has been discovered, the respective CP shall be replaced by drawing another CP in the corresponding stratum.

No (covert) audio recordings will be made during the calls for quality assurance purposes, as otherwise the corresponding consent of the CPs would have to be obtained in advance [86], which would, however, give the possibility of not participating in the study (opt-out), which in turn could lead to a selection bias and thus to a biased assessment [87,88]. Due to the detailed scenario, however, the use of a second observer is planned for each call, who should listen in on the MC's call via the loudspeaker or telephone conference function of the MC's mobile phone. One second observer will come from the family environment of one of the MCs and will be trained in the same way as the MCs. The other second observers will come from the group of the other MCs and will therefore already be trained. The MC should then complete the assessment form in writing immediately after the call with the help of the second observer, who should take notes during the call. Possible disagreements should be clarified by a discussion between the MC and the second observer. In case of unsuccessful clarification, the assessment of the second observer is decisive.

As CPs are classified as systemically relevant in Germany and therefore remain open [89], the COVID-19 pandemic should not have any impact on the implementation of the planned data collection.

2.7. Data Management and Analysis

The data are to be entered using the "four-eyes principle" (one MC enters the data, while the second observer checks the quality of the data entry) and analysed with SPSS version 26 for Windows (IBM, Armonk, NY, USA). Within the framework of descriptive statistics, frequencies and percentages are to be determined for categorical data. In addition, 95% confidence intervals will be reported for categorical data using bootstrapping. With the help of the Shapiro–Wilk test as well as the Kolmogorov–Smirnov test, it is to be tested for continuous data whether they are normally distributed. In the case of a normal distribution, the mean, standard deviation, minimum and maximum as well as the range should be reported, whereas, in the case of non-normally distributed data, the median, interquartile range, minimum and maximum as well as the range should be presented [90]. Since unconnected samples are involved, a chi-square test (or alternatively an exact test according to Fisher for expected cell frequencies below five) should be applied for categorical variables to determine correlations. Cramer's V should be reported as an effect size measure, whereby, according to Cohen, a small effect exists from 0.10, a medium effect from 0.30 and a large effect from 0.50 [91]. For continuous data, the t-test for unconnected samples should be used in the case of a normal distribution, and the Mann–Whitney U-test should be used in the case of non-normally distributed data to determine differences between the groups. If the t-test is used for independent samples, Cohen's d (from 0.20 a small effect, from 0.50 a medium effect and from 0.80 a large effect) should be used as an effect size measure [91]. If the Mann–Whitney U-test is used, the effect size should be measured with the help of the Pearson correlation coefficient r, whereby, according to Cohen, there is a small effect from 0.10, a medium effect from 0.30 and a large effect from 0.50 [91]. In all statistical analyses, a p-value less than 0.05 should be considered significant.

2.8. Performance Feedback

After evaluation of the data—as recommended internationally [59,66]—each CP should receive written, pharmacy-specific performance feedback including graphically prepared benchmarking by e-mail or letter post, whereby the improvement or deterioration with regard to the individual items is shown for each CP in comparison to the remaining, anonymously presented CPs. This provides the CPs with information about their competitive position, so that ideally—if necessary—corresponding optimisation processes can be initiated on the part of the examined CPs with the aim of sustainably improving information gathering and selecting the appropriate medicine. It would be ideal if these optimisation processes would be initiated and accompanied by the research team, but this is not possible due to time and financial restrictions. In addition, it is planned to provide the CPs with general performance feedback on the basis of the planned publication of the study results. In a German SPM study, it was reported that feedback was well accepted by the pharmacy staff [92].

2.9. Ethics and Dissemination

The study planned here has been applied for and approved by the Ethics Committee of the University of Applied Sciences Neubrandenburg, Germany (protocol code HSNB/171/21). According to the "Guideline for the Use of Mystery Research in Market and Social Research" [93], the data are processed in such a way that neither the CPs involved in the study nor their personnel can be identified. This applies to both the data collection and storage as well as the publication of the research results in a peer-reviewed journal. There is also no picture or sound recording of the calls. This ensures that the pharmacy owner or its staff are not exposed to any criminal or civil liability or that their reputation is damaged by the investigation. Nevertheless, in order to meet the CPs' need for information, a letter was sent to all participating CPs in March 2021—analogous to recommendations in the international literature [87,88] and to the implementation in numerous studies [94–96]—informing them about the background and the conduct of the study. However, in order not to jeopardise the covert study design, a correspondingly long time period (calls are planned from August to October 2021) was specified in this letter instead of a specific date, in that calls will be conducted at a time unknown to the CPs. In addition, it is planned that the persons recruited as MCs and second observers will sign a declaration stating that they agree to act as MCs and second observers, respectively.

3. Discussion

The study planned here is of enormous importance to answer the questions whether the German CPs offer information gathering including a possible recommendation of oral EC on the phone, and whether they live up to their great responsibility for continuous availability and relatively accessible prices without too great price differences. Ideally, these framework conditions should be in place so that, in such an emergency, those women are given the opportunity to prevent an unwanted pregnancy. In addition, representative nationwide results would considerably improve the rather poor study situation in Germany.

It will be interesting to see to what extent information gathering or a possible recommendation of oral EC takes place on the phone or is referred to a visit to the CP. In any case, the only national SPM study on oral EC to date has identified deficits in the provision of self-medication consultations with the help of visits in the CPs studied [60]. Regarding the availability of oral EC, international SPM studies [37–39,41,42,45] suggest that there are problems—especially with UPA. Some price differences—even between identical preparations—could also be identified, as in addition to international SPM studies on oral EC [11,12,41–47,97,98], a national SPM study on a different indication has already identified significant price differences between CPs that are even located in the same city and in some cases only a few hundred metres apart [15].

Strengths and Limitations

As far as the authors are aware, this will be the first representative nationwide study in Germany to investigate oral EC practices including information gathering, a possible recommendation, availability and pricing of CPs with the help of the internationally already frequently used [59,65,66] SPM in the form of covert mystery calls. However, as the study is planned with a cross-sectional design, interpretations of the results will be limited, i.e., no causal relation between studied variables can be established. In order to be able to determine how results change over time, it would make more sense to plan a longitudinal study, but, due to the high financial and time costs involved, we refrain from doing so.

The information provided by the pharmacy staff may also differ in calls from face-to-face situations. For example, although the actual prices are to be determined, different prices may be quoted on the phone than on the spot. Since certain MCs were recruited to carry out the planned study and are in a certain age range, it cannot be ruled out that information gathering including a possible recommendation could turn out differently for those affected from other educational strata or age groups [98]. Furthermore, other scenarios could lead to different results [99–101]. However, the scenario planned here is very comprehensive analogous to other international EC studies using a MC approach [33,34,100]. Finally, the validation based on the pilot study could have been additionally planned with other persons than the acquired MCs, which could probably improve the approach [102].

With regard to the assessment, no items are planned that could allow a subjective assessment and thus a margin of discretion in the assessment (e.g., the friendliness of the pharmacy staff). Since a second observer is planned for the quality assurance of the data collection, distortions in the study results due to possible lacking or faulty memories (recall bias) of the MCs should be minimised. Finally, pharmacy-specific performance feedback would be desirable directly after the respective call, since the pharmacy staff's memory of the specific conversation situation should be most present at that time [59]. However, there is a risk that the pharmacy staff will inform other CPs in the vicinity about the call and then the subsequent calls can only be evaluated in a distorted way.

Author Contributions: Conceptualisation, C.K., M.A.B., L.D., L.E., Y.S., N.W., B.L.; Methodology, C.K., M.A.B., L.D., L.E., Y.S., N.W., B.L.; Writing—Original draft preparation, C.K.; Writing—Review and editing, M.A.B., L.D., L.E., Y.S., N.W., B.L.; Visualisation, C.K.; Project administration, B.L.; All authors have read and agreed to the published version of the manuscript.

Funding: We acknowledge support for the Article Processing Charge from the Deutsche Forschungsgemeinschaft (DFG, German Research Foundation, 414051096) and the Open Access Publication Fund of the Hochschule Neubrandenburg (Neubrandenburg University of Applied Sciences).

Institutional Review Board Statement: The study was conducted according to the guidelines of the Declaration of Helsinki and approved by the Ethics Committee of the University of Applied Sciences Neubrandenburg (Protocol code HSNB/171/21).

Informed Consent Statement: Participant consent was waived due to the special study design (covert participant observation to avoid a "Hawthorne effect") required to achieve the study objectives. Nevertheless, in order to meet the CPs' need for information, a letter was sent to all participating CPs in March 2021 informing them about the background and the conduct of the study. In addition, it is planned that the persons recruited as MCs and second observers will sign a declaration stating that they agree to act as MCs and second observers, respectively.

Data Availability Statement: All of the study data will be available to interested researchers upon request to Bernhard Langer, who is responsible for the project. Requests will be reviewed by the research team and will require a data transfer agreement.

Conflicts of Interest: The authors declare no conflict of interest.

References

1. WHO—World Health Organization. Emergency Contraception. Available online: https://www.who.int/news-room/fact-sheets/detail/emergency-contraception (accessed on 22 February 2021).
2. Rabe, T.; Goeckenjan, M.; Ahrendt, H.-J.; Ludwig, M.; Merkle, E.; König, K.; Merki Feld, G.; Albring, C. Postkoitale Kontrazeption. Gemeinsame Stellungnahme der Deutschen Gesellschaft für Gynäkologische Endokrinologie und Fortpflanzungsmedizin (DGGEF) e.V. und des Berufsverbands der Frauenärzte (BVF) e.V. *J. Reproduktionsmed. Endokrinol.* **2011**, *8*, 390–414.
3. Rabe, T.; Albring, C.; Ahrendt, H.-J.; Mueck, A.O.; Merkle, E.; König, K.; Merki, G. Notfallkontrazeption—ein Update. *Gynäkologische Endokrinol.* **2013**, *11*, 197–202. [CrossRef]
4. Goeckenjan, M.; Rabe, T.; Strowitzki, T. Postkoitale Kontrazeption. *Gynäkologische Endokrinol.* **2012**, *10*, 45–56. [CrossRef]
5. ICEC—International Consortium on Emergency Contraception. Status & Availability Database. Available online: https://www.cecinfo.org/country-by-country-information/status-availability-database/ (accessed on 3 June 2021).
6. Bundesrat; Beschluss des Bundesrates. Vierzehnte Verordnung zur Änderung der Arzneimittelverschreibungsverordnung. Drucksache 28/15. 06.03.2015. Available online: https://www.bundesrat.de/SharedDocs/drucksachen/2015/0001-0100/28-15(B).pdf?__blob=publicationFile&v=4 (accessed on 22 February 2021).
7. AMVV. Arzneimittelverschreibungsverordnung vom 21. Dezember 2005 (BGBl. I S. 3632), die zuletzt durch Artikel 1 der Verordnung vom 21. Oktober 2020 (BGBl. I S. 2260) geändert worden ist. Available online: https://www.gesetze-im-internet.de/amvv/AMVV.pdf (accessed on 22 February 2021).
8. ECEC—European Consortium for Emergency Contraception. Emergency Contraception in Europe. Poland. Available online: https://www.ec-ec.org/emergency-contraception-in-europe/country-by-country-information-2/poland/ (accessed on 3 June 2021).
9. Amnesty International. Poland: Emergency Contraception Restrictions Catastrophic for Women and Girls. Available online: https://www.amnesty.org/en/latest/news/2017/06/poland-emergency-contraception-restrictions-catastrophic-for-women-and-girls/ (accessed on 3 June 2021).
10. ApoG. Apothekengesetz in der Fassung der Bekanntmachung vom 15. Oktober 1980 (BGBl. I S. 1993), das zuletzt durch Artikel 2 des Gesetzes vom 9. Dezember 2020 (BGBl. I S. 2870) Geändert Worden ist. Available online: https://www.gesetze-im-internet.de/apog/ApoG.pdf (accessed on 22 February 2021).
11. Chau, V.M.; Stamm, C.A.; Borgelt, L.; Gaffaney, M.; Moore, A.; Blumhagen, R.Z.; Rupp, L.; Topp, D.; Gilroy, C. Barriers to Single-Dose Levonorgestrel-Only Emergency Contraception Access in Retail Pharmacies. *Women's Health Issues* **2017**, *27*, 518–522. [CrossRef]
12. Chin, J.; Salcedo, J.; Raidoo, S. Over-The-Counter Availability of Levonorgestrel Emergency Contraception in Pharmacies on Oahu. *Pharmacy* **2020**, *8*, 20. [CrossRef]
13. Deutscher Bundestag. Achtzehntes Hauptgutachten der Monopolkommission 2008/2009. Drucksache 17/2600. Available online: http://www.monopolkommission.de/images/PDF/HG/HG18/1702600.pdf (accessed on 22 February 2021).
14. Arora, S.; Sood, N.; Terp, S.; Joyce, G. The price may not be right: The value of comparison shopping for prescription drugs. *Am. J. Manag. Care* **2017**, *23*, 410–415.
15. Langer, B.; Kunow, C. Medication dispensing, additional therapeutic recommendations, and pricing practices for acute diarrhoea by community pharmacies in Germany: A simulated patient study. *Pharm. Pract.* **2019**, *17*, 1579. [CrossRef]
16. ABDA—Federal Union of German Associations of Pharmacists. German Pharmacies. Figures, Data, Facts. Available online: https://www.abda.de/fileadmin/user_upload/assets/ZDF/ZDF_2020/ABDA_ZDF_2020_Brosch_english.pdf (accessed on 22 February 2021).
17. BAK—Federal Chamber of Pharmacists. Information und Beratung des Patienten bei der Abgabe von Arzneimitteln—Selbstmedikation. Available online: https://www.abda.de/fuer-apotheker/qualitaetssicherung/leitlinien/leitlinien-und-arbeitshilfen/ (accessed on 3 June 2021).
18. ApBetrO. Apothekenbetriebsordnung in der Fassung der Bekanntmachung vom 26. September 1995 (BGBl. I S. 1195), die zuletzt durch Artikel 3 des Gesetzes vom 9. Dezember 2020 (BGBl. I S. 2870) geändert worden ist. Available online: https://www.gesetze-im-internet.de/apobetro_1987/ApBetrO.pdf (accessed on 22 February 2021).

19. Schulz, M.; Goebel, R.; Schumann, C.; Zagermann-Muncke, P. Non-prescription dispensing of emergency oral contraceptives: Recommendations from the German Federal Chamber of Pharmacists [Bundesapothekerkammer]. *Pharm. Pract.* **2016**, *14*, 828. [CrossRef]
20. BAK—Federal Chamber of Pharmacists. Handlungsempfehlung: Rezeptfreie Abgabe von Notfallkontrazeptiva ("Pille danach"). Available online: https://www.abda.de/aktuelles-und-presse/newsroom/detail/pille-danach/ (accessed on 22 February 2021).
21. Arzbach, V. Pille Danach: Ein Jahr Rezeptfrei. PTA-Forum. Available online: https://ptaforum.pharmazeutische-zeitung.de/ausgabe-062016/ein-jahr-rezeptfrei/ (accessed on 22 February 2021).
22. Heßling, A.; Bode, H. Sexual- und Verhütungsverhalten Jugendlicher im Wandel Sexual and contraceptive behaviour of young people throughout the decades. *Bundesgesundheitsblatt-Gesundh.-Gesundh.* **2017**, *60*, 937–947. [CrossRef]
23. Von Rosen, F.T.; Von Rosen, A.J.; Muller-Riemenschneider, F.; Tinnemann, P. Awareness and knowledge regarding emergency contraception in Berlin adolescents. *Eur. J. Contracept. Reprod. Health Care* **2017**, *22*, 45–52. [CrossRef] [PubMed]
24. Burgo, C.L.-D.; Mikolajczyk, R.T.; Osorio, A.; Carlos, S.; Errasti, T.; De Irala, J. Knowledge and beliefs about mechanism of action of birth control methods among European women. *Contraception* **2012**, *85*, 69–77. [CrossRef]
25. Nappi, R.E.; Abascal, P.L.; Mansour, D.; Rabe, T.; Shojai, R.; for the Emergency Contraception Study Group. Use of and attitudes towards emergency contraception: A survey of women in five European countries. *Eur. J. Contracept. Reprod. Health Care* **2014**, *19*, 93–101. [CrossRef] [PubMed]
26. Arzbach, V. Pille Danach: Wissenslücken und Abgabehindernisse. PTA-Forum. Available online: https://ptaforum.pharmazeutische-zeitung.de/ausgabe-222018/wissensluecken-und-abgabehindernisse/ (accessed on 22 February 2021).
27. Freye, R. Immer noch viel Unwissenheit über die Pille danach. *Gynäkologie + Geburtshilfe* **2018**, *23*, 68. [CrossRef]
28. Bode, H.; Heßling, A. Jugendsexualität 2015. Die Perspektive der 14- bis 25-Jährigen. Ergebnisse einer aktuellen Repräsentativen Wiederholungsbefragung. Bundeszentrale für gesundheitliche Aufklärung, Köln. Available online: https://www.forschung.sexualaufklaerung.de/fileadmin/fileadmin-forschung/pdf/Jugendendbericht%2001022016%20.pdf (accessed on 22 February 2021).
29. Renner, I. Informationsstand zur Pille danach—Ergebnisse einer bundesweiten repräsentativen Befragung erwachsener Frauen. In *Rezeptfreie Pille danach—Abgabepraxis und Information*; pro familia Bundesverband: Berlin, Germany, 2015; pp. 11–13. Available online: https://www.profamilia.de/fileadmin/publikationen/Fachpublikationen/doku_pille__danach-2016_web.pdf (accessed on 22 February 2021).
30. Wilkinson, T.A.; Fahey, N.; Shields, C.; Suther, E.; Cabral, H.J.; Silverstein, M. Pharmacy Communication to Adolescents and Their Physicians Regarding Access to Emergency Contraception. *Pediatrics* **2012**, *129*, 624–629. [CrossRef]
31. Wilkinson, T.A.; Fahey, N.; Suther, E.; Cabral, H.J.; Silverstein, M. Access to Emergency Contraception for Adolescents. *JAMA* **2012**, *307*, 362–363. [CrossRef]
32. Wilkinson, T.A.; Vargas, G.; Fahey, N.; Suther, E.; Silverstein, M. "I'll See What I Can Do": What Adolescents Experience When Requesting Emergency Contraception. *J. Adolesc. Heal.* **2014**, *54*, 14–19. [CrossRef]
33. Wilkinson, T.A.; Clark, P.; Rafie, S.; Carroll, A.E.; Miller, E. Access to Emergency Contraception After Removal of Age Restrictions. *Pediatrics* **2017**, *140*, e20164262. [CrossRef]
34. Wilkinson, T.A.; Rafie, S.; Clark, P.D.; Carroll, A.E.; Miller, E. Evaluating Community Pharmacy Responses about Levonorgestrel Emergency Contraception by Mystery Caller Characteristics. *J. Adolesc. Heal.* **2018**, *63*, 32–36. [CrossRef]
35. Ritter, A.H.; Isaacs, C.R.; Lee, S.M.; Lee, A.J. Single-Dose Levonorgestrel Emergency Contraception and Silent Barriers to Its Access: Is It Really Just One Step? *J. Women's Health* **2018**, *27*, 646–650. [CrossRef]
36. French, V.A.; Rangel, A.V.; Mattingly, T.L. Access to emergency contraception in Kansas City clinics. *Contraception* **2018**, *98*, 482–485. [CrossRef] [PubMed]
37. French, V.A.; Mattingly, T.L.; Rangel, A.V.; Shelton, A.U. Availability of ulipristal acetate: A secret shopper survey of pharmacies in a metropolitan area on emergency contraception. *J. Am. Pharm. Assoc.* **2019**, *59*, 832–835. [CrossRef]
38. Ditmars, L.; Rafie, S.; Kashou, G.; Cleland, K.; Bayer, L.; Wilkinson, T.A. Emergency Contraception Counseling in California Community Pharmacies: A Mystery Caller Study. *Pharmacy* **2019**, *7*, 38. [CrossRef]
39. Brant, A.; White, K.; Marie, P.S. Pharmacy availability of ulipristal acetate emergency contraception: An audit study. *Contraception* **2014**, *90*, 338–339. [CrossRef]
40. Peters, J.; Desai, K.; Ricci, D.; Chen, D.; Singh, M.; Chewning, B. The power of the patient question: A secret shopper study. *Patient Educ. Couns.* **2016**, *99*, 1526–1533. [CrossRef]
41. Bullock, H.; Steele, S.; Kurata, N.; Tschann, M.; Elia, J.; Kaneshiro, B.; Salcedo, J. Pharmacy access to ulipristal acetate in Hawaii: Is a prescription enough? *Contraception* **2016**, *93*, 452–454. [CrossRef]
42. Bullock, H.; Tschann, M.; Elia, J.; Kaneshiro, B.; Salcedo, J. From Kaua'i to Hawai'i Island: Interisland Differences in Emergency Contraceptive Pill Availability. *Hawaii J. Med. Public Health* **2017**, *76*, 178–182.
43. Gaffaney, M.; Stamm, C.; Borgelt, L.; Chau, V.M.; Rupp, L.; Blumhagen, R.; Gilroy, C. 67. Barriers to Emergency Contraception Access in the State of Wyoming. *J. Adolesc. Health* **2015**, *56*, S36. [CrossRef]
44. Orr, K.K.; Lemay, V.A.; Wojtusik, A.P.; Opydo-Rossoni, M.; Cohen, L.B. Availability and Accuracy of Information Regarding Nonprescription Emergency Contraception. *J. Pharm. Pract.* **2016**, *29*, 454–460. [CrossRef]
45. Shigesato, M.; Elia, J.; Tschann, M.; Bullock, H.; Hurwitz, E.; Wu, Y.Y.; Salcedo, J. Pharmacy access to Ulipristal acetate in major cities throughout the United States. *Contraception* **2018**, *97*, 264–269. [CrossRef]

46. Uysal, J.; Tavrow, P.; Hsu, R.; Alterman, A. Availability and Accessibility of Emergency Contraception to Adolescent Callers in Pharmacies in Four Southwestern States. *J. Adolesc. Health* **2019**, *64*, 219–225. [CrossRef]
47. Bell, D.L.; Camacho, E.J.; Velasquez, A.B. Male access to emergency contraception in pharmacies: A mystery shopper survey. *Contraception* **2014**, *90*, 413–415. [CrossRef]
48. Bruhns, C. Ergebnisse einer bundesweiten Befragung zur aktuellen Abgabepraxis der Pille danach. In *Rezeptfreie Pille danach—Abgabepraxis und Information*; pro familia Bundesverband: Berlin, Germany, 2015; pp. 14–20. Available online: https://www.profamilia.de/fileadmin/publikationen/Fachpublikationen/doku_pille__danach-2016_web.pdf (accessed on 22 February 2021).
49. Dierolf, V.; Freytag, S. Zugang zur Pille danach in den Apotheken nach der Rezeptfreigabe. *Pro Fam. Magazin.* **2017**, *45*, 9–12.
50. Pro familia Bundesverband. Pille danach rezeptfrei: Zugang ohne Hürden? Nutzerrinnenbefragung zur Vergabepraxis in Apotheken. Available online: https://www.profamilia.de/fileadmin/publikationen/Fachpublikationen/Verhuetung/Pille_danach-Zugang-ohne_huerden.pdf (accessed on 22 February 2021).
51. Said, A.; Ganso, M.; Freudewald, L.; Schulz, M. Trends in dispensing oral emergency contraceptives and safety issues: A survey of German community pharmacists. *Int. J. Clin. Pharm.* **2019**, *41*, 1499–1506. [CrossRef]
52. Callegaro, M. Social Desirability. In *Encyclopedia of Survey Research*; SAGE Publications: Los Angeles, CA, USA, 2008; pp. 825–826. [CrossRef]
53. Saxena, P.; Mishra, A.; Nigam, A. Evaluation of pharmacists' services for dispensing emergency contraceptive pills in Delhi, India: A mystery shopper study. *Indian J. Community Med.* **2016**, *41*, 198–202. [CrossRef]
54. McCambridge, J.; Witton, J.; Elbourne, D.R. Systematic review of the Hawthorne effect: New concepts are needed to study research participation effects. *J. Clin. Epidemiol.* **2014**, *67*, 267–277. [CrossRef]
55. Caamaño, F.; Ruano, A.; Figueiras, A.; Gestal-Otero, J. Data collection methods for analyzing the quality of the dispensing in pharmacies. *Pharm. World Sci.* **2002**, *24*, 217–223. [CrossRef]
56. Puspitasari, H.P.; Aslani, P.; Krass, I. A review of counseling practices on prescription medicines in community pharmacies. *Res. Soc. Adm. Pharm.* **2009**, *5*, 197–210. [CrossRef]
57. Converse, L.; Barrett, K.; Rich, E.; Reschovsky, J. Methods of Observing Variations in Physicians' Decisions: The Opportunities of Clinical Vignettes. *J. Gen. Intern. Med.* **2015**, *30*, 586–594. [CrossRef]
58. Bardage, C.; Westerlund, T.; Barzi, S.; Bernsten, C. Non-prescription medicines for pain and fever—A comparison of recommendations and counseling from staff in pharmacy and general sales stores. *Heal. Policy* **2013**, *110*, 76–83. [CrossRef]
59. Xu, T.; Neto, A.C.D.A.; Moles, R.J. A systematic review of simulated-patient methods used in community pharmacy to assess the provision of non-prescription medicines. *Int. J. Pharm. Pract.* **2012**, *20*, 307–319. [CrossRef]
60. Langer, B.; Grimm, S.; Lungfiel, G.; Mandlmeier, F.; Wenig, V. The Quality of Counselling for Oral Emergency Contraceptive Pills—A Simulated Patient Study in German Community Pharmacies. *Int. J. Environ. Res. Public Health* **2020**, *17*, 6720. [CrossRef]
61. Hussainy, S.Y.; Ghosh, A.; Taft, A.; Mazza, D.; Black, K.I.; Clifford, R.; Gudka, S.; Mc Namara, K.; Ryan, K.; Jackson, J.K. Protocol for ACCESS: A qualitative study exploring barriers and facilitators to accessing the emergency contraceptive pill from community pharmacies in Australia. *BMJ Open* **2015**, *5*, e010009. [CrossRef] [PubMed]
62. STROBE Statement—Checklist of Items That Should Be Included in Reports of Cross-Sectional Studies. Available online: https://www.strobe-statement.org/fileadmin/Strobe/uploads/checklists/STROBE_checklist_v4_cross-sectional.pdf (accessed on 22 February 2021).
63. Langer, B.; Kunow, C. Do north-eastern German pharmacies recommend a necessary medical consultation for acute diarrhoea? Magnitude and determinants using a simulated patient approach [version 2; peer review: 3 approved]. *F1000Research* **2020**, *8*, 1841. [CrossRef] [PubMed]
64. Kunow, C.; Langer, B. Using the simulated patient methodology to assess the quality of counselling in german community pharmacies: A systematic review from 2005 to 2018. *Int. J. Pharm. Pharm. Sci.* **2021**, *13*, 10–19. [CrossRef]
65. Watson, M.C.; Norris, P.; Granas, A.G. A systematic review of the use of simulated patients and pharmacy practice research. *Int. J. Pharm. Pract.* **2010**, *14*, 83–93. [CrossRef]
66. Björnsdottir, I.; Granas, A.G.; Bradley, A.; Norris, P. A systematic review of the use of simulated patient methodology in pharmacy practice research from 2006 to 2016. *Int. J. Pharm. Pract.* **2020**, *28*, 13–25. [CrossRef]
67. da Costa, F.A. Covert and overt observations in pharmacy practice. In *Pharmacy Practice Research Methods*; Babar, Z.U.D., Ed.; Springer: Singapore, 2020; pp. 93–114. [CrossRef]
68. PSA—Pharmaceutical Society of Australia. Guidance for Provision of a Pharmacist Only Medicine. Levonorgestrel. Approved Indication: Emergency Contraception. Available online: https://www.familyplanningallianceaustralia.org.au/wp-content/uploads/2015/08/PSA-Guidelines-on-EC.pdf (accessed on 3 June 2021).
69. Fergusson, D.M.; Horwood, L.J.; Boden, J.M. Does abortion reduce the mental health risks of unwanted or unintended pregnancy? A re-appraisal of the evidence. *Aust. N. Z. J. Psychiatry* **2013**, *47*, 819–827. [CrossRef]
70. Steinberg, J.; Rubin, L.R. Psychological Aspects of Contraception, Unintended Pregnancy, and Abortion. *Policy Insights Behav. Brain Sci.* **2014**, *1*, 239–247. [CrossRef]
71. Abajobir, A.A.; Maravilla, J.C.; Alati, R.; Najman, J. A systematic review and meta-analysis of the association between unintended pregnancy and perinatal depression. *J. Affect. Disord.* **2016**, *192*, 56–63. [CrossRef]
72. BZgA. Contraceptive Behaviour of Adults 2011. Results of a Representative Survey. Available online: https://publikationen.sexualaufklaerung.de/fileadmin/redakteur/publikationen/dokumente/13317270.pdf (accessed on 22 February 2021).

73. David, M.; Radke, A.-M.; Pietzner, K. The Prescription of the Morning-After Pill in a Berlin Emergency Department Over a Four-Year Period—User Profiles and Reasons for Use. *Geburtshilfe Frauenheilkd.* **2012**, *72*, 392–396. [CrossRef]
74. Apotheken Umschau. Apotheken in Deutschland nach Postleitzahlbereichen suchen und finden. Available online: https://www.apotheken-umschau.de/apotheken/Deutschland (accessed on 22 February 2021).
75. Israel, G.D. Determining Sample Size. University of Florida. Available online: http://www.psycholosphere.com/Determining%20sample%20size%20by%20Glen%20Israel.pdf (accessed on 22 February 2021).
76. ICEC/FIGO—International Consortium for Emergency Contraception/International Federation of Gynecology and Obstetrics. Emergency Contraceptive Pills. Medical and Service Delivery Guidance. Available online: https://www.cecinfo.org/wp-content/uploads/2018/12/ICEC-guides_FINAL.pdf (accessed on 3 June 2021).
77. Creinin, M.D.; Schlaff, W.; Archer, D.F.; Wan, L.; Frezieres, R.; Thomas, M.; Rosenberg, M.; Higgins, J. Progesterone Receptor Modulator for Emergency Contraception. *Obstet. Gynecol.* **2006**, *108*, 1089–1097. [CrossRef] [PubMed]
78. Glasier, A.F.; Cameron, S.T.; Fine, P.M.; Logan, S.J.; Casale, W.; Van Horn, J.; Sogor, L.; Blithe, D.L.; Scherrer, B.; Mathe, H.; et al. Ulipristal acetate versus levonorgestrel for emergency contraception: A randomised non-inferiority trial and meta-analysis. *Lancet* **2010**, *375*, 555–562. [CrossRef]
79. Shen, J.; Che, Y.; Showell, E.; Chen, K.; Cheng, L. Interventions for emergency contraception. *Cochrane Database Syst. Rev.* **2019**, *2019*, CD001324. [CrossRef]
80. Lauer Taxe. LTO4.0. Available online: https://www.cgm.com/deu_de/produkte/apotheke/lauer-taxe.html (accessed on 24 April 2021).
81. Zapata-Cachafeiro, M.; Piñeiro-Lamas, M.; Guinovart, M.C.; López-Vázquez, P.M.; Vazquez-Lago, J.; Figueiras, A. Magnitude and determinants of antibiotic dispensing without prescription in Spain: A simulated patient study. *J. Antimicrob. Chemother.* **2019**, *74*, 511–514. [CrossRef]
82. Paravattil, B.; Kheir, N.; Yousif, A. Utilization of simulated patients to assess diabetes and asthma counseling practices among community pharmacists in Qatar. *Int. J. Clin. Pharm.* **2017**, *28*, 179–768. [CrossRef]
83. Saba, M.; Diep, J.; Bittoun, R.; Saini, B. Provision of smoking cessation services in Australian community pharmacies: A simulated patient study. *Int. J. Clin. Pharm.* **2014**, *36*, 604–614. [CrossRef]
84. Kippist, C.; Wong, K.K.H.; Bartlett, D.; Saini, B. How do pharmacists respond to complaints of acute insomnia? A simulated patient study. *Int. J. Clin. Pharm.* **2011**, *33*, 237–245. [CrossRef]
85. Al Qarni, H.; Alrahbini, T.; AlQarni, A.M.; Alqarni, A. Community pharmacist counselling practices in the Bisha health directorate, Saudi Arabia –simulated patient visits. *BMC Health Serv. Res.* **2020**, *20*, 745. [CrossRef]
86. StGB—Strafgesetzbuch in der Fassung der Bekanntmachung vom 13. November 1998 (BGBl. I S. 3322), das zuletzt durch Artikel 1 des Gesetzes vom 3. März 2020 (BGBl. I S. 431) geändert worden ist. Available online: https://www.gesetze-im-internet.de/stgb/StGB.pdf (accessed on 8 March 2021).
87. Rhodes, K.V.; Miller, F.G. Simulated Patient Studies: An Ethical Analysis. *Milbank Q.* **2012**, *90*, 706–724. [CrossRef]
88. Fitzpatrick, A.; Tumlinson, K. Strategies for Optimal Implementation of Simulated Clients for Measuring Quality of Care in Low- and Middle-Income Countries. *Glob. Health Sci. Pract.* **2017**, *5*, 108–114. [CrossRef]
89. BKK—Bundesamt für Bevölkerungsschutz und Katastrophenhilfe. COVID-19: Übersicht Kritischer Dienstleistungen. Sektorspezifische Hinweise und Informationen mit KRITIS-Relevanz. Available online: https://www.bbk.bund.de/SharedDocs/Downloads/BBK/DE/Sonstiges/Covid_19_Uebersicht_Kritischer_Dienstleistungen.pdf?__blob=publicationFile (accessed on 17 March 2021).
90. Habibzadeh, F. Common statistical mistakes in manuscripts submitted to biomedical journals. *Eur. Sci. Ed.* **2013**, *39*, 92–94.
91. Cohen, J. A power primer. *Psychol. Bull.* **1992**, *112*, 155–159. [CrossRef]
92. Berger, K.; Eickhoff, C.; Schulz, M. Counselling quality in community pharmacies: Implementation of the pseudo customer methodology in Germany. *J. Clin. Pharm. Ther.* **2005**, *30*, 45–57. [CrossRef]
93. BVM. Berufsverband Deutscher Markt-und Sozialforscher e.V. Richtlinie für den Einsatz von Mystery Research in der Markt- und Sozialforschung. Available online: https://www.bvm.org/fileadmin/user_upload/Verbandsdokumente/Standesregeln/RL_2006_Mystery.pdf (accessed on 22 February 2021).
94. Kashyap, K.C.; Nissen, L.; Smith, S.; Kyle, G. Management of over-the-counter insomnia complaints in Australian community pharmacies: A standardized patient study. *Int. J. Pharm. Pract.* **2014**, *22*, 125–134. [CrossRef]
95. da Rocha, C.E.; Bispo, M.L.; dos Santos, A.C.O.; Mesquita, A.; Brito, G.C.; de Lyra, D.P. Assessment of Community Pharmacists' Counseling Practices With Simulated Patients Who Have Minor Illness. *Simul. Heal. J. Soc. Simul. Heal.* **2015**, *10*, 227–238. [CrossRef]
96. Mobark, D.M.; Al-Tabakha, M.M.; Hasan, S. Assessing hormonal contraceptive dispensing and counseling provided by community pharmacists in the United Arab Emirates: A simulated patient study. *Pharm. Pract.* **2019**, *17*, 1465. [CrossRef] [PubMed]
97. Hernandez, J.H.; Mbadu, M.F.; Garcia, M.; Glover, A. The provision of emergency contraception in Kinshasa's private sector pharmacies: Experiences of mystery clients. *Contraception* **2018**, *97*, 57–61. [CrossRef] [PubMed]
98. Tavares, M.P.; Foster, A.M. Emergency contraception in a public health emergency: Exploring pharmacy availability in Brazil. *Contraception* **2016**, *94*, 109–114. [CrossRef] [PubMed]

99. Collins, J.C.; Schneider, C.R.; Naughtin, C.L.; Wilson, F.; Neto, A.C.D.A.; Moles, R.J. Mystery shopping and coaching as a form of audit and feedback to improve community pharmacy management of non-prescription medicine requests: An intervention study. *BMJ Open* **2017**, *7*, e019462. [CrossRef]
100. Hussainy, S.Y.; Stewart, K.; Pham, M.-P. A mystery caller evaluation of emergency contraception supply practices in community pharmacies in Victoria, Australia. *Aust. J. Prim. Heal.* **2015**, *21*, 310–316. [CrossRef]
101. Langer, B.; Bull, E.; Burgsthaler, T.; Glawe, J.; Schwobeda, M.; Simon, K. Assessment of counselling for acute diarrhoea in German pharmacies: A simulated patient study. *Int. J. Pharm. Pract.* **2018**, *26*, 310–317. [CrossRef] [PubMed]
102. Sharif, S.I. Peer Review Report For: Do north-eastern German pharmacies recommend a necessary medical consultation for acute diarrhoea? Magnitude and determinants using a simulated patient approach [version 1; peer review: 1 approved, 2 approved with reservations]. *F1000Research* **2019**, *8*, 1841. [CrossRef]

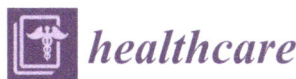

Article

Regulation Awareness and Experience of Additional Monitoring among Healthcare Professionals in Finland

Andreas Sandberg [1,*], Pauliina Ehlers [1], Saku Torvinen [2], Heli Sandberg [1] and Mia Sivén [1]

[1] Division of Pharmaceutical Chemistry and Technology, Faculty of Pharmacy, University of Helsinki, FI-00014 Helsinki, Finland; pauliina.ehlers@helsinki.fi (P.E.); heli.sandberg@helsinki.fi (H.S.); mia.siven@helsinki.fi (M.S.)

[2] MedEngine Oy, FI-00130 Helsinki, Finland; saku.torvinen@medengine.fi

[*] Correspondence: andreas.sandberg@helsinki.fi

Abstract: Background: Challenges in post-marketing adverse event reporting are generally recognized. To enhance reporting, the concept of additional monitoring was introduced in 2012. Additional monitoring aims to enhance reporting of adverse events (AE) for medicines for which the clinical evidence base is less well developed. Purpose: The purpose was to get a deeper understanding of the underlying reasons why additional monitoring has not increased AE reporting as much as initially hoped. We examined how healthcare professionals (HCPs) in Finland perceive additional monitoring, why they do or do not report AEs more readily for these medicines and how they interact with patients treated with additionally monitored medicines. Methods: An anonymous, open questionnaire was developed and made available online at the e-form portal of University of Helsinki. Physicians, nurses, and pharmacists were invited to complete the questionnaire via their respective trade or area unions. Content analysis of answers to open-ended questions was performed by two independent coders. Results: Pharmacists have the best understanding about additional monitoring but at the same time do not recognize their role in enhancing monitoring. Only 40% of HCPs working with patients knows always or often if a specific medicine is additionally monitored. Half (53%) of HCPs do not tell or tell only rarely patients about additional monitoring. 18% of HCPs reported having received additional monitoring training whereas 29% had received general AE reporting training. AE reporting was more common among HCPs who had received training. Conclusions: Additional monitoring awareness among HCPs and patients should be increased by organizing regular educational events and making additional monitoring more visible. Educational events should emphasize the significance additional monitoring has on patient safety and promote a reporting culture among HCPs.

Keywords: additional monitoring; black triangle; adverse event reporting; pharmacovigilance

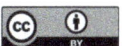

1. Introduction

The early post-marketing period is especially important for establishing a more comprehensive safety profile for new active pharmaceutical ingredients (API), which usually only have safety data about a restricted patient population in controlled experimental conditions [1–3]. Spontaneous adverse event (AE) reporting is the main source of safety information during this period although under-reporting of AEs is generally recognized [4].

To enhance AE reporting, the current EU pharmacovigilance (PV) legislation which came into effect in July 2012 introduced the concept of additional monitoring [5,6]. Medicines under additional monitoring have an inverted black triangle (▼) displayed in their package leaflet (PL) and summary of product characteristics (SmPC), together with a statement explaining what the triangle means. The aim of the triangle is to point out to healthcare professionals (HCP) and patients the medicines whose safety is particularly closely monitored by the regulatory authorities [1].

AE reporting has been studied extensively in the 21st century [7–11]. There are however only a few studies concerning additional monitoring as the concept is under a decade old. In Ireland, the awareness of the inverted black triangle symbol among HCPs who knew about additional monitoring was high among pharmacists (>86%) but relatively low among physicians ($\approx$35%) and nurses (15%) [12]. Approximately one-fourth of HCPs who knew about additional monitoring were never or rarely aware if additional monitoring applied to the medicines they used in their practice [12]. Nearly 58% of the HCPs working with patients stated that they did not inform or informed patients only rarely about additional monitoring [12].

The European Medicines Agency (EMA) conducted an EU-wide questionnaire study of additional monitoring in 2017 [13,14]. Only 69% of the HCPs answering the questionnaire reported that they had seen the black triangle and the accompanying statement before [13,14]. Some differences were observed among professions as 83% of the pharmacists, 50% of the physicians, and 42% of the nurses had seen the black triangle [13,14]. In this research, it was concluded that 45% of the pharmacists, 35% of the physicians, and 27% of the nurses had an acceptable understanding of the black triangle and additional monitoring concept [13].

The first package leaflets with the black triangle were introduced to the EU market during spring 2013. In 2019, six years after the introduction of the triangle, we conducted this cross-sectional survey of HCPs (i.e., physicians, pharmacists, and nurses) in Finland to get a more detailed understanding about how HCPs perceive additional monitoring, why they do or do not report AEs more readily for these medicines, and how they interact with patients treated with additionally monitored medicines.

In Finland, pharmacists licensed to practice the profession are Bachelors of Science (B.Sc.) in Pharmacy (1st Cycle Degree) or Masters of Science (M.Sc.) in Pharmacy (2nd cycle degree) graduates [15]. Both groups work with patients and have similar responsibilities in the patient interface. AE reporting is voluntary for HCPs in Finland.

2. Methods

2.1. Questionnaire Design

An anonymous, open questionnaire was developed and made available online at the e-form portal of University of Helsinki. The final wording of the questionnaire was agreed by an expert panel consisting of two physicians, two nurses, and five pharmacists. Members of the expert panel represented the Finnish healthcare system well as it included experts from industry, academia, hospitals, and open healthcare.

The questionnaire consisted of a cover letter including informed consent statement and a total of 26 questions. Nine questions were open-ended. Two of the 17 multiple-choice questions were designed to measure the knowledge of the respondents. A 5-point Likert scale was used in four questions concerning additional monitoring. The questionnaire is presented in the Supplementary Materials of this article.

The face validity of the questionnaire was tested in a small-scale pilot study with five HCPs. Based on the pilot study, small modifications were made to the questionnaire to improve clarity. No problems were observed with the e-form portal. It was estimated that answering the questionnaire would take 10–15 min.

2.2. Questionnaire Distribution

A convenience sample was collected by inviting physicians, nurses, and pharmacists to complete the questionnaire via their respective trade or area unions. The invitation and link to the questionnaire was sent to the respondents via email or by including it to a union newsletter. One reminder was sent in order to maximize the amount of responses. An invitation to complete the survey was also added to the HCP restricted front page of Finnish Medical Network (www.fimnet.fi). No honorarium was provided to Finnish Medical Network, unions or the respondents. Answers were collected from May 2019 to December 2019.

2.3. Analysis

2.3.1. Statistical Analysis

IBM SPSS Statistics Version 27 (IBM, Armonk, NY, USA) was used to analyse the data. In the two questions that measured the knowledge of the respondents, the average knowledge score for each HCP subgroup was calculated by summing all correct items and dividing by the total number of items. One-way Analysis of Variance (ANOVA) was used to compare mean knowledge scores between HCP subgroups and most categorical variables. Chi-square test for independence was used in two comparisons of categorical variables. A 5% significance level applies in all hypothesis testing. A Bonferroni correction was applied when multiple group comparisons were made. The Bonferroni corrected alpha level was adjusted to 0.0125 when four comparisons were made and to 0.0167 when three comparisons were made.

2.3.2. Content Analysis

Content analysis of answers to open-ended questions was performed by two independent coders. Data-driven coding approach was used [16].

Reclassification of answer categories was performed in situations where the independent coders had initially created differing categories. Reclassification of answer categories was performed in two questions for physicians and M.Sc. pharmacists, in three questions for nurses and in one question for B.Sc. pharmacists. Re-evaluation of answers in a category was performed in situations where the initial coding resulted in a difference above three answers between the two coders. All differences were discussed until a mutual opinion was reached between the coders.

3. Results

A total of 241 responses was received. The response rates could not be calculated as the trade and area unions did not reveal the exact number of email and newsletter recipients. There were 240 complete responses. Six responses did not meet the inclusion criteria (i.e., physician, pharmacist, or nurse). A total of 234 responses were analysed (38 physician, 45 nurse, 36 M.Sc. pharmacist, and 115 B.Sc. pharmacist).

3.1. Demographics

Most of the HCPs answering the questionnaire were professionally experienced. 69% ($n = 161$) of the respondents had at least 10 years of experience in their profession. Physicians were the most experienced as 92% ($n = 35$) of them had a minimum experience of 10 years.

The primary workplace was a hospital for most physicians (37%, $n = 14$) and nurses (44%, $n = 20$). Retail pharmacy was the primary workplace for most B.Sc. pharmacists (57%, $n = 66$) whereas the pharmaceutical industry was a major employer of M.Sc. pharmacists (33%, $n = 12$). Demographics are summarised in Table 1.

3.2. Adverse Event Reporting Experience

Nearly 56% ($n = 131$) of the HCPs responding to the questionnaire had not reported any AEs during their careers and 38% ($n = 89$) of the HCPs had reported an AE one to nine times. Only 6% ($n = 14$) had reported an AE over 10 times.

The majority of nurses (80%, $n = 36$) and B.Sc. pharmacists (58%, $n = 67$) had not reported any AEs. Correspondingly the majority of physicians and M.Sc. pharmacists had reported at least one AE. A statistically significant difference was observed between nurses and other HCP subgroups. A greater proportion of nurses had not reported any AEs compared to physicians ($p < 0.001$, One-way ANOVA with post-hoc Bonferroni correction) and pharmacists ($p = 0.004$, One-way ANOVA with post-hoc Bonferroni correction). The AE reporting experience is presented in Figure 1.

Table 1. Healthcare professional demographics.

Profession	Physician	Nurse	M.Sc. Pharmacist	B.Sc. Pharmacist	Total
Group size (*n*)	38	45	36	115	234
Years in practice, % (*n*)					
<5	5.3 (2)	17.8 (8)	19.4 (7)	13.9 (16)	14.1 (33)
5–9	2.6 (1)	15.6 (7)	30.6 (11)	18.3 (21)	17.1 (40)
10–19	18.4 (7)	31.1 (14)	30.6 (11)	29.6 (34)	28.2 (66)
>20	73.7 (28)	35.6 (16)	19.4 (7)	38.3 (44)	40.6 (95)
Primary workplace, % (*n*)					
Hospital	36.8 (14)	44.4 (20)	0 (0)	7.8 (9)	18.4 (43)
Private clinic	23.7 (9)	2.2 (1)	0 (0)	0 (0)	4.3 (10)
Healthcare center	18.4 (7)	20.0 (9)	0 (0)	4.3 (5)	9.0 (21)
Government	5.3 (2)	(0)	5.6 (2)	3.5 (4)	3.4 (8)
Nursing home	2.6 (1)	17.8 (8)	0 (0)	0 (0)	3.8 (9)
Retail pharmacy	0 (0)	0 (0)	36.1 (13)	57.4 (66)	33.8 (79)
Pharmaceutical industry	0 (0)	0 (0)	33.3 (12)	5.2 (6)	7.7 (18)
Hospital pharmacy	0 (0)	0 (0)	13.9 (5)	16.5 (19)	10.3 (24)
Other	13.2 (5)	15.6 (7)	11.1 (4)	5.2 (6)	9.4 (22)

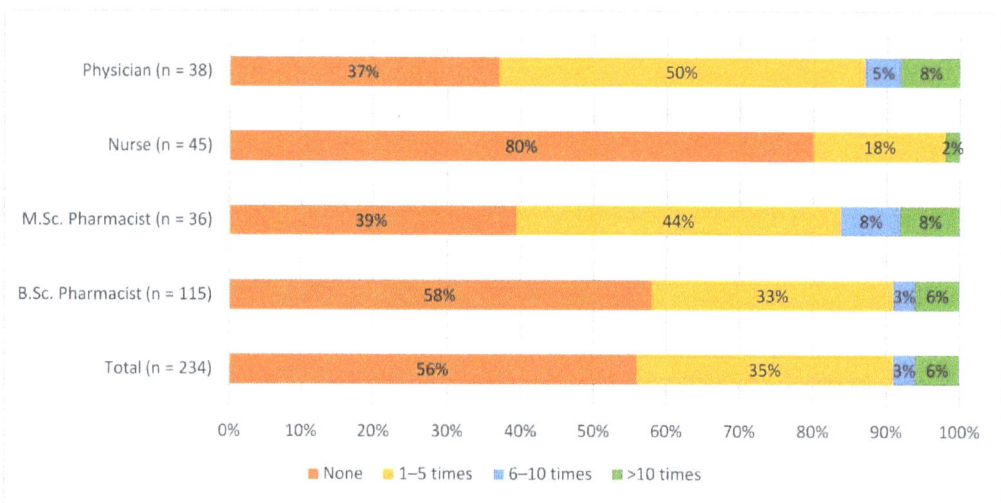

Figure 1. Adverse event reporting experience among healthcare professionals. Questionnaire question: How many times have you reported an adverse event to the local health authority (Fimea) or to the marketing authorization holder?

3.3. Adverse Event Reporting Knowledge

Pharmacists scored higher knowledge scores than physicians and nurses when asked about general AE reporting. The average knowledge scores for physicians, nurses, M.Sc. pharmacists, and B.Sc. pharmacists were 4.76, 4.60, 6.19, and 5.34, respectively, out of the possible 8.0. The average knowledge score for all HCPs was 5.24. A statistically significant difference was observed between nurses and pharmacists. Nurses have poorer AE reporting knowledge compared to pharmacists (p = 0.016, One-way ANOVA with post-hoc Bonferroni correction). Claims used to test AE reporting knowledge and the results are presented in Table 2.

Table 2. Adverse event reporting knowledge among Finnish HCPs, % correct, (n/n) correct answers/all answers.

Claim [a]	Physician (n = 38)	Nurse (n = 45)	M.Sc. Pharmacist (n = 36)	B.Sc. Pharmacist (n = 115)	Total (n = 234)
HCPs are encouraged to report AEs even if uncertain medicine is the culprit (yes)	89.5% (34/38)	57.8% (26/45)	91.7% (33/36)	82.6% (95/115)	80.3% (188/234)
HCPs are encouraged to report AEs even if they do not have all the details of the event (yes)	68.4% (26/38)	60.0% (27/45)	86.1% (31/36)	72.2% (83/115)	71.4% (167/234)
All serious AEs are known once the medicine enters the market (no)	92.1% (35/38)	80.0% (36/45)	97.2% (35/36)	94.8% (109/115)	91.9% (215/234)
AEs reported by Finnish HCPs are handled locally and do not influence safety information in other countries (no)	92.1% (35/38)	80.0% (36/45)	94.4% (34/36)	93.9% (108/115)	91.0% (213/234)
Patients themselves can report AEs to HA or MAHs (yes)	55.3% (21/38)	57.8% (26/45)	86.1% (31/36)	73.0% (84/115)	69.2% (162/234)
HCPs are also encouraged to report overdoses, misuse, and medication errors (yes)	34.2% (13/38)	62.2% (28/45)	63.9% (23/36)	37.4% (43/115)	45.7% (107/234)
HCPs are encouraged to report medicine use during pregnancy (yes)	7.9% (3/38)	17.8% (8/45)	41.7% (15/36)	24.4% (28/115)	23.1% (54/234)
HCPs should report AEs to the local HA, not to MAH (no)	36.8% (14/38)	44.4% (20/45)	58.3% (21/36)	55.7% (64/115)	50.9% (119/234)
I do not know [b]	7.9% (3/38)	15.6% (7/45)	2.8% (1/36)	5.2% (6/115)	7.3% (17/234)
Total amount of right answers	59.5% (181/304)	57.5% (207/360)	77.4% (223/288)	66.7% (614/920)	65.4% (1225/1872)
Average knowledge score per responder	4.76 (181/38)	4.6 (207/45)	6.19 (223/36)	5.34 (614/115)	5.24 (1225/234)

AE adverse event, HCP healthcare professional, HA health authority, MAH marketing authorization holder. [a] Correct answer is presented in brackets after the claim. [b] "I do not know" was an option to HCPs who could not answer the claims. The answers of HCPs who chose "I do not know" were considered as wrong answers in the analysis of results.

The Finnish HCPs scored the lowest score on questions concerning topics such as pregnancy and off-label use that were introduced to the EU PV legislation in 2012 [17]. Approximately 70% (n = 162) of HCPs knew that patients can report AEs themselves and 51% (n = 119) knew that HCPs can report AEs also to the marketing authorization holder (MAH).

Up to 56% (n = 132) of the HCPs do not feel that they have enough information on how to report AEs. A prominent share of nurses (73%, n = 33) and B.Sc. pharmacists (60%, n = 69) would want to have more information about AE reporting.

3.4. Additional Monitoring Knowledge

Approximately 87% (n = 203) of the HCPs were aware that some medicines were under additional monitoring before answering the questionnaire.

Questions measuring additional monitoring knowledge rendered the same result as the questions measuring general AE reporting knowledge. Pharmacists scored higher knowledge scores than physicians and nurses. The average knowledge scores for physicians, nurses, M.Sc. pharmacists, and B.Sc. pharmacists were 2.68, 2.16, 3.44, and 3.03, respectively out of the possible 4.0. The average knowledge score for all HCPs was 2.87. A statistically significant difference was observed between nurses and pharmacists. Nurses have poorer additional monitoring knowledge compared to pharmacists ($p < 0.001$, One-way ANOVA with post-hoc Bonferroni correction). Claims used to test additional monitoring knowledge and the results are presented in Table 3.

Table 3. Additional monitoring knowledge among Finnish HCPs: Why are some medicines additionally monitored? % correct, (n/n) correct answers/all answers.

Claim [a]	Physician (n = 38)	Nurse (n = 45)	M.Sc. Pharmacist (n = 36)	B.Sc. Pharmacist (n = 115)	Total (n = 234)
These medicines have more serious AEs (No)	50.0% (19/38)	35.6% (16/45)	69.4% (25/36)	57.4% (66/115)	53.9% (126/234)
AEs are more common with these medicines (No)	68.4% (26/38)	44.4% (20/45)	88.9% (32/36)	77.4% (89/115)	71.4% (167/234)
Safety information has not yet been collected as much as desired for these medicines (Yes)	73.7% (28/38)	60.0% (27/45)	94.4% (34/36)	82.6% (95/115)	78.6% (184/234)
No reason. All medicines will be additionally monitored after the transition period (No)	76.3% (29/38)	75.6% (34/45)	91.7% (33/36)	85.2% (98/115)	82.9% (194/234)
I do not know [b]	21.1% (8/38)	24.4% (11/45)	5.6% (2/36)	11.3% (13/115)	14.5% (34/234)
Total amount of right answers	67.1% (102/152)	53.9% (97/180)	86.1% (124/144)	75.7% (348/460)	71.7% (671/936)
Average knowledge score per responder	2.68 (102/38)	2.16 (97/45)	3.44 (124/36)	3.03 (348/115)	2.87 (671/234)

AE adverse event, HCP healthcare professional. [a] Correct answer is presented in brackets after the claim. [b] "I do not know" was an option to HCPs who could not answer the claims. The answers of HCPs who chose "I do not know" were considered as wrong answers in the analysis of results.

Approximately 78% (n = 184) of the HCPs knew that the reason for additional monitoring is that for these medicines safety information has not yet been collected as much as desired. Almost 15% (n = 34) of the HCPs could not answer the true–false statements concerning additional monitoring.

3.5. Black Triangle Requirement and Noticeability

Overall, 70% (143/203) of the Finnish HCPs who knew about the additional monitoring concept before answering the questionnaire knew that additionally monitored medicines must have a black triangle in the SmPC, PL, and marketing materials. The black triangle requirement was well-known among pharmacists as 86% (118/138) knew about it. Among other professions this requirement was not that familiar as less than half of the physicians (45%, 14/31) and one-third of the nurses (32%, 11/34) knew about the requirement. A statistically significant difference among all responders was observed between pharmacists and other HCP subgroups. A greater proportion of pharmacists knew about the black triangle requirement compared to physicians ($p < 0.001$, One-way ANOVA with post-hoc Bonferroni correction) and nurses ($p < 0.001$, One-way ANOVA with post-hoc Bonferroni correction). Results are presented in Table 4.

Table 4. Percentage of HCPs who knew about the additional monitoring concept and black triangle requirement.

Profession	Knew about Additional Monitoring	Knew about Black Triangle Requirement	Knew about Additional Monitoring and Black Triangle Requirement
Physician	81.6% (31/38)	36.8% (14/38)	45.2% (14/31)
Nurse	75.6% (34/45)	24.4% (11/45)	32.4% (11/34)
M.Sc. pharmacist	97.2% (35/36)	86.1% (31/36)	88.6% (31/35)
B.Sc. pharmacist	89.6% (103/115)	75.7% (87/115)	84.5% (87/103)
Total	86.8% (203/234)	61.1% (143/234)	70.4% (143/203)

HCP healthcare professional.

One-fourth (26%, 60/234) of the HCPs had never noticed the black triangle. A breakdown between professions revealed that approximately 40% of physicians (15/38) and nurses (18/45) had not noticed the triangle whereas the corresponding numbers where 8% (3/36) and 21% (24/115) for M.Sc. pharmacists and B.Sc. pharmacists, respectively. In all professions, the majority of responders would prefer that the black triangle and information of additional monitoring is available electronically, preferably in the electronic interface they are using in their everyday tasks.

3.6. Effect of Additional Monitoring on Daily Work

Out of the 234 HCPs, 185 worked with patients in their current position. 40% (63/157) of HCPs who worked with patients and knew about the additional monitoring concept stated that they knew always, or often which medicines were under additional monitoring. Correspondingly one-fourth (26%, 41/157) of HCPs did not know or did only rarely know if additional monitoring applied to the medicines.

Half (50%, 101/203) of the HCPs who knew about the additional monitoring concept stated that they report AEs more readily for these medicines compared to other medicines. The most common reason for more active reporting was the desire to increase safety information about the medicine. A significant amount of HCPs emphasized that they report all AEs according to same principles regardless of the medicine. There were responders in all professions who admitted that they do not report AEs more readily as they do not recognize these medicines or do not know how to report AEs.

A quarter (27%) of the HCPs who knew about the additional monitoring concept and worked with patients stated to be always or often more cautious with medicines under additional monitoring whereas 17% stated they are never more cautious. Thirty-five percent of the physicians and 45% of the nurses stated being always or often more cautious whereas only 18% of the pharmacists felt the same. For physicians and nurses, the main reason for being more cautious was the low amount of information available about the medicine. Approximately one-fifth of pharmacists (19%) stated that they are never more cautious. The main reason for not exercising additional caution was that they felt that it was the responsibility of the person prescribing the medicine.

Even 53% of the HCPs who worked with patients and knew about the additional monitoring concept do not tell or tell only rarely the patient about additional monitoring. A quarter (26%) tell the patient always or often. Pharmacists are the most reluctant to tell about additional monitoring as 61% stated that they do not tell or tell only rarely. For pharmacists, the most common reason for not telling was that the information of additional monitoring was considered to be harmful or useless to the patient. 44% of physicians, 28% of nurses, and 19% of pharmacists tell always or often the patient about additional monitoring. For physicians, the most common reason for telling the patient was to get the patient involved in the treatment whereas many nurses felt that telling the patient was their duty.

Only 9% (21/234) of the HCPs answering the questionnaire have received additional monitoring related questions from patients. Most of the questions have concerned the meaning of the inverted black triangle and if it were safe to use the medicine.

3.7. Enhancing Adverse Event Reporting of APIs under Additional Monitoring

The Finnish HCPs feel that making AE reporting easier and instructions more clear is most important when trying to enhance AE reporting of APIs under additional monitoring. Many hoped for a simple and fast electronic reporting system that was integrated to the programs used by the HCPs in their everyday practice. Especially nurses wished that the responsibilities and guidelines around AE reporting would be more clear so that it would be easier decide who reports the AEs.

The second most important factor in enhancing AE reporting is to increase communication about additional monitoring and reminding HCPs which medicines are additionally monitored. Several HCPs felt that education around additional monitoring should be increased.

3.8. Pharmacovigilance Training of HCPs

Sixty-eight out of the 234 (29%) HCPs have received AE reporting training. The percentage drops to 23% (46/202) when HCPs working in the pharmaceutical industry, academia, and government are excluded. Correspondingly 41 out of the 234 (18%) have received training concerning additional monitoring. The percentage drops to 12% (25/202) when HCPs working in the pharmaceutical industry, academia and government, are excluded. No differences in AE reporting or additional monitoring training prevalence were observed between HCP subgroups (Chi-square test for independence). The PV training prevalence among HCP subgroups is presented in Figure 2.

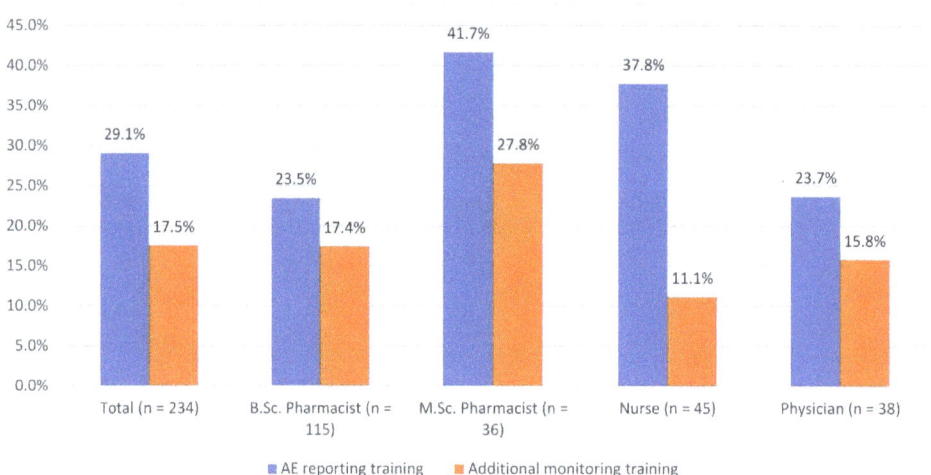

Figure 2. Percentage of healthcare professionals who have received pharmacovigilance training.

AE reporting is more common among HCPs who have received AE reporting training ($p = 0.009$, Chi-square test for independence). Sixty-eight percent (15/22) of HCPs who had reported five or more AEs during their career had received general AE reporting training. The corresponding percentages were 38% (39/103) for HCPs who had reported at least one AE and 22% (29/131) for HCPs who had not reported any AEs.

4. Discussion

Challenges in post-marketing AE reporting are generally recognized. It is estimated that even 94% of all AEs are not reported [4]. Based on previous research, it seems that making AE reporting mandatory by law does not either increase reporting [18]. In 2012, EU introduced additional monitoring to tackle this gap for medicines for which the clinical evidence base is less well developed. Based on an analysis by EMA, it seems however that reporting activity has not increased significantly [14,19]. Our research revealed some of the underlying reasons why additional monitoring has failed to increase AE reporting in the EU as much as initially hoped. Our research is a first-in-kind to study AE reporting knowledge and experience in Finland.

Our results concerning HCP knowledge about additional monitoring and the inverted black triangle are mostly aligned with previously conducted studies. As in the Irish research, our results suggest that among HCPs pharmacists are best aware that authorities are performing additional monitoring and that the black triangle symbolizes this monitoring. Similar to the EU-wide research conducted by EMA, it is evident that pharmacists have the best understanding about what additional monitoring is and why it is performed. The percentage of HCPs who know about the black triangle requirement is slightly higher in Finland compared to Ireland, especially for physicians (45% vs. ~35%) and nurses (32% vs. 15%) [12]. Correspondingly the percentage of HCPs who have never noticed the black triangle is a bit lower in Finland compared to the EU-wide research (26% vs. 29%) [13,14]. The two-year gap between our research and these two other studies might explain the difference as the number of additionally monitored medicines has increased together with opportunities to notice the triangle.

Based on our results, it is clear that additional monitoring and the black triangle must be made more visible to HCPs working with patients. Only 40% of HCPs who know about additional monitoring and work with patients can always or often tell if additional monitoring applies to the medicine they are giving to the patient. Exactly the same result was observed in the Irish research [12]. The list of additionally monitored medicines contains already hundreds of APIs and for HCPs to remember this list by heart is impossible [20]. It is now clear that HCPs prefer to get information about additional monitoring via the electronic interface they use while working with patients. Adding a notification in the interface before prescribing, administering, or dispensing the medicine would make sure the information is at hand when needed.

Half of Finnish HCPs state to report AEs more readily for additionally monitored medicines if they are aware of additional monitoring. It was reassuring to discover that a big portion of these HCPs report AEs because they want to increase knowledge about the medicines and improve patient safety. It is nevertheless troublesome to notice that some HCPs still do not see the value of single AE reports and neglect reporting entirely for example because it is too laborious.

Our research revealed that unlike physicians and nurses, a big part of pharmacists do not see the significance of their efforts in the additional monitoring process. The majority feel that telling the patient about additional monitoring and being more cautious with these treatments is the responsibility of the physician or nurse prescribing the medicine. Whereas for physicians the most common reason for telling the patient about additional monitoring was to get the patient involved in the treatment; the pharmacists refrained from informing the patient. In many instances, pharmacists see the patients much more often than the nurse or physician. With this in mind, we can argue that pharmacists actually have a pivotal role in the process as they can readily disseminate information about additional monitoring and also collect new safety information.

Our results suggest that over half (53%) of HCPs do not tell or tell only rarely the patient about additional monitoring. At the same time, it was made clear that less than 10% of the HCPs have received additional monitoring or black triangle-related questions from patients. Currently the black triangle and the accompanying statement are only present in the SmPC and PL. Previous research suggest that many patients find PLs hard to comprehend and have difficulties in finding the information they are looking for [21–23]. Many patients do not either read the PL [21–23]. Adding the additional monitoring information also to outer packaging might help in raising awareness especially among the public. This could in turn increase discussion among patients and their HCPs and ultimately enhance AE reporting.

Based on our research, AE reporting of APIs under additional monitoring could be enhanced by increasing awareness among HCPs via frequent information campaigns and active training. A statistical significance between training combined with PV information campaigns and increased AE reporting rate was found in a Portuguese study [24]. Training without information campaigns failed to show statistical significance [24]. Only a fraction of the Finnish HCPs working with patients reported to having received AE reporting or additional monitoring training. It is therefore of utmost importance to get HCPs educated about PV and keep PV on display e.g., by making educational events recurring. Based on our results and previous research, the training should be designed to change erroneous beliefs and promote a reporting culture among HCPs [25].

The majority HCPs answering our questionnaire were professionally experienced as 69% had at least 10 years of experience. This may be a source of bias as HCPs receiving their basic education after additional monitoring implementation are underrepresented in our sample. Correspondingly M.Sc. pharmacists working in the pharmaceutical industry or the government are overrepresented in our sample as nearly 40% of M.Sc. pharmacist responders belonged to this group and are probably better trained on the current legislation and AE reporting guidelines. This effect is however diluted in the whole pharmacist group as only 16% of the pharmacists worked in the industry or the government.

Non-response bias is the main limitation of this research. Response rates could not be calculated due to the method of questionnaire distribution but based on previous research, it is expected that the response rate is low [12]. In this research, HCPs reflected their past actions and knowledge, which is the second most important source of possible bias as answers depended on own recollection and honesty. Although sources of bias must be taken into consideration, our results are well aligned with previous research and with this sample size largely generalisable to other European countries with similar regulation and HCP educational criteria.

5. Conclusions

In conclusion, pharmacists were found to be best aware of additional monitoring but at the same time they did not recognize their role in the additional monitoring process. Like other HCPs, pharmacists could also serve an important role in getting the patient involved in treatment and tell them about the importance of additional monitoring. This discovery requires confirmation in future research but it is nevertheless certain that additional monitoring awareness among HCPs working with patients should be increased to avoid any possible misconceptions. Clarification of roles and responsibilities between different healthcare professions should also be emphasized. Locations where many different HCPs are in contact with the same patient (e.g., hospitals) are especially vulnerable and require in-house procedures stating when AEs are reported and by whom. Finally we recommend that health authorities look into the benefits and risks associated with adding the black triangle also to the outer packaging of additionally monitored medicines. We believe that making additional monitoring more visible to HCPs and patients will increase AE reporting and thereby promote patient safety.

Supplementary Materials: The following are available online at https://www.mdpi.com/article/10.3390/healthcare9111540/s1. A questionnaire concerning adverse event reporting of medicines.

Author Contributions: All authors participated in the conception and development of this article. A.S. designed the research with P.E., M.S. and H.S. A.S. performed the content analysis of answers to open-ended questions. S.T. performed the statistical analysis. All authors have read and agreed to the published version of the manuscript.

Funding: Open access funding provided by Helsinki University Library.

Institutional Review Board Statement: The research was approved by the University of Helsinki Ethical Review Board in the Humanities and Social and Behavioural Sciences on 25 April 2019 (statement 22/2019). No other institutional statements were needed [26].

Informed Consent Statement: Informed consent was obtained from all subjects involved in the study.

Data Availability Statement: Data is not available online.

Acknowledgments: The authors acknowledge The Finnish Pharmacists' Association, The Finnish Pharmacists' Society, The Finnish Nurses Association, Physician union of Helsinki, Physician union of Northern Savonia, Finnish Physician union of Pediatrics and Finnish Medical Network for distributing the questionnaire. The authors acknowledge Minna Parhiala (University of Helsinki) for performing duplicate content analysis of answers to open-ended questions.

Conflicts of Interest: A.S. is an employee of Takeda Oy. P.E. is an employee of Novartis Finland Oy. S.T. is an employee of MedEngine Oy. H.S. is an employee of GlaxoSmithKline Oy. The views expressed are entirely those of the authors and do not necessarily reflect the policy of the companies they are working for.

References

1. European Medicines Agency (EMA). Guideline on Good Pharmacovigilance Practices (GVP) Module X—Additional Monitoring. 2013. Available online: https://www.ema.europa.eu/en/documents/scientific-guideline/guideline-good-pharmacovigilance-practices-module-x-additional-monitoring_en.pdf (accessed on 1 October 2021).
2. World Health Organization. *Safety of Medicines: A Guide to Detecting and Reporting Adverse Drug Reactions: Why Health Professionals Need to Take Action*; World Health Organization: Geneva, Switzerland, 2002.
3. Sharrar, R.G.; Dieck, G.S. Monitoring product safety in the postmarketing environment. *Ther. Adv. Drug Saf.* **2013**, *4*, 211–219. [CrossRef] [PubMed]
4. Hazell, L.; Shakir, S.A. Under-reporting of adverse drug reactions: A systematic review. *Drug Saf.* **2006**, *29*, 385–396. [CrossRef] [PubMed]
5. European Parliament. Directive. 2010/84/EU of the European parliament and of the Council. *Off. J. Eur. Union* **2010**, *53*, L348/75.
6. Fornasier, G.; Francescon, S.; Leone, R.; Baldo, P. An historical overview over Pharmacovigilance. *Int. J. Clin. Pharm.* **2018**, *40*, 744–747. [CrossRef] [PubMed]
7. Dos Santos Pernas, S.I.; Herdeiro, M.T.; Lopez-Gonzalez, E. Attitudes of portuguese health professionals toward adverse drug reaction reporting. *Int. J. Clin. Pharm.* **2012**, *34*, 693–698. [CrossRef] [PubMed]
8. Pirmohamed, M.; James, S.; Meakin, S.; Green, C.; Scott, A.K.; Walley, T.; Farrar, K.; Park, B.K.; Breckenridge, A.M. Adverse drug reactions as cause of admission to hospital: Prospective analysis of 18820 patients. *BMJ* **2004**, *329*, 15–19. [CrossRef] [PubMed]
9. Margraff, F.; Bertram, D. Adverse drug reaction reporting by patients: An overview of fifty countries. *Drug Saf.* **2014**, *37*, 409–441. [CrossRef] [PubMed]
10. Irujo, M.; Beitia, G.; Bes-Rastrollo, M.; Figueiras, A.; Hernández-Díaz, S.; Lasheras, B. Factors that influence under-reporting of suspected adverse drug reactions among community pharmacists in a Spanish region. *Drug Saf.* **2007**, *30*, 1073–1082. [CrossRef] [PubMed]
11. Stergiopoulos, S.; Brown, C.A.; Felix, T.; Grampp, G.; Getz, K.A. A survey of adverse event reporting practices among US healthcare professionals. *Drug Saf.* **2016**, *39*, 1117–1127. [CrossRef] [PubMed]
12. O'Callaghan, J.; Griffin, B.T.; Morris, J.M.; Bermingham, M. Knowledge of adverse drug reaction reporting and the pharmacovigilance of biological medicines: A survey of healthcare professionals in Ireland. *BioDrugs* **2018**, *32*, 267–280. [CrossRef] [PubMed]
13. Januskiene, J.; Segec, A.; Slattery, J.; Genov, G.; Plueschke, K.; Kurz, X.; Arlett, P. What are the patients' and health care professionals' understanding and behaviors towards adverse drug reaction reporting and additional monitoring? *Pharmacoepidemiol. Drug Saf.* **2021**, *30*, 334–341. [CrossRef] [PubMed]
14. European Medicines Agency (EMA). European Medicines Agency and Member States Joint Report to the European Commission on the Experience with the List of Products Subject to Additional Monitoring. 2018; EMA/385597/2019. Available online: https://www.ema.europa.eu/en/documents/report/european-medicines-agency-member-states-joint-report-european-commission-experience-list-products_en.pdf (accessed on 27 September 2021).
15. Hirvonen, J.; Salminen, O.; Vuorensola, K.; Katajavuori, N.; Huhtala, H.; Atkinson, J. Pharmacy practice and education in Finland. *Pharmacy* **2019**, *7*, 21. [CrossRef] [PubMed]
16. Gibbs, G.R. *Analyzing Qualitative Data*, 1st ed.; SAGE Publications Ltd.: London, UK, 2007.
17. Borg, J.-J.; Aislaitner, G.; Pirozynski, M.; Mifsud, S. Strengthening and rationalizing pharmacovigilance in the EU: Where is Europe heading to? A review of the new EU legislation on pharmacovigilance. *Drug Saf.* **2011**, *34*, 187–197. [CrossRef] [PubMed]
18. Srba, J.; Descikova, V.; Vlcek, J. Adverse drug reactions: Analysis of spontaneous reporting system in Europe in 2007–2009. *Eur. J. Clin. Pharmacol.* **2012**, *68*, 1057–1063. [CrossRef] [PubMed]
19. Segec, A.; Slattery, J.; Morales, D.R.; Januskiene, J.; Kurz, X.; Arlett, P. Does additional monitoring status increase the reporting of adverse drug reactions? An interrupted time series analysis of EudraVigilance data. *Pharmacoepidemiol. Drug Saf.* **2021**, *30*, 350–359. [CrossRef] [PubMed]

20. European Medicines Agency (EMA). List of Medicinal Products under Additional Monitoring. 21 May 2021. EMA/245297/2013 Rev. 89. Available online: https://www.ema.europa.eu/en/documents/additional-monitoring/list-medicinal-products-under-additional-monitoring_en-0.pdf (accessed on 27 September 2021).
21. Hammar, T.; Nilsson, A.L.; Hovstadius, B. Patients' views on electronic patient information leaflets. *Pharm. Pract.* **2016**, *14*, 702. [CrossRef] [PubMed]
22. Salgueiro, E.; Gurruchaga, C.; Jimeno, F.J.; Martinez-Mugica, C.; Martin Arias, L.H.; Manso, G. What can we learn from the public's understanding of drug information and safety? A population survey. *Int. J. Pharm. Pract.* **2019**, *27*, 96–104. [CrossRef] [PubMed]
23. van Beusekom, M.M.; Grootens-Wiegers, P.; Bos, M.J.W.; Guchelaar, H.J.; van den Broek, J.M. Low literacy and written drug information: Information-seeking, leaflet evaluation and preferences, and roles for images. *Int. J. Clin. Pharm.* **2016**, *38*, 1372–1379. [CrossRef] [PubMed]
24. Duarte, M.; Ferreira, P.; Soares, M.; Cavaco, A.; Martins, A.P. Community pharmacists attitudes towards adverse drug reaction reporting and their knowledge of the new pharmacovigilance legislation in the southern region of Portugal: A mixed methods study. *Drugs Ther. Perspect.* **2015**, *31*, 316–322. [CrossRef]
25. Herdeiro, M.T.; Figueiras, A.; Polonia, J. Influence of pharmacists' attitudes on adverse drug reaction reporting: A case-control study in Portugal. *Drug Saf.* **2006**, *29*, 331–340. [CrossRef] [PubMed]
26. Finnish National Board on Research Integrity. Finnish National Board on Research Integrity TENK Guidelines 2019: The Ethical Principles of Research with Human Participants and Ethical Review in the Human Sciences in Finland (TENK 3/2019). Available online: https://tenk.fi/sites/default/files/2021-01/Ethical_review_in_human_sciences_2020.pdf (accessed on 1 November 2021).

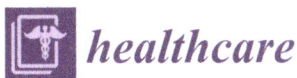

Review

Biosensing Technology to Track Adherence: A Literature Review

Cody K. Dukes [1] and Elizabeth A. Sheaffer [2,*]

[1] Alumnus, McWhorter School of Pharmacy, Samford University, Birmingham, AL 35229, USA; cdukes@samford.edu
[2] Department of Pharmaceutical, Social, and Administrative Sciences, McWhorter School of Pharmacy, Samford University, Birmingham, AL 35229, USA
* Correspondence: esheaffe@samford.edu; Tel.: +1-205-726-2896

Abstract: Tracking adherence can be a useful means of identifying opportunities to provide educational intervention to nonadherent patients. The aim of this study was to evaluate the ability of biosensing technology to track medication adherence. Searches of PubMed and Ovid IPA were conducted. The criteria for inclusion were studies that tracked and reported ingestion events. Studies that did not track ingestion events were excluded from this review. Titles and abstracts were assessed for relevance, and full-text reviews were performed on all potentially relevant studies. References from the studies retrieved from the literature searches were assessed for additional applicable articles. Overall, ingestion events were detected 91.3% of the time, with many of the failed detections being related to patients not using or inappropriately using the system. In the studies that looked at the latency time, the overall mean time to detection by the wearable sensor was between 1.1 and 5.1 min. With medication nonadherence being a persistent problem in healthcare, biosensing technology presents an innovative approach to tracking adherence. The technology has been shown to be accurate in its ability to track actual medication use in patients. It has also been shown to detect ingestions with a minimal delay after administration. Accessibility may be an issue with this technology in the future, and further studies may be necessary to access the viability of biosensing technology.

Keywords: biosensing technology; digital medicine system; medication adherence; medication event monitoring system; nonadherence; pharmacy

1. Introduction

Medication adherence is of critical importance in today's healthcare system. Adherence can be described simply as the extent to which a patient follows through in sticking to a planned regimen for his/her treatment from a health care provider [1]. This follow-through can often be the linchpin in a patient's health. It is generally accepted that an adherence rate of at least 80% is required to achieve optimal therapeutic outcomes [2]. However, medication nonadherence is very prevalent in the United States. It is estimated that nonadherence accounts for up to 50% of failures in treatment, about 125,000 deaths, and around 25% of hospitalizations each year [2].

The responsibility of adherence is not solely a patient-based issue. This problem falls on the shoulders of patients and practitioners alike. Patients are ultimately responsible (in most cases) for the administration of their medication, but there are other steps in the healthcare process that are important in reducing nonadherence. Doctors can explain the necessity of consistently using a medication regimen when prescribing to patients. Nurses can emphasize adherence and ensure patient understanding during transitions of care and discharges. Pharmacists can educate patients on how the medications work, why they are being used, and how often they are to use them. A breakdown at any of these stages or others in the healthcare system can be the cause of medication nonadherence.

New technologies are frequently being implemented to try to curtail this problem. The subjective and often inaccurate feedback associated with pill counts and self-reports has not been very successful in achieving adherence in patients. Healthcare has begun to look at utilizing technology as a path to possible solutions. The advent of mobile technology has allowed for a variety of ways to help with medication adherence. This makes sense as most adult Americans now own a cell phone. Mobile devices have several functions that lend themselves to healthcare, such as phone calls, text messaging, and mobile applications. Due to this functionality, we have seen the utilization of these functions in the effort to increase medication adherence. Some institutions practice automated calling to serve as reminders for patients to take their medications or show up for appointments. Others have implemented automated text messaging to provide a similar reminder to patients. Various applications have been created to help with adherence. Some practitioners will suggest these applications to their patients, or the patients will find one that they find convenient of their own volition. Many of these have shown effective results in previous studies, but medication nonadherence is still an issue, and the healthcare system still seeks to find ways to improve adherence.

Numerous other methods currently exist to directly and/or objectively assess adherence, including pill counts, Medication Event Monitoring System (MEMS) bottle caps, pharmacy refill records, and biological assays from bodily fluids [3]. However, they all have limitations, and none provide an actual measure of medication ingestion. Therefore, the ability to precisely and objectively assess medication adherence in patients is a significant unmet need [3].

A newer technological advancement that may have a profound effect on increasing (or at least monitoring) adherence is biosensing technology. This technology works by having patients consume medication in a special formulation that allows it to be tracked outside of the body. This technology also includes the use of mobile technology and may be of great use in nonadherent patients. This technology not only allows the patients to track their own administration habits, but it also allows prescribers to track the patient's adherence to medication regimens in order to make changes to the regimen and/or counsel patients on the need to be adherent. This technology has the potential to eliminate the guesswork associated with whether a patient is taking his or her medications.

Digital medicine systems (DMSs) are a newly designed technology that has been developed for the purpose of tracking the ingestion of medication. They provide a more accurate and objective measure for tracking adherence than a patient's self-reporting or pill counting. "DMSs combine the proven safety and efficacy of orally administered medications with the ability to electronically confirm medication ingestion and send feedback to the patient, health care provider, and elected others such as caregivers or family members" [4].

The digital medicine system consists of three integrated components: an ingestible sensor in tablet form, a wearable sensor, and a mobile/cloud-based computing system [4]. See Figure 1 for a visualization of the data flow. The system works by a dose of medication preformulate with the ingestible sensor being placed in a tablet. Once the tablet is ingested and activated in the stomach, the data is transmitted to the wearable sensor. The wearable sensor relays the ingestion to the application on the patient's mobile device, which records the ingestion event on the cloud server. This allows for the information to be accessed by providers.

There are important aspects of this technology that must exist for it to serve as a viable strategy to affect adherence rates:

- Accuracy: The system must be able to accurately track ingestion events (adherence).
- Tablet to Sensor Latency: The system must be able to relay a tablet ingestion to the wearable system in a reasonable amount of time.
- Sensor to Mobile Application/Cloud Server Latency: The system must be able to communicate the data received by the wearable sensor to the mobile device or cloud-based server in a reasonable amount of time.

For a digital medicine system to serve as a worthwhile response to nonadherence, it must ensure that all three of the above-mentioned requirements are met, or it would not warrant the trouble of using such a technology as it would not be cost-effective [4].

The objective of this review is to assess the ability of the DMS to track adherence by examining available data pertaining to its capability to track ingestion events. Like many other new technologies, the DMS comes with a steep price tag. A currently available DMS, the Abilify Mycite®, costs approximately $2000 for a month's supply.

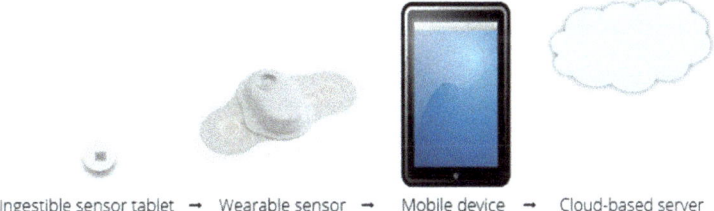

Ingestible sensor tablet → Wearable sensor → Mobile device → Cloud-based server

Figure 1. Digital medicine system data flow.

2. Methods

A systematic literature review and analysis was performed for this study. To identify relevant publications, PubMed and Ovid International Pharmaceutical Abstracts (IPA) were searched for all articles relevant to the study regardless of the publication date. First, a search of PubMed MeSH terms was conducted. The search terms were as follows: Medication Adherence AND (Biosensing Techniques OR Radio Waves OR Radio Frequency Identification Device). Then, a free-text search of PubMed was conducted. The search terms were as follows: Medication adherence AND (Biosensing techniques OR Radio waves OR Radio frequency identification device). Then, the same free-text search was conducted on the Ovid IPA database. The search terms were as follows: Medication adherence AND (Biosensing techniques OR Radio waves OR Radio frequency identification device). Titles and abstracts were assessed for relevance, and full-text reviews were performed on all potentially relevant studies. References from the studies retrieved from the literature searches were assessed for additional applicable articles.

Studies that tracked and reported ingestions using a DMS were included. Studies that did not track and report ingestions of a DMS were not included. As there is not much literature that exists on the subject, studies meeting inclusion criteria were identified and included. Two studies that returned from the search were excluded from this review as they did not track ingestions of a DMS. The extracted data included the clinical setting, purpose, methods, population, accuracy of the digital medicine system in tracking ingestion events, and the latency of the data transmission.

3. Results

The search of the literature produced four total studies that met the criteria for inclusion and two that did not meet the inclusion criteria. In the four studies that were included, biosensing technology was found to capture 86.3% of ingestions events. When accounting for a transmission issue in one of the studies, 91.3% of tablets formulated with the digital medicine system were captured in the studies. See Table 1 for the study comparisons, including the purpose, methods, population, accuracy, and latency.

Ten participants were included in a study conducted at an emergency department where oxycodone was the medication within the digital medicine system. A pill count was used to verify the fidelity of the system. Of the 110 pills that were taken, 96 ingestion events were recorded by the system (87.3% accuracy) [5]. The 14 missed events were accounted for by two participants, both of whom refused to use the system [5]. Therefore, these 14 missed events were considered as nonadherence by two of the ten participants. It can be inferred that the system would have otherwise detected 100% of the ingestion events. In this study, the system received a 90% acceptance rate from participants [5].

A similar study was conducted in an emergency room that also used oxycodone as the medication within the digital medicine system. Sixteen individuals consented to participate in this study, but only fifteen completed the study. A pill count was also used to verify the fidelity of the system in this study. The digital medicine system recorded 112 ingestion events, while the pill counts suggested 134 total pills ingested (83.6% accuracy) [6]. Similar to the other study, all missed doses were accounted for by two participants who failed to properly use the system [6]. It can similarly be inferred that the detection rate would have been 100% otherwise.

Two sub-studies were conducted as part of a study examining the aripiprazole digital medicine system. These studies not only looked at accuracy but also latency. In the first sub-study, 30 participants were enrolled and completed the study. Participants were taking one of the digital medicine system tablets at four time points. The tablet at the first time point contained aripiprazole, and the tablets at the other three time points contained a placebo. The overall accuracy (overall ingestion detections at the four time points) was 78.3% (94/120 events detected) [4]. However, a post hoc analysis of the information transmission at each stage showed that the wearable sensor had a much higher rate of detection at 98.3% (118/120 events detected) [4]. This implies that somewhere between the transmission from the wearable sensor to the mobile application to the cloud-based server, there was a breakdown that caused the ingestion event not to be recorded at every step. It should be noted that this breakdown was the product of two factors: (1) an early version of the application used in this sub-study did not properly check for a complete data transfer from the wearable sensor to the application, and (2) the protocol for this sub-study did not emphasize to patients the option of a forced data upload from the wearable sensor before the removal of the sensor after each ingestion event [4].

In the other sub-study, 29 individuals enrolled in and completed the study. In this study, the results from the previous sub-study were used to update the software and improve the outcomes. Participants were similarly using the digital medicine systems at four time points. The wearable sensor detected ingestion events between 93.1% and 100% for all four time points [4]. The overall accuracy of detected ingestions was 96.6% (112/116 events detected) [4]. This was consistent with the accuracy reported in the previous study.

The mean latency time from the actual ingestion events to signal detection by the wearable sensor at the four time points was between 1.1 and 1.3 min. Seventy-seven point six percent (77.6%) of ingestions (90/116 ingestion events) were detected between 1 and 3 min, with 16.4% (19/116) of ingestions detected in less than 1 min [4]. The mean latency time from the wearable sensor detection of an ingestion event to the cloud-based server detection of that same ingestion event at the four time points was between 6.2 and 10.3 min [4]. "50% of transmissions from the wearable sensor to the server were completed in less than 2 min, and approximately 90% (105/116) of all ingestion events were registered by the mobile application within 30 min from ingestion." [4]. In both sub-studies, the mean times of latency between the sensor ingestion and detection by the wearable sensor were 1.1 and 5.1 min for sensors in the placebo and aripiprazole tablets, respectively [3].

Overall, 86.3% (414/418) of ingestion events were detected in all studies. This rate is increased to 91.3% if adjusted for the detections with incomplete transmissions recorded in the first sub-study of the aripiprazole trials.

Table 1. Biosensing Study Comparisons.

	Digital Pills to Measure Opioid Ingestion Patterns in Emergency Dept. Patients with Acute Fracture Pain: A Pilot Study [6]	Oxycodone Ingestion Patterns in Acute Fracture Pain with Digital Pills [5]	Developing a Digital Medicine System in Psychiatry: Ingestion Detection Rate and Latency Period, Substudy A [3]	Developing a Digital Medicine System in Psychiatry: Ingestion Detection Rate and Latency Period, Substudy B [4]
Study				
Purpose	Determine feasibility of a digital medication system (DMS); patients needing as-needed pain medication after fractures	Measure as-needed pain medication utilization after acute fractures	Measure accuracy and latency of detections by a DMS	Measure accuracy and latency of detections by a DMS
Methods	Patients received a DMS containing oxycodone; use was tracked for one week	Patients received a DMS containing oxycodone; use was tracked for one week	Patients received a DMS containing aripiprazole/placebo; detection and latency were measured	Patients received a DMS containing aripiprazole/placebo; detection and latency were measured
Population	10 participants	15 participants	30 participants	29 participants
Accuracy	96/110 (87.3%) ingestion events detected	112/134 (83.6%) ingestion events detected	94/120 (78.3%) ingestion events detected	112/116 (96.6%) ingestion events detected
Latency	Not tracked	Not tracked	Mean latency time of 1.1 (placebo) minutes and 5.1 (aripiprazole) minutes by wearable sensor [118/120 ingestions detected by wearable sensor]	

4. Discussion

The digital medicine system is a new and exciting technology that might serve as a method to help improve therapeutic outcomes by improving adherence. Biosensing technology gives both prescribers and patients the ability to accurately determine the level of adherence to a specific medication regimen. It has shown accuracy in detecting ingestion events in two different drug classes where adherences to a medication regimen are pivotal in order to reach positive therapeutic outcomes. In opioids, where monitoring a patient's medication usage could be vital to pain control and avoiding overuse, it has proven to be a viable option in accurately detecting adherence. Likewise, in the antipsychotic drug class where a near-perfect adherence is necessary in order to remain effectively treated but where 40–50% of patients being treated for serious mental illnesses are estimated to be nonadherent, the digital medicine system has been demonstrated to be an option for providers to be able to ensure that their patients are sticking to their treatment plans [4].

It is suggested that an adherence rate of at least 80% is generally necessary to reach desired therapeutic outcomes [2]. In all the studies reviewed, more than 80% of ingestions were detected. Many of the failed detections were a result of a user error, and it could be inferred that if not for the user error the digital medicine system would have detected more than 90% of all ingestions in each of the studies reviewed. Despite this fact, ingestions were detected at an overall rate of 91.3%. Therefore, the DMS consistently demonstrated the ability to track adherence rates that were congruent with positive outcomes in therapy.

In the two sub-studies examining the aripiprazole DMS, the mean latency times were reported at 1.1 and 5.1 min [3]. This demonstrated that biosensing technology not only provided a consistent accuracy needed to track adherence but also provided a short latency time that allowed the technology to be viable as a means of tracking adherence. However, further studies evaluating the latency times of digital medication systems are necessary in the future in order to prove consistently short latency times with the use of digital medication systems.

While the accuracy and latency of the biosensing technology would make a digital medicine system favorable (if not preferable) in the setting of treating patients with non-adherence issues or prescribing drugs that require consistent administration, there still remains the issue of cost. Because this is a fairly new technology, it is not marketed for many drugs, and it is likely to be expensive. The Abilify Mycite® (aripiprazole DMS) tablet is approximately $66 per DMS (about $2000 per month). It is unlikely that insurances would cover it and even more unlikely that patients would be willing to pay for it out-of-pocket. Thus, while this technology has brought medication monitoring a long way in its ability to accurately and promptly detect adherence, it still has a long way to go before the population at large will have access to it.

In a recent study [7], the ethical nature of the DMS has been questioned and is still a concern that should be considered before making a tablet containing a sensor a common practice in healthcare. Another consideration is whether or not a technology that relies on a patch is optimal for tracking adherence. Patches tend toward user errors and therefore could render the DMS less reliable.

Another study [8] calls into question whether or not enough rigorous evidence is available to justify the use of the DMS. The authors' primary concern is the use of this new delivery system as a means to repackage and extend the life cycle of a drug nearing the end of its patent-protected exclusivity without any noticeable improvement in outcomes.

The studies included in this review were appropriate as they all used a DMS and reported on actual ingestions. This limitation of this review is the apparent lack of available studies conducted using the DMS technology, which may not provide a great deal of evidence for the mainstream applicability of this technology.

5. Conclusions

The advent of the digital medication system utilizing biosensing technology can have a significant impact on monitoring and tracking adherence, especially in certain at-risk medication classes. It has shown both a good accuracy and acceptable latency in the detection of actual ingestions in patients administering medications that require close monitoring (opioids and antipsychotics). If properly used, this technology can be helpful in the monitoring of other high-risk medication classes (anticoagulants, antiretrovirals, etc.). Limited data exist on latency times, and while more research needs to be completed relating to the overall viability of this technology, it currently appears to be a promising advancement in the healthcare system to help tackle the issue of medication nonadherence.

The lack of existing data on the ability of the DMS to track adherence is likely a sign of the need for more studies before the technology is used more commonly. This lack of data could also be a sign of a couple of obstacles to the commonplace use of the technology: the cost and necessity (cost vs. benefit). Increasing cost to the healthcare system might not be worth the ability to more closely monitor adherence when there is always the option to count pills as was done in the past.

Author Contributions: Conceptualization, C.K.D.; methodology, C.K.D.; software, C.K.D. and E.A.S.; validation, C.K.D.; formal analysis, C.K.D.; investigation, C.K.D.; resources, E.A.S.; data curation, C.K.D.; writing—original draft preparation, C.K.D.; writing—review and editing, E.A.S.; visualization, C.K.D. and E.A.S.; supervision, E.A.S.; project administration, C.K.D.; funding acquisition, not applicable. All authors have read and agreed to the published version of the manuscript.

Funding: This research received no external funding.

Institutional Review Board Statement: Not applicable.

Informed Consent Statement: Not applicable.

Data Availability Statement: Not applicable.

Conflicts of Interest: The authors declare no conflict of interest.

References

1. Sabaté, E. *Adherence to Long-Term Therapies: Evidence for Action*; World Health Organization: Geneva, Switzerland, 2003. Available online: https://apps.who.int/iris/handle/10665/42682 (accessed on 10 September 2021).
2. Kim, J.; Combs, K.; Downs, J.; Tillman, F., III. Medication Adherence: The Elephant in the Room. *US Pharm.* **2018**, *43*, 30–34. Available online: https://www.uspharmacist.com/article/medication-adherence-the-elephant-in-the-room (accessed on 13 August 2021).
3. Rohatagi, S.; Profit, D.; Hatch, A.; Zhao, C.; Docherty, J.P.; Peters-Strickland, T.S. Optimization of a Digital Medicine System in Psychiatry. *J. Clin. Psychiatry* **2016**, *77*, e1101–e1107. [CrossRef] [PubMed]
4. Profit, D.; Rohatagi, S.; Zhao, C.; Hatch, A.; Docherty, J.P.; Peters-Strickland, T.S. Developing a Digital Medicine System in Psychiatry: Ingestion Detection Rate and Latency Period. *J. Clin. Psychiatry* **2016**, *77*, e1095–e1100. [CrossRef] [PubMed]
5. Chai, P.R.; Carreiro, S.; Innes, B.J.; Rosen, R.K.; O'Cleirigh, C.; Mayer, K.H.; Boyer, E.W. Digital Pills to Measure Opioid Ingestion Patterns in Emergency Department Patients with Acute Fracture Pain: A Pilot Study. *J. Med. Internet Res.* **2017**, *19*, e19. [CrossRef] [PubMed]
6. Chai, P.R.; Carreiro, S.; Innes, B.J.; Chapman, B.; Schreiber, K.L.; Edwards, R.R.; Carrico, A.W.; Boyer, E.W. Oxycodone Ingestion Patterns in Acute Fracture Pain with Digital Pills. *Anesthesia Analg.* **2017**, *125*, 2105–2112. [CrossRef] [PubMed]
7. Martani, A.; Geneviève, L.D.; Poppe, C.; Casonato, C.; Wangmo, T. Digital Pills: A Scoping Review of the Empirical Literature and Analysis of the Ethical Aspects. *BMC Med. Ethics.* **2020**, *21*, 3–13. [CrossRef] [PubMed]
8. Egilman, A.C.; Ross, J.S. Digital Medicine Systems: An Evergreening Strategy or an Advance in Medication Management? *BMJ Evid.-Based Med.* **2019**, *24*, 203–204. [CrossRef] [PubMed]

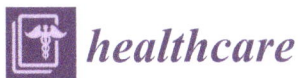

Review

Clinical and Humanistic Outcomes of Community Pharmacy-Based Healthcare Interventions Regarding Medication Use in Older Adults: A Systematic Review and Meta-Analysis

Christina Malini Christopher [1], Bhuvan KC [1,*], Ali Blebil [1], Deepa Alex [2], Mohamed Izham Mohamed Ibrahim [3], Norhasimah Ismail [4] and Alian A. Alrasheedy [5,*]

1. School of Pharmacy, Monash University Malaysia, Subang Jaya 47500, Malaysia; christina.christopher@monash.edu (C.M.C.); aliblebil@yahoo.com (A.B.)
2. Jeffrey Cheah School of Medicine and Health Sciences, Monash University Malaysia, Subang Jaya 47500, Malaysia; deepa.alex@monash.edu
3. Clinical Pharmacy and Practice Department, College of Pharmacy, QU Health Qatar University, Doha 2713, Qatar; mohamedizham@qu.edu.qa
4. Bayan Lepas Health Clinic, Bayan Lepas 11900, Malaysia; asmak4468@gmail.com
5. Department of Pharmacy Practice, College of Pharmacy, Qassim University, Buraidah 51452, Saudi Arabia
* Correspondence: bhuvan.kc@monash.edu (B.K.); aarshiedy@qu.edu.sa (A.A.A.)

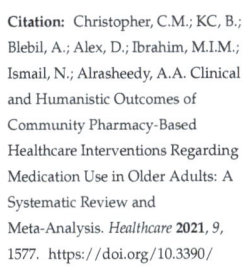

Citation: Christopher, C.M.; KC, B.; Blebil, A.; Alex, D.; Ibrahim, M.I.M.; Ismail, N.; Alrasheedy, A.A. Clinical and Humanistic Outcomes of Community Pharmacy-Based Healthcare Interventions Regarding Medication Use in Older Adults: A Systematic Review and Meta-Analysis. *Healthcare* 2021, 9, 1577. https://doi.org/10.3390/healthcare9111577

Academic Editor: Georges Adunlin

Received: 18 September 2021
Accepted: 15 November 2021
Published: 18 November 2021

Publisher's Note: MDPI stays neutral with regard to jurisdictional claims in published maps and institutional affiliations.

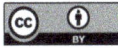

Copyright: © 2021 by the authors. Licensee MDPI, Basel, Switzerland. This article is an open access article distributed under the terms and conditions of the Creative Commons Attribution (CC BY) license (https://creativecommons.org/licenses/by/4.0/).

Abstract: This review and meta-analysis aimed to determine the clinical and humanistic outcomes of community pharmacy-based interventions on medication-related problems of older adults at the primary care level. We identified randomized controlled trials (RCTs) examining the impact of various community pharmacy-based interventions from five electronic databases (namely, MEDLINE (Ovid), EMBASE (Ovid), CINAHL, APA PSYInfo, and Scopus) from January 2010 to December 2020. Consequently, we assessed these interventions' clinical and humanistic outcomes on older adults and compared them with non-intervention. We included 13 RCTs in the current review and completed a meta-analysis with six of them. The included studies had a total of 6173 older adults. Quantitative analysis showed that patient education was significantly associated with an increase in the discontinuation of sedative–hypnotics use (risk ratio 1.28; 95% CI (1.20, 1.36) I2 = 0%, $p < 0.00001$). Moreover, the qualitative analysis showed that medication reviews and education with follow-ups could improve various clinical outcomes, including reducing adverse drug events, reducing uncontrolled health outcomes, and improving appropriate medication use among the elderly population. However, medication review could not significantly reduce the number of older adults who fall (risk ratio 1.25; 95% CI (0.78, 1.99) I2 = 0%, $p = 0.36$) and require hospitalization (risk ratio 0.72; 95% CI (0.47, 1.12) I2 = 45%, $p = 0.15$). This study showed that community pharmacy-based interventions could help discontinue inappropriate prescription medications among older adults and could improve several clinical and humanistic outcomes. However, more effective community pharmacy-based interventions should be implemented, and more research is needed to provide further evidence for clinical and humanistic outcomes of such interventions on older adults.

Keywords: community pharmacy; intervention; older adults; outcomes; systematic review

1. Introduction

There is an ever-increasing need for healthcare services for older adults because of the increase in the aging population. The population of older adults (65 and above) was estimated to be 8.5% of the total population (i.e., 617.1 million) in 2015 and is expected to reach 12% in 2050 (i.e., 1 billion) [1]. The prevalence of multiple chronic illnesses that require comprehensive and complex care is higher in this population. Accordingly, older adults consume a high proportion of prescription medicines and over-the-counter (OTC) medicines and take multiple medicines to manage their chronic illnesses [2–4]. Health-related problems arise when older adults do not take medicines as prescribed, self-consume medicines, or consume the wrong medicines for various reasons [5].

Medication-use problems of older adults are complex and multifaceted and cause an enormous public health, social, and financial burden to the economy [6,7]. Medication usage problems of older adults can affect the optimal therapeutic outcomes and cause adverse drug events and serious harm. The problems related to medication usage in older adults happen at both secondary/tertiary and primary care levels. In the hospital setting, the involvement of multiple healthcare professionals, via a collaborative care model, and the focus on medication safety can help identify and minimize medication-related problems of older adults. In contrast, in primary care settings, the approach of healthcare delivery mostly focuses on preventing illness and promoting health [8]. In general, the primary care level lacks a geriatric-focused care delivery that can identify complex healthcare and medication usage need of older adults and support them adequately.

Medication usage for the older adults at the primary care level is coordinated via general practitioners (both private and government primary health clinics), community nurses, and community pharmacists. Furthermore, the transition of care for older adults happens from secondary and tertiary healthcare to primary healthcare facilities [9]. Consequently, community pharmacies are a pivotal junction in this entire paradigm, responsible for delivering medications and ensuring appropriate use of medications among older adults.

Several studies have examined the problems of medication use of older adults and the potential for community pharmacists to contribute to appropriate medication use at the primary care level. Studies have reported a post-discharge medication review by community pharmacists and its impact on the aging population [10–12]. A study by Kayyali et al. [13] in the UK has reported problems among older adults such as difficulty in medication administration (40%), lack of monitoring of patients with diabetes, and risk of falling (14.3%). Another study by Foubert et al. [14] conducted among community-dwelling older adults (patients) with polypharmacy and those receiving home health care with medication schemes' altercation (review) by community pharmacists showed that pharmacists' interventions enabled more complete and accurate medication schemes. Several reviews have highlighted the improvement in medication adherence among older adults following an intervention by community pharmacists [15–17]. Apart from medication adherence, there was improved quality of life and reduced drug-related problems from these reviews.

Overall, several studies have reported improved health outcomes from various pharmacists' interventions on older adults' medication use [18,19]. Some of these interventions were delivered by pharmacists during the transition of care as a collaborative care model with community pharmacists, while some are delivered solely via community pharmacy-based interventions. A systematic review by Cooper et al. [20] regarding pharmacists' interventions to improve appropriate use of polypharmacy among older adults did not find significant clinical improvements. However, the systematic review evaluated pharmacists' interventions from both primary and secondary care settings. Likewise, another systematic review by Clyne et al. [21] on pharmacists' interventions to address potentially inappropriate prescribing in community-dwelling older adults reported that such interventions were beneficial in reducing potentially inappropriate prescribing but with modest effect size. This systematic review included pharmacist's intervention from different settings, not just the community pharmacy [21]. Thus, from a health system perspective, there is still a need for studies that thoroughly evaluate community pharmacy-based services' impact with an exclusive focus on older adults' medication usage problems and relevant clinical and humanistic outcomes. Therefore, this systematic review and meta-analysis aimed to determine the clinical and humanistic outcomes of community pharmacy-based interventions for older adults to solve their medication usage problems. We believe this review will provide evidence for creating and funding a community pharmacy-based appropriate medicine usage support program for older adults.

2. Materials and Methods

The study protocol has been registered at PROSPERO 2021 CRD42021229948 and was developed based on the Cochrane Handbook for Systematic Reviews of Interventions and the Preferred Reporting Items for Systematic Reviews and Meta-Analyses (PRISMA) guidelines [22].

2.1. Eligibility Criteria

Studies which specifically included population of older adults aged 65 years and above were eligible for the review. Moreover, community pharmacy-based interventions were the main inclusion criteria. Comparator or control was based on non-intervention or not receiving community pharmacy-based services. The outcome was based on interventions regarding medication use among older adults. Study designs of included studies were randomized controlled studies. The exclusion criteria were studies published in a language other than in English and before the year 2010, studies that are not randomized controlled studies, and studies that are not community pharmacy-based interventions.

2.2. Search Strategy

The electronic search was performed in MEDLINE (Ovid), Ovid EMBASE, CINAHL, APA PSY Info, and Scopus. The search was for original articles describing community pharmacy-based interventions for older adults regarding medication use from January 2010 to December 2020. (Refer supplementary material, Table S1). The search process was taken in three steps. The initial search was completed using Scopus and Medline to explore the literature and become more familiar with the terms and current studies—including analyzing each word/term in the titles and abstracts and identifying index terms in each article. After that, in the second step, a comprehensive search was completed by using all index terms and identifying key terms by using the selected databases. In the third step, references of key articles were searched for additional studies. Studies were restricted to the English language. In addition, grey literature was explored to find any potential studies relevant to the study objectives and eligibility criteria. The entire actual search is available in Table S1.

2.3. Study Selection

Two reviewers (C.M.C. and B.K.C.) screened and reviewed the titles and abstracts of identified studies using the search strategy and those from additional sources (i.e., references of retrieved articles, grey literature, and websites from professional pharmacy societies such as Malaysian Pharmaceutical society) to identify studies that meet the inclusion criteria mentioned earlier. Full-text articles were also screened in the same manner. Any disagreements were resolved by consensus through another reviewer (A.B.). Interventions were included if they were community pharmacy-based, and the study design was a randomized controlled trial. Consequently, other studies not meeting these criteria were excluded, including review articles and conference abstracts.

2.4. Data Extraction

The first author (C.M.C.) extracted data using a standardized form and was checked by the second author (B.K.C.). Data extracted included publication details (author, year of publication, and journal name); study design characteristics (study design, sample size, objectives, country); study characteristics (type of intervention, method of intervention, and outcome of intervention); and the main results of the study.

2.5. Risk of Bias (Quality Assessment)

Two authors (C.M.C and B.K.C.) independently assessed the risk of bias using Cochrane Risk of Bias (ROB 2.0) for randomized controlled trials, which is a revised Cochrane tool [23]. The main domains where bias could arise and judgment of risk of bias needed to be completed include randomization process, deviation from intended interventions, missing outcome data, measurement of outcome, and the selection of reported results. Consequently, based on the risk-of-bias judgment of each domain in the clinical trial, the overall risk of bias can be judged as low risk of bias, some concerns, or high risk of bias. During the judgment of risk of bias, if there were any discrepancies, both reviewers discussed and resolved them. Moreover, we used the GRADE criteria to assess the quality of evidence for each outcome reported [24].

2.6. Data Analysis

Studies were eligible for the meta-analysis if at least two outcomes were comparable. Cochrane handbook was used as a guide to analyzing our data [25]. Statistical heterogeneity was assessed using the I^2 statistic, one of the statistical tools to be present in the meta-analysis study [26]. Heterogeneity was defined as high if $I^2 > 75\%$ and low if $I^2 < 25\%$ [27]. We used a random-effect model in our meta-analysis, assuming that heterogeneity exists within the samples. Results were presented with a risk ratio for the dichotomous variable with a confidence interval of 95%. As a priori, we performed subgroup analyses by the duration of follow-up to review the number of older adults hospitalized. All analyses were performed using Cochrane Review Manager version 5.4. (The Nordic Cochrane Centre, Copenhagen, Denmark).

3. Results

A total of 6917 articles were identified through the selected databases. Another nine articles were retrieved from other sources such as Google Scholar for grey literature, manual search in the key references retrieved, and other websites particularly the Ministry of Health Malaysia and the Malaysian Pharmaceutical Society website. After removing duplications ($n = 1337$), a total of 5589 articles were identified for the title and abstract screening, and 108 articles were included for further review by accessing the full texts and assessing them against the inclusion criteria. Most full texts were excluded because of a non-randomized controlled study design ($n = 49$) and non-community pharmacy-based intervention ($n = 17$). Consequently, 13 randomized controlled trials (RCT) were included in this systematic review. Reasons for the exclusion of full texts and the flow of studies are described in Figure 1. In this review, the inter-rater reliability for the final extraction between two reviewers was 0.918.

3.1. Characteristics of Included Studies

Among the 13 randomized controlled trials, 7 were cluster randomized control trials, 1 was a double-blind RCT, 1 was a single-blind RCT, 3 were RCTs, and 1 was a pilot RCT, as summarized in Table 1. Trials were carried out in Croatia (two studies), the Netherlands (two studies), the USA (two studies), Canada (two studies), Spain (two studies), New Zealand (one study), Denmark (one study), and Finland (one study) The interventions were conducted by community pharmacists either in a community pharmacy or at patient's home or medical center clinics or home care unit. The included studies had a total of 6173 older adults with a sample size ranging from 39 to 715 participants. In terms of the type of interventions provided, most of the community pharmacy-based interventions were medication review ($n = 7$), education ($n = 4$), pharmaceutical care ($n = 1$), and electronic device reminder ($n = 1$). In terms of the type of measured outcomes, there were various outcomes reported by studies. Some studies reported the impact on hospitalization ($n = 4$), number of potentially inappropriate medicines (PIM) ($n = 3$), rate of sedative–hypnotics use ($n = 2$), time in warfarin therapeutic range ($n = 1$), quality of life ($n = 1$), medication appropriateness ($n = 1$), drug burden ($n = 1$), rate of discontinuing fall-risk inducing drug ($n = 1$), number of adverse drug events ($n = 2$), mortality ($n = 1$), medication adherence ($n = 2$), and uncontrolled health problems ($n = 1$). The details are presented in Table 1.

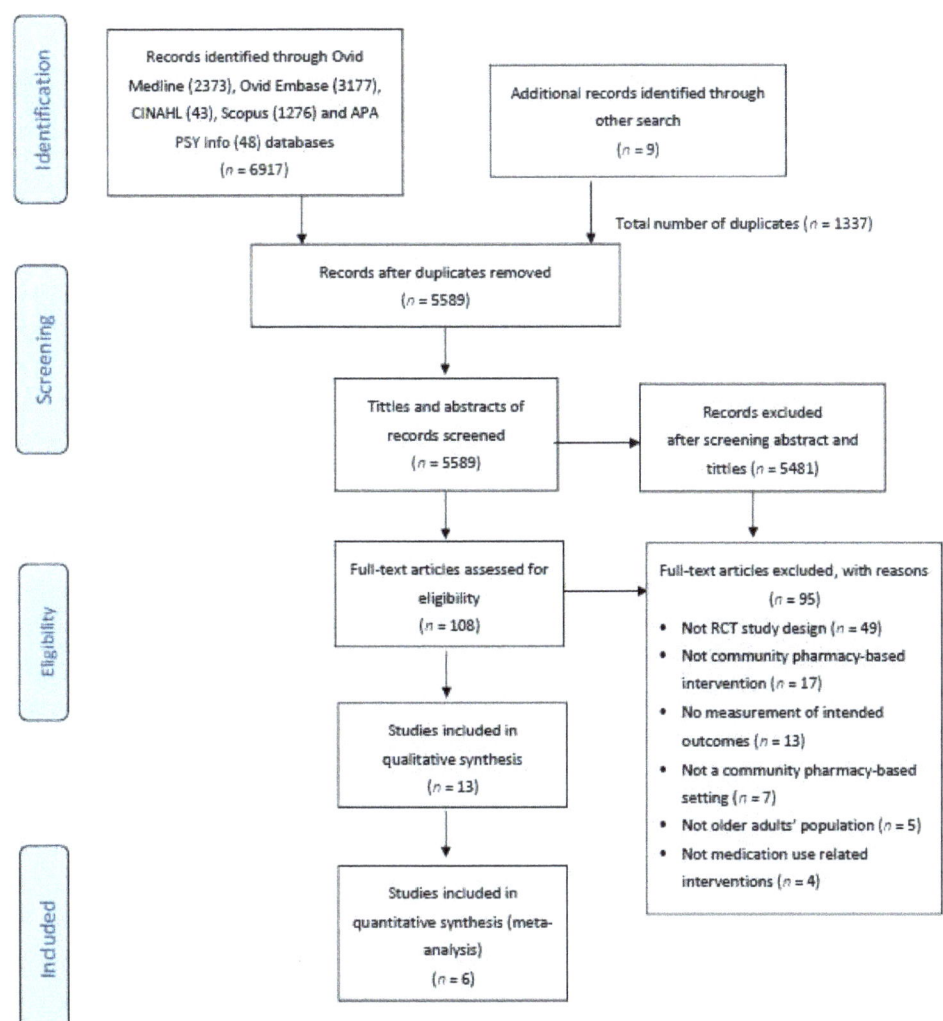

Figure 1. PRISMA flowchart of the selection process.

Table 1. Characteristics of included studies.

Author, Year, Country	Study Design, Settings	Interventions	Control Sample Size	Intervention Sample Size	Follow-Up Period	Outcomes	Conclusion
Bryant et al. [28] (2010) New Zealand	Randomized, controlled trial, Community pharmacy	IG: Medication review was completed with the access of medical records from GP. A care plan was prepared, and discussions were completed among CP and GP. Follow-up consultations with patients were completed after taking action on the care plan. CG: Usual care	143	207	6 months and 12 months	Quality of Life (SF-36) and Medication Inappropriateness Index (MAI), number of inappropriate medications	Medication review improved MAI and reduced the number of potentially inappropriate medicines at 6 months follow-up. However, this intervention did not produce a significant improvement in quality of life.
Falamic et al. [29] (2019) Croatia	Randomized, controlled trial, Community pharmacy	IG: Education with follow-up plan (given pillbox and plan form) CG: Standard GP-managed care	66	65	6 months	The incidence and type of adverse drug reactions caused by warfarin	The cumulative incidence of adverse drug reactions was significantly lower in the intervention group.
Mott et al. [30] (2016) United States	Cluster-randomized, controlled trial, Community pharmacy	IG: Medication therapy management with follow-up CG: Received mailed pamphlet describing medication use and falls	41	39	6 months	Rate of discontinuing the fall-risk inducing drug	Medication review significantly improved the rate of discontinuation of fall-risk-inducing drugs among older adults and reduced the number of falls.
Touchette et al. [31] (2012) United States	Randomized, controlled trial, Academic medical center, community pharmacies, and family medicine clinics	IG: Medication therapy management (MTM) with follow-up (enhanced MTM) CG: Usual care	208	Basic MTM = 211 Enhanced MTM = 218	6 months	Frequency of adverse drug events and hospitalization	Medication review did not have a beneficial impact on adverse drug events and hospitalization.

Table 1. *Cont.*

Author, Year, Country	Study Design, Settings	Interventions	Control Sample Size	Intervention Sample Size	Follow-Up Period	Outcomes	Conclusion
Varas–Doval et al. [32] (2020) Spain	Open-label, multi-center, cluster-randomized, controlled trial, Community pharmacy	IG: Medication review with follow-up CG: Usual care	715	688	6 months	Uncontrolled health problems	Medication review benefited, with a significant reduction in the number of uncontrolled health problems.
Olesen et al. [33] (2014) Denmark	Cluster-randomized, controlled trial, Patient's home	IG: Pharmaceutical care (examining medication list of older adults, answering any questions on their medications, providing leaflets and motivational adherence support) CG: Usual care	264	253	3, 6, 9, and 24 months	Medication adherence, hospitalization, and mortality	Pharmaceutical care did not bring a beneficial impact on medication adherence, hospitalization, and mortality among older adults.
Toivo et al. [34] (2019) Finland	Cluster-randomized, controlled trial, Community pharmacy, homecare units, public health care center	IG: Collaborative coordination of care (medication review and triage meeting) CG: Standard home care	87	104	12 months	Potentially inappropriate medication	No significant findings were found on the impact of coordination of care on outcomes of older adults' health.
Malet-Larrea et al. [35] (2016) Spain	Cluster-randomized, controlled trial, Community pharmacy	IG: Medication review with follow-up CG: Usual care	715	688	6 months	Hospitalization	The probability of being hospitalized was 3.7 times higher in the non-intervention group. Thus, medication review had reduced the number of older adults hospitalized.

Table 1. *Cont.*

Author, Year, Country	Study Design, Settings	Interventions	Control Sample Size	Intervention Sample Size	Follow-Up Period	Outcomes	Conclusion
Tannenbaum et al. [36] (2014) Canada	Cluster-randomized, controlled trial. Community pharmacy	IG: Patient education (materials which also contained benzodiazepine safety and tapering dose) CG: Usual care	155	148	6 months	Benzodiazepine therapy discontinuation	Patient education improved the benzodiazepine discontinuation rate among older adults.
Van Der Meer et al. [37] (2018) Netherlands	Single-blind, randomized, controlled trial, Community pharmacy	IG: Medication review with follow-up CG: Usual care	82	75	3 months	Drug burden index, hospitalization	Medication review did not have significant effects on the number of falls and hospitalization. Moreover, it did not produce an impact on the difference in drug burden index between groups.
Martin et al. [38] (2018) Canada	Cluster-randomized, controlled trial, Community pharmacy	IG: Patient education (education materials were distributed), and education materials were given to prescribers CG: Usual care	241	248	6 months	Sedative-hypnotics (benzodiazepine therapy discontinuation) and potentially inappropriate medication	Patient education reduced the number of benzodiazepine users and reduced the number of inappropriate medications among older adults.
Falamic et al. [39] (2018) Croatia	Prospective, double-blind, randomized, controlled trial, Community pharmacy	IG: Education and follow-up plan with medication review (given a form containing lab values, INR, and pillbox. CG: Usual GP care	66	65	6 months	Time in therapeutic range of warfarin	Patient education improved time in the therapeutic range of warfarin.

3.2. Risk of Bias Assessment

Figure 2 shows the risk of bias of all the included studies in each domain. Overall, four studies were judged to have a low risk of bias, seven studies were judged to have some concerns regarding the level of risk, and two studies had a high risk of bias. Five studies raise some concerns regarding potential biases in the randomization process [28–32]. All studies did not deviate from intended interventions. Only one study reported some concerns regarding biases on missing outcome data [33]. Two studies did not report a measurement of outcome [32,34]. Some studies were judged to have a selection of reporting biases but were judged to have "some concerns" [28–33,35,36].

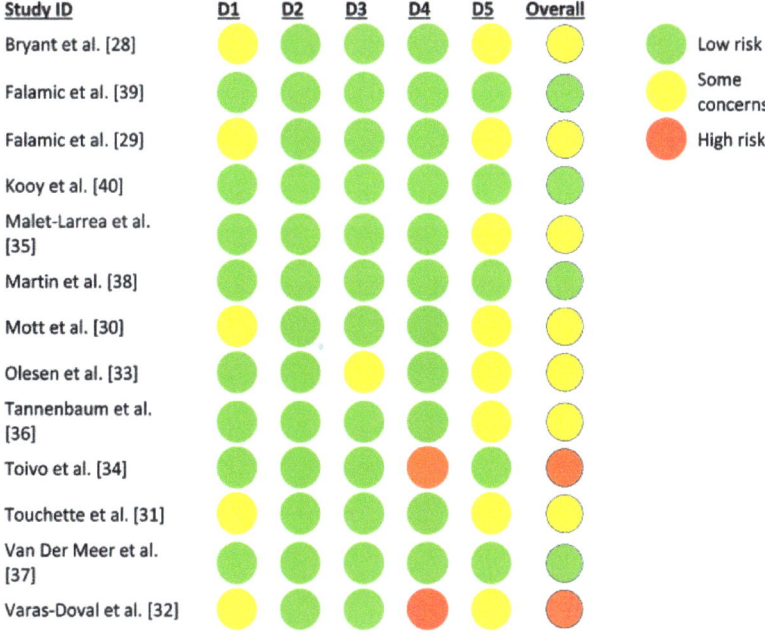

D1	Randomisation process
D2	Deviations from the intended interventions
D3	Missing outcome data
D4	Measurement of the outcome
D5	Selection of the reported result

Figure 2. Risk of bias assessment of included studies.

3.3. Types of Community Pharmacists' Interventions

3.3.1. Medication Review

Most of the studies ($n = 7$) performed medication reviews as their main intervention. Comprehensive medication reviews were initiated by interviewing older adults; screening their medication list, lab values, and complementary medicines; and a pharmacotherapeutic plan was decided [28,30–32,34,35,37]. Then, the plan was discussed with prescribers and patients. Finally, the plan was executed with follow-up monitoring by the community pharmacist [28,30–32,34,35,37]. One study had implemented medication review as their main intervention under the coordination of care with other primary health care providers [34].

The study by Touchette et al. [31] included two groups as interventions: basic medication review care and medication review enhanced care. The difference between both is that the latter group had access to clinical information regarding laboratory values of patients, and the former did not have access to the information. In this review, we included the medication review enhanced care as the intervention since it included a comprehensive review with patient lab findings and usual care as a control group.

3.3.2. Educational Intervention

Four RCTs examined the impact of educational intervention [29,36,38,39]. Under this intervention, two studies included a follow-up plan. Participants were provided with a form containing lab values, INR, and important education points and were given a pillbox [29,39]. Tannenbaum et al. [36] provided patient education materials that also contained a tapering benzodiazepine dose in a separate study. Martin et al. [38] mentioned that their study included education materials, including on tapering benzodiazepine dose, distributed to patients and prescribers provided with basic educational materials.

3.3.3. Pharmaceutical Care

This intervention was undertaken by a community pharmacist initially examining the medication list of older adults, answering any questions on their medications, and providing leaflets and motivational adherence support [33]. Older adults would then be followed up after 3, 6, and 9 months, and any drug-related problems involved consultation with prescribers. This intervention differs from a comprehensive medication review because it includes no pharmacotherapeutic plan to be discussed with the prescribers before dispensing the medications to older adults.

3.3.4. Electronic Reminder Device

Only one study implemented this intervention with brief counseling to assess whether it improved refill adherence and persistence for statin treatment in non-adherent older adults [40].

3.4. The Outcomes of the Interventions

3.4.1. Hospitalization

Three studies specifically examined the impact of medication review on the hospitalization of older adults [31,35,37]. In one of the studies, Touchette et al. [31] reported outcomes based on a shorter follow-up duration of three months and a longer duration of six months. The quantitative analysis showed that these three pooled studies did not show a statistically significant impact of medication review on the probability of hospitalization (risk ratio 0.72; 95% confidence interval (0.47, 1.12) $I^2 = 45\%$, $p = 0.15$) (Figure 3).

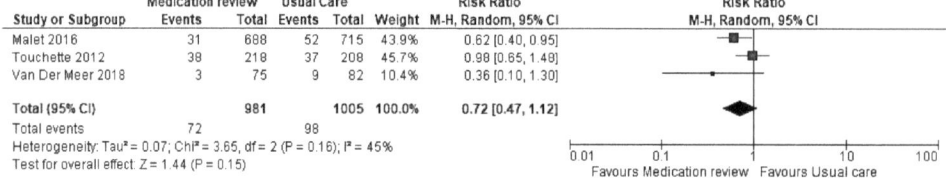

Figure 3. Forest plot showing the risk ratio of older adults hospitalized after medication review.

3.4.2. Sedative–Hypnotics Users

Two studies were using sedative–hypnotics (benzodiazepines) as their outcome assessment drug [36,38]. Both studies were pooled, and patient education was statistically significant for reducing the number of sedative–hypnotic users (risk ratio 1.28; 95% confidence interval (1.20, 1.36) $I^2 = 0\%$, $p < 0.00001$). (Figure 4).

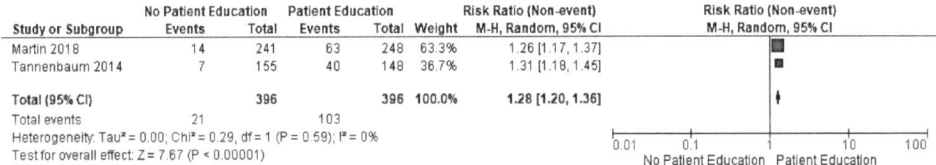

Figure 4. Forest plot showing risk ratio of older adults ceasing benzodiazepine after the patient education intervention.

3.4.3. Number of Older Adults Who Fall

Two studies were pooled to assess the medication review intervention on the number of older adults' falls [30,37]. Both studies were not statistically significant for reducing the number of older adults who fall (risk ratio 1.25; 95% confidence interval (0.78, 1.99) I^2 = 0%, p = 0.36) (Figure 5).

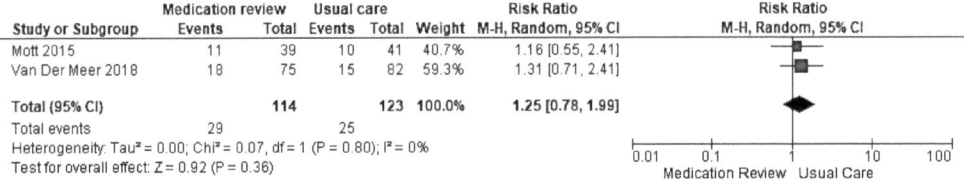

Figure 5. Forest plot showing risk ratio of older adults falls after medication review intervention.

3.4.4. Potentially Inappropriate Medications

Three studies reported the number of potentially inappropriate medicines as the outcome of the intervention. Martin et al. [38] reported that at 6 months, 43% in the intervention group did not have prescriptions for inappropriate medicines compared with only 12% in the control group. Moreover, Bryant et al. [28] reported that the mean number of inappropriate medicines per patient was higher for the intervention group at baseline (2.5) and reduced after 6 months of intervention (2.5 versus 1.6, respectively, p < 0.001) compared to the control group (2.1 versus 2.1, respectively, p = 0.991). Another study by Toivo et al. [34] did not have significant findings based on their intervention on the potentially inappropriate medication. However, the role of pharmacists in this study was part of coordinated care involving other healthcare professionals. The results are summarized in Table 1.

3.4.5. Medication Adherence

One RCT that examined the impact of one type of pharmaceutical care did not report a significant impact on medication adherence as per the study by Olesen et al. [33]. Similarly, with the electronic reminder device intervention, no improvement of refill adherence was found in the older adults" population [40].

3.4.6. Adverse Drug Events

Two studies measured the impact of the interventions in terms of adverse drug events. One study by Falamic et al. [29] highlighted that adverse drug reactions were significantly lower in the group of older adults who were prescribed warfarin and were receiving an educational intervention. The author described that providing patient education on warfarin, pillbox, and a follow-up plan reduced the risk of bleeding as an adverse drug event. Meanwhile, Touchette et al. [31] mentioned no significant impact on adverse drug events after providing medication reviews. However, overall, community-pharmacy-based interventions managed to reduce the number of adverse drug events through patient education.

3.4.7. Other Outcomes

A study by Bryant et al. [28] stated that through medication review, the medication appropriateness index improved, but it did not improve the quality of life in the intervention group. Meanwhile, Mott, Martin [30] described that the intervention group had a significant impact by leading to a higher rate of discontinuing fall-risk-inducing drugs among older adults after medication review completed by the community pharmacist. Another study by Varas–Doval et al. [32] had a significant reduction in the number of uncontrolled health problems after the same intervention. Despite that, Olesen et al. [33] reported no significant improvement in mortality rate after medication adherence was completed. As for educational interventions, Falamic et al. [39] pointed out that it improved warfarin's therapeutic time range in older adults. As a whole, various community pharmacy-based interventions show improvement in clinical outcomes among older adults. However, evidence is lacking regarding patient satisfaction and quality of life in these studies.

3.5. Sensitivity Analysis

Moderate heterogeneity, $I^2 = 45\%$, was found in the outcome of hospitalization. Thus, a one-on-one removal of studies in the meta-analysis was completed by removing a study by Touchette et al. [31] in the hospitalization outcome, and subsequently, no heterogeneity was found. This analysis reported that medication review was significant for reducing hospitalization of older adults (risk ratio 0.59; 95% confidence interval (0.39, 0.88) $I^2 = 0\%$, $p = 0.01$. (Figure 6)

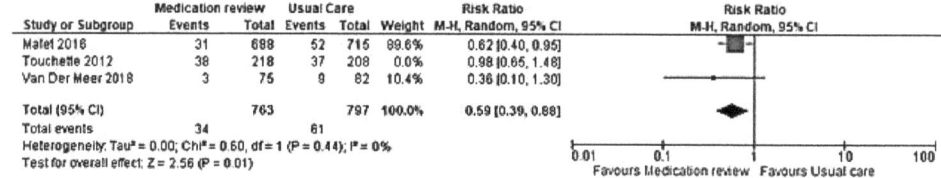

Figure 6. Forest plot of sensitivity analysis showing risk ratio of older adults hospitalized after medication review intervention.

3.6. Subgroup Analysis

Subgroup analysis comparing studies that reported hospitalization after three months and six months medication reviews were completed (Table 2). The effect of the intervention was not statistically significant between the duration of follow-up of subgroups (risk ratio 0.74; 95% confidence interval (0.54, 1.00) $I^2 = 18\%$, $p = 0.05$ (Figure 7).

Table 2. Subgroup analysis according to the duration of follow-up.

Outcome	Number of Studies	Number of Participants	Statistical Method	Effect Size 95% (CI)
Hospitalization	3 [31,35,37]	1986	Risk ratio (M–H, random, 95% CI)	0.74 (0.54,1.00)
3 months	2 [31,35]	583	Risk ratio (M–H, random, 95% CI)	0.62 (0.35,1.11)
6 months	2 [31,37]	190	Risk ratio (M–H, random, 95% CI)	0.78 (0.50,1.23)

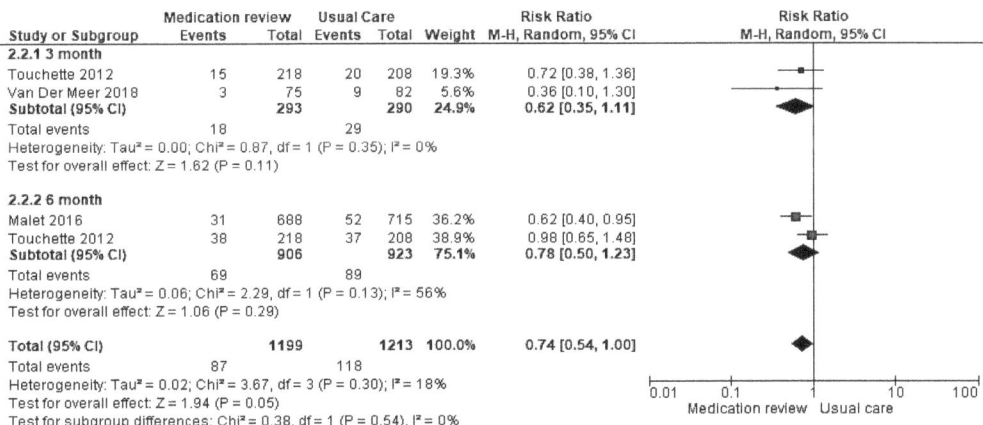

Figure 7. Forest plot showing subgroup analysis of the risk ratio in older adults' hospitalization according to the duration of follow-up after medication review intervention.

3.7. Certainty of Evidence

Based on GRADE criteria, the certainty of the evidence was rated as moderate for the outcome of hospitalization. Outcomes of the number of older adults who fell and ceased benzodiazepine were rated as high-quality based on GRADE criteria.

4. Discussion

To the best of our knowledge, this meta-analysis is probably the first study that focused exclusively on the impact of community pharmacy-based interventions on medication use and related clinical and humanistic outcomes among the older population (i.e., 65 years and over). Previous studies have focused on a particular intervention that was carried out within and outside community pharmacy settings and focused on medications usage problems of both the general population and older adults [41–44]. This review focused on various community pharmacy-based services/interventions for medications usage problems of older adults and its impact based on the best available evidence (i.e., RCTs).

Previous reviews (systematic review and meta-analysis) have focused on various interventions by pharmacists regarding medication usage problems. However, they looked at the outcomes of pharmacists' interventions regarding medication usage problems of both the general population and older adults (i.e., mixed populations) and reviewed interventions that were carried out by pharmacists working in both primary and secondary care settings (i.e., different settings) [45–48]. These reviews focused on all types of community pharmacy-based services, and these were not exclusively focused on any specific sub-group of the population. Thus, so far, only one systematic review by Tasai et al. [16] focused on the medication usage problems of the elderly population; however, it also only looked at the impact of medication review on one service (i.e., polypharmacy) in the elderly population. The current systematic review and meta-analysis are different from other studies and reviews as they critically review all the eligible community pharmacy-based services, focusing on medication usage problems of older adults in particular.

Community pharmacy-based interventions were regarded as one of the most accessible primary services by the older population. Most of the interventions were provided by community pharmacies in collaboration with other healthcare professionals, including physicians, general practitioners, and nurses. As a whole, there is evidence in the literature that community pharmacy-based interventions impacted several clinical outcomes among older adults, including reducing inappropriate medicine use (including that of sedative–hypnotics); reducing uncontrolled health problems; and potentially reducing ADRs. However, evidence was lacking in terms of the impact on patient satisfaction and quality of life. Consequently, given the limited literature for studies focused on the elderly population in the community pharmacy setting (i.e., RCTs), more research is needed in this area.

The current review showed that patient education delivered by community pharmacists increased the number of older adults who benefited from the pharmacists' interventions and discontinued their sedative–hypnotic drugs. For example, we found that patient education improved the cessation of benzodiazepine among older adults. This is in line with a previous review in which education improved the number of older adults who ceased benzodiazepine [49]. However, Reeve, Ong [50], in their review, reported that the rate of benzodiazepine discontinuation was lower with patient education compared with other interventions. However, the differences could be explained by the fact that patient education could be provided in different ways, and hence its impact could be different depending on the type, structure, and nature of the educational intervention. We have noted that the patient education included in our review was thorough and innovative. For example, it was provided together with the visual tapering dose, which is a method of effective intervention leading to the reduced use of benzodiazepine. Brochures on educational materials have also influenced the choices of hypnotic–sedative users. In addition, patient education helps provide knowledge on sedative–hypnotic medication, including its risks and side effects for patients. Consequently, this information provides evidence for supporting this professional service and could be further expanded as part of a collaborative health care model in the primary care setting.

Various community pharmacy-based interventions were identified in this systematic review and meta-analysis. Among various interventions, medication review was the most common intervention carried out by the community pharmacists and was evaluated in RCTs. Varas–Doval et al. [32] reported that medication review with follow-up resulted in a significant reduction in the number of uncontrolled health problems over 6 months in the intervention group compared to no change in the control group. Moreover, it was shown that medication reviews and education by community pharmacists targeting elderly patients resulted in better outcomes in terms of appropriate medication use [28,38]. However, medication reviews by community pharmacists did not reduce the probability of hospitalization among older adults, in contrast with the previous findings of Tasai, Kumpat et al. [16] and Jokanovic et al. [17] on this outcome. However, our findings were on par with several other reviews [51–53]. This is possibly because there are only limited studies with moderate heterogeneity in the literature, which cause a non-significance impact; however, significant findings were noted when sensitivity analysis was completed in our review. In the literature, similar to the hospitalization outcomes, mixed results were reported regarding the impact of medication reviews on the risk of falls. Our current study showed that medication reviews did not reduce the number of older adults falling. Similar to our findings, Hart, Phelan [54], and colleagues pointed out that medication review did not reduce the number of older adults who fall in their review. However, another study by Huiskes et al. [51] indicated that medication review decreased the number of older adults falling. Several factors could explain the differences among the results, including self-reporting. The two studies included in our meta-analysis were based on patient self-reporting findings [30,37]. Thus, the possibility of not accurately revealing the number of older adults who fall is high due to old-aged patients' frail conditions. Moreover, the study by Mott et al. [30] was a pilot study, and the sample size was limited. Thus, this might explain the non-significance results. Consequently, we believe more research is needed to further investigate the impact of community pharmacists' intervention on these outcomes. In addition, more structured and tailored interventions are needed to be established at the community pharmacies to provide quality services to the elderly population.

There was evidence of a reduction in the inappropriate medications in one of the included studies through patient education on other outcomes [38]. Moreover, Falamic et al. [29] provided education with a pillbox, and adverse drug events were significantly reduced among older adults prescribed warfarin. Kallio et al. [15] justified that most studies showed improvement in medication adherence and reduced drug-related problems among older patients after medication review intervention is completed by community pharmacists. Our systematic review shows some evidence of improvement in medication adherence because of community pharmacy-based interventions. However, when it comes to long term impact, such as the effect of community-pharmacy-based interventions on quality of life, we found limited evidence, with one study by Bryant et al. [28] not showing an impact, which is similar to the results from Huiskes et al. [51]. Several recent studies have investigated telephone calls and automated telephonic prompts as a digital tool, and medication adherence was the most included topic in the digital conversation between community pharmacists and patients [55]. However, these studies did not include any specific population, and there were no studies found on social media platforms as a digital tool, especially involving the older adult population.

Overall, our findings revealed that community pharmacy services are beneficial to older adults to optimize proper medication use, reduce unnecessary benzodiazepine use, reduce uncontrolled health problems, and ADRs among older adults. Therefore, evidence-based educational interventions should be encouraged in community pharmacies to achieve rational medication use among older adults visiting community pharmacies and to provide further improvements in their health.

4.1. Strengths and Limitation

The current review has some points of strength. First, we have only considered randomized, controlled trials in our review, and this increased the robustness of the study [56]. Furthermore, we have assessed the outcomes of quantitative analysis through GRADE criteria and only included moderate- and high-quality studies. Heterogeneity across studies was also assessed with sensitivity analysis, and we have reported the homogeneity of studies after removing one study. Our search narrowed to community pharmacy-based interventions, focusing on the older population, which was an added advantage to review older adults' health care outcomes. However, there are several limitations to this review. Firstly, the search articles for this review were restricted to the English language. Thus, we acknowledge that there might be a limitation to the search in non-English native regions. Secondly, the age limit for older adults in this review was 65 years and above. Therefore, we could not have captured studies that included older adults in the range of 60 years and above. Thirdly, our review resulted in various interventions with different features in terms of the duration, nature, and components of the intervention. Lastly, we could not determine the pooled estimates for other outcomes—medication adherence, quality of life, potentially inappropriate medication, and adverse drug events—because of different outcomes with various interventions. In addition, there were limited RCTs on several outcomes of interest such as adherence, quality of life, etc. However, overall, we believe the current review and meta-analysis provided useful data for future guidance to improve the pharmaceutical care services provided to the older population at community pharmacies.

4.2. Implications for Research and Practice

It is well known that community pharmacy is one of the most accessible health care resources and could play a fundamental role in the health care of older adults in a community [16]. However, there are limited RCTs that evaluated the impact of interventions and services in community pharmacies on the health outcomes of populations aged 65 years and over. Consequently, given the rapid surge in the aging population, more future research is needed to implement pharmacists' interventions and evaluate their clinical, humanistic, and economic outcomes among older adults. In addition, more qualitative exploration focusing on older adults' mobility, hearing, etc., and other access problems at community pharmacies should be explored. The role of a community pharmacy in certain lower- and middle-income countries (LMICs) still lacks the recognition as primary health care providers. Many older adults in these regions still access tertiary health care as their first point of care. Therefore, this review will help provide an evidence for the development of community pharmacy-based interventions focused on reducing medication-related problems of older adults in the LMICs. Furthermore, future research should look at the integration of pharmacists in the primary care system so that they can provide long-term support for older adults, focusing on the appropriate use of medicines among older adults. It will ease the rising burden of general practitioners in primary care settings and establish pharmacists' services as an integral element of geriatric-focused primary care service.

5. Conclusions

The current review showed that there are several healthcare interventions conducted by community pharmacists for the elderly population. The most common interventions evaluated by RCTs included medication reviews and educational interventions. Moreover, there is evidence in the literature that community pharmacy-based interventions have a beneficial impact on clinical outcomes among older adults, including a reduction in inappropriate medicine use (e.g., sedative–hypnotic drugs), reduction in uncontrolled health problems, and reduction of ADRs. There is limited or inconclusive evidence on the impact of community pharmacists' interventions on hospitalization, quality of life, and other outcomes from RCTs. Consequently, we believe more research is needed to further investigate the impact of community pharmacists' intervention on these outcomes. In addition, more structured and tailored interventions are needed to be established at community pharmacies to provide quality services to the elderly population in collaboration with other healthcare professionals (i.e., medical practitioners and nurses) and in an integrated manner within the primary care system.

Supplementary Materials: The following are available online at https://www.mdpi.com/article/10.3390/healthcare9111577/s1, Table S1: Search Strategy.

Author Contributions: Conceptualization, C.M.C., B.K. and A.B.; methodology, C.M.C., B.K. and D.A.; validation, A.B. and D.A.; formal analysis, C.M.C. and B.K.; Writing—original draft preparation, C.M.C., B.K., and A.A.A.; writing—review and editing, B.K., A.B., D.A., M.I.M.I., N.I., and A.A.A. supervision, B.K.; project administration, B.K. and A.A.A. All authors have read and agreed to the published version of the manuscript.

Funding: This research received no external funding.

Institutional Review Board Statement: Not applicable.

Informed Consent Statement: Not applicable.

Data Availability Statement: The authors confirm that data supporting the findings of this study are available within the article and its Supplementary Materials.

Acknowledgments: The authors would like to thank Sunil Shrestha for his invaluable contributions in providing inputs on data extraction and assessing the quality of included studies.

Conflicts of Interest: The authors declare no conflict of interest.

References

1. He, W.; Goodkind, D.; Kowal, P.R. *An Aging World, International Population Reports*; U.S. Government Printing Office: Washington, DC, USA, 2015.
2. Amoako, E.P.; Richardson-Campbell, L.; Kennedy-Malone, L. Self-Medication with Over-The-Counter Drugs Among Elderly Adults. *J. Gerontol. Nurs.* **2003**, *29*, 10–15. [CrossRef] [PubMed]
3. Kim, J.; Parish, A.L. Polypharmacy and Medication Management in Older Adults. *Nurs. Clin. N. Am.* **2017**, *52*, 457–468. [CrossRef] [PubMed]
4. Scott, I.A.; Hilmer, S.N.; Reeve, E.; Potter, K.; Le Couteur, D.; Rigby, D.; Gnjidic, D.; Del Mar, C.B.; Roughead, E.E.; Page, A.; et al. Reducing Inappropriate Polypharmacy. *JAMA Intern. Med.* **2015**, *175*, 827–834. [CrossRef]
5. Balbuena, F.R.; Aranda, A.B.; Figueras, A. Self-Medication in Older Urban Mexicans. *Drugs Aging* **2009**, *26*, 51–60. [CrossRef]
6. Chiatti, C.; Bustacchini, S.; Furneri, G.; Mantovani, L.G.; Cristiani, M.; Misuraca, C.; Lattanzio, F. The Economic Burden of Inappropriate Drug Prescribing, Lack of Adherence and Compliance, Adverse Drug Events in Older People. *Drug Saf.* **2012**, *35*, 73–87. [CrossRef]

7. Aparasu, R.R.; Mort, J.R. Prevalence, correlates, and associated outcomes of potentially inappropriate psychotropic use in the community-dwelling elderly. *Am. J. Geriatr. Pharmacother.* **2004**, *2*, 102–111. [CrossRef]
8. Bennett, J.A.; Flaherty-Robb, M.K. Issues affecting the health of older citizens: Meeting the challenge. *Online J. Issues Nurs.* **2003**, *8*, 2.
9. Baillie, L.; Gallini, A.; Corser, R.; Elworthy, G.; Scotcher, A.; Barrand, A. Care transitions for frail, older people from acute hospital wards within an integrated healthcare system in England: A qualitative case study. *Int. J. Integr. Care* **2014**, *14*, e009. [CrossRef]
10. Ramsbottom, H.; Rutter, P.; Fitzpatrick, R. Post discharge medicines use review (dMUR) service for older patients: Cost-savings from community pharmacist interventions. *Res. Soc. Adm. Pharm.* **2018**, *14*, 203–206. [CrossRef] [PubMed]
11. Ramsbottom, H.F.; Fitzpatrick, R.; Rutter, P. Post discharge medicines use review service for older patients: Recruitment issues in a feasibility study. *Int. J. Clin. Pharm.* **2016**, *38*, 208–212. [CrossRef] [PubMed]
12. Rutter, P.; Ramsbottom, H.; Fitzpatrick, R. Community pharmacist perceptions of delivering post-hospital discharge Medicines Use Reviews for elderly patients. *Int. J. Clin. Pharm.* **2017**, *39*, 33–36. [CrossRef] [PubMed]
13. Kayyali, R.; Funnell, G.; Harrap, N.; Patel, A. Can community pharmacy successfully bridge the gap in care for housebound patients? *Res. Soc. Adm. Pharm.* **2019**, *15*, 425–439. [CrossRef]
14. Foubert, K.; Mehuys, E.; Claes, L.; Abeele, D.V.D.; Haems, M.; Somers, A.; Petrovic, M.; Boussery, K. A shared medication scheme for community dwelling older patients with polypharmacy receiving home health care: Role of the community pharmacist. *Acta Clin. Belg.* **2018**, *74*, 326–333. [CrossRef]
15. Kallio, S.E.; Kiiski, A.; Airaksinen, M.S.; Mäntylä, A.T.; Kumpusalo-Vauhkonen, A.E.; Järvensivu, T.P.; Pohjanoksa-Mäntylä, M.K. Community Pharmacists' Contribution to Medication Reviews for Older Adults: A Systematic Review. *J. Am. Geriatr. Soc.* **2018**, *66*, 1613–1620. [CrossRef]
16. Tasai, S.; Kumpat, N.; Dilokthornsakul, P.; Chaiyakunapruk, N.; Saini, B.; Dhippayom, T. Impact of Medication Reviews Delivered by Community Pharmacist to Elderly Patients on Polypharmacy: A Meta-analysis of Randomized Controlled Trials. *J. Patient Saf.* **2021**, *17*, 290–298. [CrossRef]
17. Jokanovic, N.; Tan, E.; Sudhakaran, S.; Kirkpatrick, C.; Dooley, M.J.; Ryan-Atwood, T.E.; Bell, J.S. Pharmacist-led medication review in community settings: An overview of systematic reviews. *Res. Soc. Adm. Pharm.* **2017**, *13*, 661–685. [CrossRef] [PubMed]
18. Banning, M. A review of interventions used to improve adherence to medication in older people. *Int. J. Nurs. Stud.* **2009**, *46*, 1505–1515. [CrossRef]
19. Loganathan, M.; Singh, S.; Franklin, B.D.; Bottle, A.; Majeed, A. Interventions to optimise prescribing in care homes: Systematic review. *Age Ageing* **2011**, *40*, 150–162. [CrossRef]
20. Cooper, J.A.; Cadogan, C.A.; Patterson, S.M.; Kerse, N.; Bradley, M.C.; Ryan, C.; Hughes, C.M. Interventions to improve the appropriate use of polypharmacy in older people: A Cochrane systematic review. *BMJ Open* **2015**, *5*, e009235. [CrossRef]
21. Clyne, B.; Fitzgerald, C.; Quinlan, A.; Hardy, C.; Galvin, R.; Fahey, T.; Smith, S. Interventions to Address Potentially Inappropriate Prescribing in Community-Dwelling Older Adults: A Systematic Review of Randomized Controlled Trials. *J. Am. Geriatr. Soc.* **2016**, *64*, 1210–1222. [CrossRef] [PubMed]
22. Liberati, A.; Altman, D.G.; Tetzlaff, J.; Mulrow, C.; Gøtzsche, P.C.; Ioannidis, J.P.; Clarke, M.; Devereaux, P.; Kleijnen, J.; Moher, D. The PRISMA statement for reporting systematic reviews and meta-analyses of studies that evaluate health care interventions: Explanation and elaboration. *J. Clin. Epidemiol.* **2009**, *62*, e1–e34. [CrossRef]
23. Sterne, J.A.C.; Savović, J.; Page, M.J.; Elbers, R.G.; Blencowe, N.S.; Boutron, I.; Cates, C.J.; Cheng, H.-Y.; Corbett, M.S.; Eldridge, S.M.; et al. RoB 2: A revised tool for assessing risk of bias in randomised trials. *BMJ* **2019**, *366*, l4898. [CrossRef] [PubMed]
24. Guyatt, G.; Oxman, A.D.; Akl, E.A.; Kunz, R.; Vist, G.; Brozek, J.; Norris, S.; Falck-Ytter, Y.; Glasziou, P.; DeBeer, H.; et al. GRADE guidelines: 1. Introduction—GRADE evidence profiles and summary of findings tables. *J. Clin. Epidemiol.* **2011**, *64*, 383–394. [CrossRef]
25. Higgins, J.P.; Thomas, J.; Chandler, J.; Cumpston, M.; Li, T.; Page, M.J.; Welch, V.A. *Cochrane Handbook for Systematic Reviews of Interventions*, 2nd ed.; John Wiley & Sons: Hoboken, NJ, USA, 2019.
26. Higgins, J.P.T.; Thompson, S.G. Quantifying heterogeneity in a meta-analysis. *Stat. Med.* **2002**, *21*, 1539–1558. [CrossRef]
27. Higgins, J.P.T.; Thompson, S.G.; Deeks, J.J.; Altman, D.G. Measuring inconsistency in meta-analyses. *Br. Med. J.* **2003**, *327*, 557–560. [CrossRef]
28. Bryant, L.J.; Coster, G.; Gamble, G.; McCormick, R.N. The General Practitioner–Pharmacist Collaboration (GPPC) study: A randomised controlled trial of clinical medication reviews in community pharmacy. *Int. J. Pharm. Pract.* **2011**, *19*, 94–105. [CrossRef]
29. Falamić, S.; Lucijanic, M.; Ortner-Hadžiabdić, M.; Marušić, S.; Bačić-Vrca, V. Pharmacists' influence on adverse reactions to warfarin: A randomised controlled trial in elderly rural patients. *Int. J. Clin. Pharm.* **2019**, *41*, 1166–1173. [CrossRef] [PubMed]
30. Mott, D.A.; Martin, B.; Breslow, R.; Michaels, B.; Kirchner, J.; Mahoney, J.; Margolis, A. Impact of a medication therapy management intervention targeting medications associated with falling: Results of a pilot study. *J. Am. Pharm. Assoc.* **2016**, *56*, 22–28. [CrossRef] [PubMed]
31. Touchette, D.R.; Masica, A.L.; Dolor, R.; Schumock, G.T.; Choi, Y.K.; Kim, Y.; Smith, S.R. Safety-focused medication therapy management: A randomized controlled trial. *J. Am. Pharm. Assoc.* **2012**, *52*, 603–612. [CrossRef]

32. Varas-Doval, R.; Gastelurrutia, M.A.; Benrimoj, S.I.; García-Cárdenas, V.; Sáez-Benito, L.; Martinez-Martínez, F. Clinical impact of a pharmacist-led medication review with follow up for aged polypharmacy patients: A cluster randomized controlled trial. *Pharm. Pract.* **2020**, *18*, 2133. [CrossRef] [PubMed]
33. Olesen, C.; Harbig, P.; Buus, K.M.; Barat, I.; Damsgaard, E.M. Impact of pharmaceutical care on adherence, hospitalisations and mortality in elderly patients. *Int. J. Clin. Pharm.* **2013**, *36*, 163–171. [CrossRef] [PubMed]
34. Toivo, T.; Airaksinen, M.; Dimitrow, M.; Savela, E.; Pelkonen, K.; Kiuru, V.; Suominen, T.; Uunimäki, M.; Kivelä, S.-L.; Leikola, S.; et al. Enhanced coordination of care to reduce medication risks in older home care clients in primary care: A randomized controlled trial. *BMC Geriatr.* **2019**, *19*, 332. [CrossRef] [PubMed]
35. Malet-Larrea, A.; Goyenechea, E.; García-Cárdenas, V.; Calvo, B.; Arteche, J.M.; Aranegui, P.; Zubeldia, J.J.; Gastelurrutia, M.A.; Martínez-Martínez, F.; Benrimoj, S. The impact of a medication review with follow-up service on hospital admissions in aged polypharmacy patients. *Br. J. Clin. Pharmacol.* **2016**, *82*, 831–838. [CrossRef]
36. Tannenbaum, C.; Martin, P.; Tamblyn, R.; Benedetti, A.; Ahmed, S. Reduction of Inappropriate Benzodiazepine Prescriptions Among Older Adults Through Direct Patient Education. *JAMA Intern. Med.* **2014**, *174*, 890–898. [CrossRef]
37. Van der Meer, H.; Wouters, H.; Pont, L.G.; Taxis, K. Reducing the anticholinergic and sedative load in older patients on polypharmacy by pharmacist-led medication review: A randomised controlled trial. *BMJ Open* **2018**, *8*, e019042. [CrossRef]
38. Martin, P.; Tamblyn, R.; Benedetti, A.; Ahmed, S.; Tannenbaum, C. Effect of a pharmacist-led educational intervention on inap-propriate medication prescriptions in older adults: The D-PRESCRIBE randomized clinical trial. *JAMA* **2018**, *320*, 1889–1898. [CrossRef]
39. Falamić, S.; Lucijanic, M.; Hadžiabdić, M.O.; Marušić, S.; Vrca, V.B. Pharmacist's interventions improve time in therapeutic range of elderly rural patients on warfarin therapy: A randomized trial. *Int. J. Clin. Pharm.* **2018**, *40*, 1078–1085. [CrossRef]
40. Kooy, M.; Van Wijk, B.L.; Heerdink, E.R.; De Boer, A.; Bouvy, M.L. Does the use of an electronic reminder device with or without counseling improve adherence to lipid-lowering treatment? The results of a randomized controlled trial. *Front. Pharmacol.* **2013**, *4*, 69. [CrossRef]
41. Gudi, S.K.; Kashyap, A.; Chhabra, M.; Rashid, M.; Tiwari, K.K. Impact of pharmacist-led home medicines review services on drug-related problems among the elderly population: A systematic review. *Epidemiol. Health* **2019**, *41*, e2019020. [CrossRef] [PubMed]
42. Tecklenborg, S.; Byrne, C.; Cahir, C.; Brown, L.; Bennett, K. Interventions to Reduce Adverse Drug Event-Related Outcomes in Older Adults: A Systematic Review and Meta-analysis. *Drugs Aging* **2020**, *37*, 91–98. [CrossRef] [PubMed]
43. Thiruchelvam, K.; Hasan, S.S.; Wong, P.S.; Kairuz, T. Residential Aged Care Medication Review to Improve the Quality of Medication Use: A Systematic Review. *J. Am. Med. Dir. Assoc.* **2017**, *18*, 87.e1–87.e14. [CrossRef]
44. Yuan, C.; Ding, Y.; Zhou, K.; Huang, Y.; Xi, X. Clinical outcomes of community pharmacy services: A systematic review and meta-analysis. *Health Soc. Care Community* **2019**, *27*, e567–e587. [CrossRef] [PubMed]
45. Al-Babtain, B.; Cheema, E.; Hadi, M.A. Impact of community-pharmacist-led medication review programmes on patient outcomes: A systematic review and meta-analysis of randomised controlled trials. *Res. Soc. Adm. Pharm.* **2021**, in press. [CrossRef] [PubMed]
46. Dawoud, D.M.; Haines, A.; Wonderling, D.; Ashe, J.; Hill, J.; Varia, M.; Dyer, P.; Bion, J. Cost Effectiveness of Advanced Pharmacy Services Provided in the Community and Primary Care Settings: A Systematic Review. *PharmacoEconomics* **2019**, *37*, 1241–1260. [CrossRef] [PubMed]
47. Milosavljevic, A.; Aspden, T.; Harrison, J. Community pharmacist-led interventions and their impact on patients' medication adherence and other health outcomes: A systematic review. *Int. J. Pharm. Pract.* **2018**, *26*, 387–397. [CrossRef]
48. Varas-Doval, R.; Sáez-Benito, L.; Gastelurrutia, M.A.; Benrimoj, S.I.; Garcia-Cardenas, V.; Martinez-Martínez, F. Systematic review of pragmatic randomised control trials assessing the effectiveness of professional pharmacy services in community pharmacies. *BMC Health Serv. Res.* **2021**, *21*, 156. [CrossRef] [PubMed]
49. Dou, C.; Rebane, J.; Bardal, S. Interventions to improve benzodiazepine tapering success in the elderly: A systematic review. *Aging Ment. Health* **2018**, *23*, 411–416. [CrossRef]
50. Reeve, E.; Ong, M.; Wu, A.; Jansen, J.; Petrovic, M.; Gnjidic, D. A systematic review of interventions to deprescribe benzodiazepines and other hypnotics among older people. *Eur. J. Clin. Pharmacol.* **2017**, *73*, 927–935. [CrossRef]
51. Huiskes, V.J.B.; Burger, D.M.; van den Ende, C.H.M.; van den Bemt, B.J.F. Effectiveness of medication review: A systematic review and meta-analysis of randomized controlled trials. *BMC Fam. Pract.* **2017**, *18*, 5. [CrossRef]
52. Holland, R.; Desborough, J.; Goodyer, L.; Hall, S.; Wright, D.; Loke, Y.K. Does pharmacist-led medication review help to reduce hospital admissions and deaths in older people? A systematic review and meta-analysis. *Br. J. Clin. Pharmacol.* **2008**, *65*, 303–316. [CrossRef]
53. Wallerstedt, S.M.; Kindblom, J.; Nylén, K.; Samuelsson, O.; Strandell, A. Medication reviews for nursing home residents to reduce mortality and hospitalization: Systematic review and meta-analysis. *Br. J. Clin. Pharmacol.* **2014**, *78*, 488–497. [CrossRef] [PubMed]
54. Hart, L.A.; Phelan, E.A.; Yi, J.Y.; Marcum, Z.A.; Gray, S.L. Use of Fall Risk–Increasing Drugs Around a Fall-Related Injury in Older Adults: A Systematic Review. *J. Am. Geriatr. Soc.* **2020**, *68*, 1334–1343. [CrossRef] [PubMed]
55. Crilly, P.; Kayyali, R. A Systematic Review of Randomized Controlled Trials of Telehealth and Digital Technology Use by Community Pharmacists to Improve Public Health. *Pharmacy* **2020**, *8*, 137. [CrossRef] [PubMed]
56. Barton, S. Which clinical studies provide the best evidence? The best RCT still trumps the best observational study. *BMJ* **2000**, *321*, 255–256. [CrossRef] [PubMed]

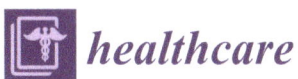

Article

Factors Affecting Pharmacy Students' Decision to Study in Pharmacy Colleges in Saudi Arabia: A Cross-Sectional Questionnaire-Based Analysis

Ahmed M. Alshehri [1,*], Lara A. Elsawaf [1], Shaikah F. Alzaid [1], Yasser S. Almogbel [2], Mohammed A. Alminggash [3], Ziyad S. Almalki [1] and Majed A. Algarni [4]

1. Clinical Pharmacy Department, College of Pharmacy, Prince Sattam bin Abdulaziz University, Al Kharj 16273, Saudi Arabia; Lara.ayman.elsawaf@gmail.com (L.A.E.); shaikah.f.alzaid@gmail.com (S.F.A.); Z.almalki@psau.edu.sa (Z.S.A.)
2. Department of Pharmacy Practice, College of Pharmacy, Qassim University, Buraidah 51452, Saudi Arabia; y.almogbel@qu.edu.sa
3. Ministry of Interior, Medical Services Headquarters, Riyadh 6389, Saudi Arabia; malshehri@moimsd.gov.sa
4. Clinical Pharmacy Department, College of Pharmacy, Taif University, P.O. Box 11099, Taif 21944, Saudi Arabia; m.alqarni@tu.edu.sa
* Correspondence: Ah.alshehri@psau.edu.sa; Tel.: +966-11-588-6055

Abstract: (1) Background: Many factors may play a role in deciding to opt for pharmacy as a major. However, no previous studies have been conducted in Saudi Arabia to explore these factors. This study aims to identify the potential factors that prompted students to join the pharmacy program. (2) Methods: A cross-sectional questionnaire was distributed among undergraduate pharmacy students in Saudi Arabia, addressing areas such as reasons that encourage them to choose pharmacy as a major, and students' socio-demographic characteristics. Descriptive statistics were used to describe the study variables, and a simple logistic regression analysis was performed to identify the potential factors. (3) Results: A total of 491 students completed the questionnaire. Around 40% of them had chosen to study pharmacy as their first choice. Only gender, current GPA, and reasons related to the pharmacy field were found to have a statistically significant association with students selecting pharmacy as their first choice. (4) Conclusions: This study shows that pharmacy students have a future-oriented outlook and selected pharmacy as their first choice because it will develop them professionally, financially, and intellectually. Educating high school students about the characteristic of pharmacy would help attract more talented students to the pharmacy carrier.

Keywords: pharmacy education; decision to study in pharmacy; selecting pharmacy as a first choice

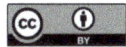

1. Introduction

By increasing the world population, high demand for healthcare professionals, such as pharmacists, is needed to manage people's health. According to the World Healthcare Organization, in 2010, in developed countries, such as France and the United States (US), there are on average 117 and 93 pharmacists per 100,000, while in developing countries such as the Kingdom of Saudi Arabia there were only 54 pharmacists per 100,000 people [1]. This indicated the need for more pharmacists to accommodate the increase in the population.

The Kingdom of Saudi Arabia has experienced rapid progress in the profession of pharmacy. This is demonstrated by the increasing number of pharmacy colleges and pharmacy graduates. In 1959, King Saud University established Saudi's first pharmacy college in Riyadh. Four decades later, King Abdulaziz University was established in Jeddah in the western region. A few years later, the course was introduced at King Faisal University, Al-Ahsa in the Eastern region, and King Khalid University, Abha in the Southern region [2,3]. Since then, according to a report published by the Saudi Commission for Health Specialties (SCFHS) in 2018, the number of public and private pharmacy colleges has increased and reached 27, with more than 14,004 pharmacy students enrolled [4]. Thus, the number of graduate pharmacists increased from 150–250 in 2000 to 1157 graduates in 2016 and is expected to increase by 7–10% every year [5,6]. In addition, with the Saudi government's National Transformation Program (Saudi Vision 2030), the need for pharmacists is increased [7].

Pharmacy degrees provided by these colleges have changed over time. King Saud University's College of Pharmacy used to offer a Bachelor's degree in Pharmacy (BPharm) after successful completion of five and a half years; while after its establishment in 2001, King Abdulaziz University's College of Pharmacy offers a Doctor of Pharmacy (PharmD) degree in six years [8]. Now, almost all colleges offer only PharmD, or are in the transition from BPharm to PharmD, or offer both degrees based on the student's preferred track. These two programs have slightly different characteristics. The PharmD degree programs reduced some of the basic pharmaceutical sciences such as pharmacognosy and medicinal chemistry and added more clinical studies and rotations [5]. Therefore, these two programs may have prompted students to select pharmacy as their first choice after graduating from high school. However, it is worth mentioning that all colleges of pharmacy in Saudi Arabia allowed students to enter pharmacy directly after graduating from high school, which is different than the admission requirements for pharmacy school in western countries [9,10].

Many studies conducted worldwide have examined the reasons and motivations for students to choose pharmacy as a major. Some studies have shown that students chose pharmacy schools as their first choice, while others have found that students chose it as their second choice. For example, studies in Sudan, Ethiopia, the US, and South Africa have examined students' selection of pharmacy as the major and shown that the majority of students (79.3%, 67.6%, 53%, and 52.3%, respectively) chose pharmacy as the first choice [11–15].

The reasons why students pick a pharmacy school as their first choice differ from one country to another. For example, in the US and Ethiopia, students were encouraged by a family member, a pharmacist, or a pharmacy student [11,14]. In a western county such as the United Kingdom (UK), students related their decision to study pharmacy to its being a science-based course [16], while in Australia, students related their decision to self-employment and salary [17]. In the South African study, the most important reasons were that they enjoy working with people, want to help poor people and advise them on different types of diseases, and earn decent wages [12]. In the Sudanese study, viewing the career of pharmacy as an excellent option for the future and pharmacists as having a good social image led students to select pharmacy as their first choice [13]. Contrastingly, a study conducted in a Jordanian university showed that almost 61% of all pharmacy students stated that pharmacy school was not their first choice; however, the desire to work in a health-related field led the majority (83.8%) to enroll in a pharmacy college [18]. Receiving encouragement from other people who share the same characteristics was shown to be one of the reasons to study pharmacy [11].

A similar study was conducted in Saudi Arabia at Taif University, and it was found that 62.3% of students (n = 398) had applied for the pharmacy program (PharmD) as their second choice after medicine. The same study found that the students were selecting pharmacy as their second choice because they wanted to work in a health-related field (83.4%), had excellent high school grades (73.4%), sought good job opportunities (72.1%), loved to work with patients (70.4%), liked flexible working hours (67.8%), and had received family encouragement (66.6%) [19]. Pharmacists' basic salary in Saudi Arabia ranged on average from $1979 to $7782 per month and more depending on their practice area, where pharmacists who worked in community pharmacies tend to receive low salaries compared to those who work in hospital pharmacies. However, since Saudi universities offer two pharmacy programs (PharmD and BPharm), examining students' preferences regarding these two programs is very important.

Students' reasons for choosing pharmacy as their first choice varied among the studies, thereby identifying different factors that may affect students' choices. It is important to know why students choose pharmacy school as their first choice after graduating from high school. To our knowledge, no previous studies have been conducted across all regions of Saudi Arabia to explore pharmacy students' reasons for studying pharmacy and making it their first choice. Therefore, this study aims to identify pharmacy students' (PharmD and BPharm) reasons for joining the pharmacy program and their career plans.

2. Materials and Methods

2.1. Study Design, Population, and Samples

A cross-sectional online questionnaire was distributed among a convenient sample of undergraduate pharmacy students in different colleges across Saudi Arabia between January 2021 until July 2021. Since there are 27 colleges of pharmacy located in different universities across Saudi Arabia, and more than 14,000 students are studying pharmacy, two methods were used to distribute the survey and to increase the study participants. First, the questionnaire link was sent to different pharmacy school clubs, and they were asked to distribute it among their undergraduate pharmacy students. Second, the authors sent the questionnaire to pharmacy students at their respective colleges and asked them to share the link with their classmates and other pharmacy students across Saudi Arabia. These two methods were repeated after two months of sending the survey to increase student participation, especially with pharmacy colleges with low response rates.

2.2. Study Ethics

Participants were informed at the beginning of the online survey that their participation would be completely voluntary and anonymous, so they could stop the survey at any time and be sure that their information was unidentifiable. In addition, participants were informed that they consented to being included in the study by accepting to complete the survey. The Research Ethics Committee in Health and Science Disciplines (REC-HSD) at Prince Sattam bin Abdulaziz University approved the study.

2.3. Survey Instrument

The survey questionnaire was created by modifying various surveys found in the literature [11,18,20–22], and it consisted of two parts. The first part focused on the reasons that encouraged the students to choose pharmacy as a major. It included 18 items, and each item needed to be ranked by the student based on its importance. These items were rated using a 5-point Likert scale ranging from "not very important" (1) to "very important" (5). This first part of the survey is divided into three sections. The first section included six items to measure students' reasons for career advice, such as advice from a high school teacher, a university faculty member, or a pharmacist, and receiving advice while attending events or browsing social media. The second section evaluated personal factors, such as receiving advice from family members or friends, previous pharmacy work experience, desire to work in the healthcare sector or to improve people's health and well-being, and their grades in high school. The last section included reasons related to the pharmacy field: work flexibility, high salary, ability to run a pharmacy business, high job demand, having a job with important knowledge, and respect.

The second part contained items that asked about students' socio-demographics variables, such as age, gender, current study year, marital status, university region, current Grade Point Average (GPA), and pharmacy degree program. Additionally, this part asked students whether they had any relatives or friends who worked in health-related fields and whether they had chosen to study Pharmacy as their first choice or not.

The survey was first formed in the English language and then translated to Arabic. To validate the translation, the Arabic version was then translated back to English. Then, the survey was sent to five pharmacy faculty members and 10 pharmacy students to validate the survey. Study item internal consistency reliability was measured through Cronbach's alpha.

2.4. Data Analysis

The study used the G power analysis to determine the required sample size, and the STATA software program to analyze the data produced by the survey. First, various assumptions were utilized to compute the needed sample size: odds ratio, 1.3; power, 0.8; alpha level, 0.05. Based on these assumptions, the required sample size was 473. Next in the Stata analysis, descriptive, simple, and multivariate logistic regression analyses were used to assess the study objectives. Descriptive statistics, including the mean and frequency distribution, were used to describe the study variables. A simple logistic regression analysis was used to determine the association between the independent study variables (age, gender, marital status, pharmacy degree program, first-degree family, current GPA, job advice, personal advice, pharmacy factors) and dependent variable (students' selecting pharmacy as their first choice after high school). A multivariate logistic regression analysis was used to identify which factors were associated with students selecting pharmacy school as their first choice. A p-value of less than 0.05 was considered significant.

3. Results

A total of 491 pharmacy students participated in this study. Participants' average age was 22.26 ($\pm$2.31) years, and the majority were female (73.12%) and single (94.50%). The participants' average GPA was 4.28 ($\pm$0.61) on a 5-point scale, and 64.15% were enrolled in a PharmD program while 35.23% were enrolled in a BPharm program. Two-thirds of participants were studying in universities located in the middle region of Saudi Arabia. Most of them (58.65%) had relatives working in health-related fields, and less than half of the participants (41.54%) had selected Pharmacy as their first choice (see Table 1).

Table 1. Students' socio-demographic characteristics (n = 491).

Characteristic	n	%
Age (years); mean $\pm$ SD	22.26 ($\pm$2.31)	
Gender		
Male, n (%)	132	26.88
Female, n (%)	359	73.12
Marital status		
Single, n (%)	464	94.50
Married, n (%)	23	4.68
Divorced, n (%)	0	0
Separated, n (%)	4	0.81
Widowed, n (%)	0	0
Current Grade Point Average (GPA); mean $\pm$ SD	4.29 ($\pm$0.61)	
Region of the university		
Northern region, n (%)	39	7.94
Southern region, n (%)	55	11.20
Middle region, n (%)	326	66.40
Eastern region, n (%)	23	4.68
Western region, n (%)	61	12.42
Pharmacy degree program		
BPharm, n (%)	173	35.23
PharmD, n (%)	315	64.15
Both (PharmD and BPharm), n (%)	3	0.61

Table 1. Cont.

Characteristic	n	%
Pharmacy as a choice		
First choice, n (%)	204	41.55
Second choice, n (%)	171	34.83
Third choice, n (%)	74	15.07
Fourth choice, n (%)	7	1.43
Fifth choice, n (%)	5	1.02
Not a choice, n (%)	36	7.33
Pharmacy year		
First year, n (%)	6	1.22
Second year, n (%)	82	16.70
Third year, n (%)	118	24.03
Fourth year, n (%)	112	22.81
Fifth year, n (%)	106	21.59
Sixth year, n (%)	67	13.65
Relatives/friends working in a health-related field		
Father, n (%)	24	4.89
Mother, n (%)	14	2.85
Sister, n (%)	109	22.20
Brother, n (%)	82	16.70
Husband, n (%)	1	0.20
Relatives, n (%)	288	58.66

3.1. Students' Reasons for Choosing Pharmacy

Table 2 shows students' reasons for studying in a pharmacy school. Among the three types of reasons, pharmacy students rated reasons related to the pharmacy field as their biggest reason for studying Pharmacy (3.96 ± 0.80), followed by personal factors (3.66 ± 0.78), and lastly, career advice (3.05 ± 0.97). Among reasons related to career advice, participants rated advice from a pharmacist as neutral to important in selecting pharmacy (3.65 ± 1.37), while they rated advice from a schoolteacher as a not important to neutral reason (2.59 ± 1.32). Among reasons related to personal factors, the desire to work in the healthcare sector was perceived as an important to very important reason (4.36 ± 0.99), and indeed, it was the highest-rated reason. Contrastingly, advice from a friend was rated as the least important among reasons related to personal factors (3.04 ± 1.24). Lastly, students rated viewing pharmacy as a leading to a respectable job and a job with important knowledge as an important to very important reason for studying pharmacy (4.30 ± 0.96 and 4.30 ± 1.24, respectively). Subsequently, students rated the ability to run a pharmacy business as neutral to important (3.23 ± 1.28). All the previous domains showed good reliability, ranging from 0.67 to 0.83.

Table 2. Students' reasons for choosing pharmacy as a major ($n = 491$).

Items	Mean ($\pm SD$)	Frequency n (%)				
		Not Very Important	Not Important	Neutral	Important	Very Important
Career Advice						
Advice from a schoolteacher	2.59 (± 1.32)	149 (30.35)	83 (16.90)	113 (23.01)	111 (22.61)	35 (7.13)
Advice from a university faculty member	3.17 (± 1.44)	105 (21.38)	56 (11.41)	83 (16.9)	143 (29.12)	104 (21.18)
Advice from a pharmacist	3.65 (± 1.37)	68 (13.85)	34 (6.92)	62 (12.63)	161 (32.79)	166 (33.81)
Advice received while attending a recruitment event	3.07 (± 1.32)	96 (19.55)	53 (10.79)	132 (26.88)	139 (28.31)	71 (14.46)
Self-directed career advice from internet searches	2.96 (± 1.23)	88 (17.92)	74 (15.07)	146 (29.74)	138 (28.11)	45 (9.16)
Advice from social media	2.85 (± 1.25)	102 (20.77)	71 (14.46)	165 (33.60)	105 (21.38)	48 (9.78)
Domain Total	3.05 (± 0.97)	Cronbach's alpha = 0.83				
Personal Factors						
Advice from a family member	3.42 (± 1.35)	74 (15.07)	46 (9.37)	87 (17.72)	168 (34.22)	116 (23.63)
Advice from a friend	3.04 (± 1.24)	88 (17.92)	59 (12.02)	138 (28.11)	159 (3238)	47 (9.57)
Previous pharmacy work experience	3.25 (± 1.53)	115 (23.42)	47 (9.57)	63 (12.83)	132 (26.88)	134 (27.29)
Desire to improve people's health and well-being	4.11 (± 1.18)	39 (7.94)	10 (2.04)	52 (10.59)	148 (30.14)	242 (49.29)
Desire to work in the healthcare sector	4.36 (± 0.99)	21 (4.28)	8 (1.63)	32 (6.52)	144 (29.33)	286 (58.25)
High school grades	3.79 (± 1.25)	45 (9.16)	28 (5.70)	88 (17.92)	152 (30.96)	178 (36.25)
Domain Total	3.66 (± 0.78)	Cronbach's alpha = 0.67				
Pharmacy Factors						
Flexible work hours	3.68 (± 1.17)	40 (8.15)	34 (6.92)	97 (19.76)	194 (39.51)	126 (25.66)
High salary after graduation	4.07 (± 1.03)	20 (4.07)	23 (4.68)	55 (11.20)	200 (40.73)	193 (39.31)
Ability to run pharmacy business	3.23 (± 1.28)	59 (12.02)	84 (17.11)	126 (25.66)	128 (26.07)	94 (17.14)
Good job opportunities	4.16 (± 1.45)	25 (5.09)	11 (2.24)	52 (10.59)	177 (36.97)	226 (46.03)
A job with important knowledge	4.30 (± 1.24)	23 (4.68)	9 (1.83)	41 (8.35)	145 (29.53)	273 (55.60)
Respectable job	4.30 (± 0.96)	19 (3.87)	8 (1.63)	38 (7.74)	168 (34.22)	258 (52.55)
Domain Total	3.96 (± 0.80)	Cronbach's alpha = 0.83				

3.2. Factors Predicting the Selection of Pharmacy Schools as the First Choice

Simple and multivariate logistic regression analyses were used to determine which factors predicted whether pharmacy students had selected pharmacy school as their first choice after graduation from high school. First, a simple logistic regression analysis examined the association between selecting pharmacy school as the first choice and age, gender, marital status, current GPA, pharmacy degree program, relatives/friends working in the healthcare sector, reasons related to career advice, personal advice, and pharmacy field. Only gender, current GPA, and reasons related to the pharmacy field were found to have a statistically significant association with students selecting pharmacy as their first choice ($\beta = 0.45, p < 0.001; \beta = 2.47, p < 0.001; \beta = 1.04; p < 0.035$, respectively).

The multivariant logistic regression identified which factors among gender, current GPA, and reasons related to the pharmacy field predicted students' selection of pharmacy as the first choice after graduating high school. The analysis showed that there was a statistically significant relationship between the variables ($\chi^2 (3, 491) = 0.619, p < 0.001$). It showed that there was a significant relationship between students' selection of pharmacy school as their first choice and their current GPA ($p < 0.001$) and the pharmacy field factors ($p = 0.017$). As a student's current GPA increased by one unit, the odds of the student selecting pharmacy school as their first choice increased by 2.52 (OR = 2.52, 95% CI = 1.55–4.08, $p < 0.001$). Moreover, as a student's reasons related to the pharmacy-field factors increased by one unit, the odds of the student selecting pharmacy school as their first choice increased by 2.52 (OR = 1.07, 95% CI = 1.01–1.13, $p = 0.017$) (see Table 3).

Table 3. Simple and multivariate logistic regression analysis of factors predicting pharmacy students' selecting pharmacy school as their first choice ($n = 491$).

Variable	p-Value	Odds Ratio	95% Confidence Interval	
			Lower	Upper
Simple Logistic Regression				
Age	0.921	1.14	0.90	1.12
Gender	<0.000 *	0.45	0.30	0.70
Marital status	0.293	1.57	0.68	3.63
Pharmacy degree program	0.352	0.84	0.58	1.22
First-degree family	0.363	1.19	0.82	1.72
Current GPA^2	<0.000 *	2.47	1.54	3.96
Job advice	0.760	1.48	0.97	1.04
Personal advice	0.583	1.01	0.97	1.05
Pharmacy factors	0.035 *	1.04	1.311	1.09
Multivariate Logistic Regression				
Gender	0.354	0.76	0.43	1.35
Current GPA^2	<0.001 *	2.52	1.55	4.08
Pharmacy field factors	0.017 *	1.07	1.01	1.13

Note: p-value < 0.05 indicated with asterisk.

4. Discussion

To the best of our knowledge, this is the first study involving the investigation of pharmacy students' reasons behind studying pharmacy as a first choice in Saudi universities. By conducting simple and multivariate logistic regression analyses, we found a positive association between GPA, factors related to the pharmacy field (good job opportunities, a job providing important knowledge, flexible working hours, a good salary, a respectable job, and the ability to run a pharmacy business) and the preference of pharmacy as a first choice.

The study sample's socio-demographics are slightly different from those of similar studies. The majority of participating students were female (73.12%), which was similar to the proportion of female students in the pharmacy colleges in the United States [23–25] and other Arab countries [13,18,26], and different from what was found in the earlier Saudi study [19]. More than half of the participants are currently studying in the central-region universities, most likely because the central region of Saudi Arabia has the highest population density and the highest number of pharmacy colleges [4,27]. Regarding students' GPA, we found that majority of students had a GPA ranging from 4 to 4.50, or "very good," which is similar to other studies conducted in Saudi Arabia and Ethiopia [14,19].

Opting for pharmacy after graduation from high school has become one of the common directions for Saudi students in recent years. In our study, 41.5% of the respondents had chosen to study Pharmacy as their first choice, followed by 34.8% and 15.1% who selected it as their second and third choice, respectively. The percentage of students selecting pharmacy school as their first choice was lower than the percentages found in Sudan (79.3%) [13], Ethiopia (67.6%) [14], the United States (53%) [11], and South Africa (52.3%) [12]. On the other hand, although the current study was conducted across different pharmacy schools and among both PharmD and BPharm students, the study's findings were similar to another study conducted in Saudi Arabia, wherein 37.7% of pharmacy students (PharmD) at Taif University revealed that they had chosen pharmacy school as their first choice [19]. In addition, the present findings were similar to those of other studies conducted in Jordan and South Africa, where only 39% of students had chosen pharmacy as their first choice [15,18]. This highlights the importance of identifying and clarifying the importance and the impact of pharmacists in the community.

Many factors could affect high school graduates' decisions to study pharmacy in Saudi Arabia. In our study, students rated reasons related to the pharmacy field as the biggest factor that influenced their decision to study Pharmacy. This indicated that students were careful in selecting their careers and were little affected by other factors. Regarding the field of pharmacy-related factors, more than 85% of students perceived having a respectable job with important knowledge as an important to very important reason to choose to study Pharmacy. This indicated students' interest in keeping up with developments in the pharmacy field and expanding their knowledge even after graduating and getting a job, which was not measured in other studies. However, viewing pharmacy as a respectable job has been reported in the US, since 71% of Americans in 2020 rated pharmacist honesty and ethical standards as "high" or "very high" [28].

A study investigating the factors influencing Sudanese pharmacy students to study pharmacy found that 30.5% of participants who chose pharmacy as their first choice did so because it offered a good future; whereas, only 1.9% of them preferred it because it provided a good social image [13]. In our study, among personal factors, around 80% of students rated their desire to work in the healthcare sector and improve people's health and well-being as "important" to "very important" factors in their decision to study pharmacy. It is very important to note that these two factors could lead students to keep pharmacy as one of the options in the healthcare sector.

Among factors related to career advice, about two-thirds of students rated the advice received from a pharmacist as important to very important, while 47% rated the advice from a schoolteacher as not very important to not important. This indicates that to attract more talented high-school students, pharmacists and pharmacy schools, in general, need to increase their visits to high schools to educate and encourage students to choose pharmacy as a career and to encourage teachers to depict it as an important profession in society. A study showed that students who decided to enter pharmacy school before starting high school were more likely to pursue their plan than students who decided to enter pharmacy while there are in pharmacy school [17]. Contrastingly, another study of pharmacy students at the University of Sierra Leone found that students cited a subject or teacher at school as their primary motivator (66.7%) in opting for pharmacy. In the present study, students considered family and friends as the most significant contributors (61.1%) to their choice. Similar to another study which found that pharmacy students encouraged to study pharmacy school due to a recommendation from their parents and other high-school students who shared similar race [11]. A job with good career opportunities (27.8%), an opportunity for self-employment (27.8%), and working in the healthcare profession with patients (16.7%) were the most valuable career-oriented factors that influenced students' choice [29]. Having a high salary after graduation was perceived as important by students, similar to the other study [17]. However, it was perceived as less important than perceiving pharmacy as a respectable job with important knowledge.

This study has several limitations. First, the study survey was self-administered; therefore, students' responses cannot be validated. Next, since taking the survey was voluntary, some students did not mention their GPA, which they may have perceived as private information. Although the survey was distributed to all universities across the country, students in the central-region universities had the maximum participation, and some pharmacy colleges were not represented because none of their students participated in the survey. Thus, the results cannot be generalized for all universities in the country.

5. Conclusions

This study shows that pharmacy students in Saudi Arabia have various reasons to enroll in pharmacy colleges. Students chose pharmacy as their first choice because it would give them good career opportunities and a respectable job with important knowledge, a high salary, and flexible working hours, in addition to the possibility of running a private pharmacy business. The study also shows that pharmacy students have a future-oriented view and desire to obtain a job that will develop them professionally, financially, and intellectually. To improve the future of pharmacy as a career option, faculties pharmacy schools need to visit high schools and provide details regarding the benefits of studying pharmacy and the future of the profession. Future studies may study the effect of pharmacy school visits to high school on students' understanding of pharmacist-related factors and the impact of these visits on their intention to study pharmacy. Additionally, using a theoretical model like the theory of planned behavior would help identify better the salient factors for studying pharmacy.

Author Contributions: Conceptualization, A.A.M., L.A.E., S.F.A., Y.S.A., M.A.A. (Mohammed A. Alminggash), Z.S.A. and M.A.A. (Majed A. Algarni); Data curation, A.A.M., L.A.E., S.F.A. and Y.S.A.; Formal analysis, A.A.M. and Y.S.A.; Funding acquisition, A.A.M.; Methodology, A.A.M., L.A.E. and S.F.A.; Software, Y.S.A.; Supervision, A.A.M.; Validation, A.A.M., L.A.E. and S.F.A.; Writing—original draft, A.A.M., L.A.E., S.F.A., Y.S.A., M.A.A. (Mohammed A. Alminggash), Z.S.A. and M.A.A. (Majed A. Algarni); Writing—review and editing, A.A.M., Y.S.A., M.A.A. (Mohammed A. Alminggash), Z.S.A. and M.A.A. (Majed A. Algarni). All authors have read and agreed to the published version of the manuscript.

Funding: This research received no external funding.

Institutional Review Board Statement: The study was conducted according to the guidelines of the Declaration of Helsinki, and approved by Research Ethics Committee of prince Sattam bin Abdulaziz University (REC-HSD-85-2021).

Informed Consent Statement: Informed consent was obtained from all participants involved in the study at the commencement of the online anonymous survey.

Data Availability Statement: The data that support the findings of this study are available from the corresponding author.

Acknowledgments: We thank the university for using their computers and software to conduct the study.

Conflicts of Interest: The authors declare that they have no conflict of interests.

References

1. Substantially Increase Health Financing and the Recruitment, Development, Training and Retention of the Health Workforce in Developing Countries, Especially in Least Developed Countries and Small Island Developing STATES. Available online: https://www.who.int/data/gho/data/indicators/indicator-details/GHO/pharmacists-(per-10-000-population) (accessed on 13 November 2021).
2. Al-Wazaify, M.; Matowe, L.; Albsoul-Younes, A.; Al-Omran, O.A. Pharmacy education in Jordan, Saudi Arabia, and Kuwait. *Am. J. Pharm. Educ.* **2006**, *70*, 18. [CrossRef] [PubMed]

3. Alhamoudi, A.; Alnattah, A. Pharmacy education in Saudi Arabia: The past, the present, and the future. *Curr. Pharm. Teach. Learn.* **2018**, *10*, 54–60. [CrossRef]
4. Alomran, S.; Alhosni, A.; Alzahrani, K.; Alamodi, A.; Alhazmi, R. The Reality of The Saudi Health Workforce During The Next Ten Years 2018–2027. *Saudi Comm. Health Spec.* **2017**, *1*, 17–19.
5. Al-Jedai, A.; Qaisi, S.; Al-Meman, A. Pharmacy practice and the health care system in Saudi Arabia. *Can. J. Hosp. Pharm.* **2016**, *69*, 231. [CrossRef]
6. Saudi Ministry of Health. *Statistical Yearbook 1438H*; Saudi Ministry of Health: Riyadh, Saudi Arabia, 2016.
7. Saudi Arabia's Vision 2030. Available online: https://www.vision2030.gov.sa/ (accessed on 13 November 2021).
8. Almaghaslah, D.A.M. An evaluation of the global pharmacy workforce highlighting pharmacy human resource issues within countries in the Gulf Cooperation Council (Doctoral dissertation). *UCL* **2016**. Available online: https://discovery.ucl.ac.uk/id/eprint/1498905/1/PhD%20thesis%20.pdf (accessed on 13 November 2021).
9. Pharmacy School Admission Requirements. Available online: https://www.aacp.org/resource/pharmacy-school-admission-requirements (accessed on 13 November 2021).
10. Pharmacy Entry Requirements. Available online: https://www.pharmacyschoolscouncil.ac.uk/study/entry-requirements/ (accessed on 13 November 2021).
11. Anderson, D.C.; Sheffield, M.C.; Hill, A.M.; Cobb, H.H. Influences on Pharmacy Students' Decision to Pursue a Doctor of Pharmacy Degree. *Am. J. Pharm. Educ.* **2008**, *72*, 22. [CrossRef] [PubMed]
12. Truter, I. Motivation and career prospects of pharmacy students at Nelson Mandela Metropolitan University: A preliminary study. *Jordan J. Pharm. Sci.* **2009**, *2*, 159–166.
13. Eldalo, A.; Albarraq, A.; Sirag, N.; Ibrahim, M. Pharmacy students' perception about education and future career. *Arch. Pharm. Pract.* **2014**, *5*, 72. [CrossRef]
14. Woldekidan, N.A.; Mohammed, A.S.; Belachew, E.A. Pharmacy Students Motivation, Preparation and Factors Affecting Pursuing Postgraduate Education in Ethiopian University. *Adv. Med. Educ. Pract.* **2020**, *11*, 429–436. [CrossRef]
15. Modipa, S.I.; Dambisya, Y.M. Profile and career preferences of pharmacy students at the University of Limpopo, Turfloop Campus, South Africa. *Educ. Health Chang. Learn. Pract.* **2008**, *21*, 21.
16. Willis, S.C.; Shann, P.; Hassell, K. Who will be tomorrow's pharmacists and why did they study pharmacy? *Pharm. J.* **2006**, *277*, 107–108.
17. Roller, L. Intrinsic and extrinsic factors in choosing pharmacy as a course of study at Monash University 1999–2004. In Proceedings of the 13th International Social Pharmacy Workshop, Msida, Malta; 2004; pp. 19–23. Available online: https://www.um.edu.mt/library/oar/handle/123456789/13430 (accessed on 13 November 2021).
18. Abdelhadi, N.; Wazaify, M.; Elhajji, F.D.; Basheti, I. Doctor of Pharmacy in Jordan: Students' Career Choices, Perceptions and Expectations. *J. Pharm. Nutr. Sci.* **2014**, *4*, 213–219. [CrossRef]
19. Alhaddad, M.S. Undergraduate pharmacy students' motivations, satisfaction levels, and future career plans. *J. Taibah Univ. Med Sci.* **2018**, *13*, 247–253. [CrossRef] [PubMed]
20. Keshishian, F.; Brocavich, J.M.; Boone, R.T.; Pal, S. Motivating Factors Influencing College Students' Choice of Academic Major. *Am. J. Pharm. Educ.* **2010**, *74*, 46. [CrossRef] [PubMed]
21. Hanna, L.-A.; Askin, F.; Hall, M. First-Year Pharmacy Students' Views on Their Chosen Professional Career. *Am. J. Pharm. Educ.* **2016**, *80*, 150. [CrossRef] [PubMed]
22. Bin Saleh, G.; Rezk, N.L.; Laika, L.; Ali, A.; El-Metwally, A. Pharmacist, the pharmaceutical industry and pharmacy education in Saudi Arabia: A questionnaire-based study. *Saudi Pharm. J.* **2015**, *23*, 573–580. [CrossRef]
23. Taylor, D.A.; Patton, J.M. The pharmacy student population: Applications received 2009-10, degrees conferred 2009-10, fall 2010 enrollments. *Am. J. Pharm. Educ.* **2011**, *75*, S3. [CrossRef]
24. Taylor, J.N.; Taylor, D.A.; Nguyen, N.T. The Pharmacy Student Population: Applications Received 2014-15, Degrees Conferred 2014-15, Fall 2015 Enrollments. *Am. J. Pharm. Educ.* **2016**, *80*, S3. [CrossRef] [PubMed]
25. Taylor, J.N.; Taylor, D.A.; Nguyen, N.T. The Pharmacy Student Population: Applications Received 2015-16, Degrees Conferred 2015-16, Fall 2016 Enrollments. *Am. J. Pharm. Educ.* **2017**, *81*, S8. [CrossRef] [PubMed]
26. Kheir, N.; Zaidan, M.; Younes, H.; El Hajj, M.; Wilbur, K.; Jewesson, P.J. Pharmacy education and practice in 13 Middle Eastern countries. *Am. J. Pharm. Educ.* **2008**, *72*, 133. [CrossRef] [PubMed]
27. ALA. Worldometers. Available online: https://www.worldometers.info/world-population/saudi-arabia-population/ (accessed on 13 November 2021).
28. U.S. Ethics Ratings Rise for Medical Workers and Teachers. Available online: https://news.gallup.com/poll/328136/ethics-ratings-rise-medical-workers-teachers.aspx (accessed on 13 November 2021).
29. James, P.B.; Batema, M.N.P.; Bah, A.J.; Brewah, T.S.; Kella, A.T.; Lahai, M.; Jamshed, S.Q. Was Pharmacy Their Preferred Choice? Assessing Pharmacy Students' Motivation to Study Pharmacy, Attitudes and Future Career Intentions in Sierra Leone. *Health Prof. Educ.* **2018**, *4*, 139–148. [CrossRef]

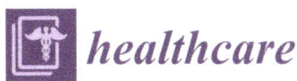

Article

Assessment of Pharmacists Prescribing Practices in Poland—A Descriptive Study

Agnieszka Zimmermann [1], Jakub Płaczek [2], Natalia Wrzosek [1] and Artur Owczarek [3,*]

1. Department of Medical and Pharmacy Law, Medical University of Gdańsk, 80-210 Gdańsk, Poland; agnieszka.zimmermann@gumed.edu.pl (A.Z.); natalia.wrzosek@gumed.edu.pl (N.W.)
2. Department of Pharmacoeconomics and Pharmacy Law, Collegium Medicum in Bydgoszcz Nicolaus Copernicus University in Torun, 85-089 Bydgoszcz, Poland; jakub.placzek@cm.umk.pl
3. Department of Drug Form Technology, Wroclaw Medical University, 50-556 Wroclaw, Poland
* Correspondence: artur.owczarek@umw.edu.pl

Abstract: Pharmacists play a beneficial role in supplying medicines to patients. Pharmacist prescribing practices were introduced into law in Poland in 2002, permitting pharmacists to prescribe medications in emergency situations and in 2020 the new law allowed to prescribe in all situation where it is needed because of the health risks reasons. Our aim was to analyze pharmacist prescribing practices in Poland and confirm the useful of pharmacists' activity in this area. Additionally, pharmacists were also authorized to issue reimbursed prescriptions for themselves or their family members. Since January 2020, only e-prescriptions are allowed in Poland. A retrospective analysis of the inspection written reports from 842 community pharmacies in the representative region of Poland with a population of two million, carried out in the time period from 2002 to 2016 was performed (2189 prescriptions) to assess the emergency pharmacist prescribing practices in Poland. The second part of the research was based on digital data on pharmacists prescriptions (18,529) provided by the e-Health Centre (a governmental organization under the Ministry of Health responsible for the development of health care information systems in Poland), enabling to conduct the analysis of pharmacist's prescribing from 1 of April 2020 to 31 of October 2020. The analysis gave the insight of the evolution of the pharmacy prescribing patterns. In general, pharmaceutical prescriptions were issued in cities with more than 100,000 inhabitants, in town- or city center pharmacies, and in pharmacies in residential areas. The most common reason for a pharmaceutical prescription was that the patient was running out of a medicine and was unable to contact their physician. Cardiovascular, respiratory, dermatological, and digestive medications were most frequently prescribed. An analysis of pharmacists' prescribing data from 1 April 2020 to 31 October 2020 confirmed the rapid increase of pharmaceutical prescriptions following implementation of the new legislative act during the COVID-19 epidemic.

Keywords: prescriptions; community pharmacy services; emergency prescribing; pharmacy practice; pharmacy law and regulation; COVID-19

1. Introduction

In its classic sense, a prescription is a specific message conveyed by a person authorized to issue such a document to a person who fills it in a pharmacy. It contains information on the medicines prescribed to the patient, data identifying both the patient and the author of the prescription, as well as the place and date of issue. In Poland, the right to prescribe belongs to physicians, nurses, midwifes and, pharmacists [1].

Pharmacist prescribing was legislated in Poland on 1 October 2002. It was limited only to emergency situations. Prior to this date, medical dispensing was determined by the type of medicine. A professional pharmacy employee (either the pharmacist or the pharmacy technician) was permitted to dispense a single packet of a medicine, which was reserved for medical prescribing, provided it was allocated to an adequate dispensing category, i.e., Rp. (Rp with a dot). However, patients have to pay 100% costs of the drug. Pharmacist emergency prescribing was possible only if "immediate risk to patient health" appeared. However, in Polish Pharmaceutical Law this term was inadequately defined. Instead, a de facto definition, derived from other regulations governing medical emergency services, became commonplace based on the assumption that "immediate risk" means the sudden onset of symptoms associated with serious damage to bodily functions, bodily injury or death, which may require an immediate or emergency medical response. Polish case law also added additional context to a health hazard, which included the need to demonstrate an imminent threat and therefore the significant probability of personal injury and risk of mortality, whether immediate or impending. In the pharmacy, the pharmacist assesses each case and determines whether there is an imminent health risk. The problem of defining what an immediate need is in pharmaceutical practice is also reviewed in the literature [2]. "Emergency prescribing" in exceptional cases, for instance, when there is an immediate risk to patient health, was introduced in several countries including the UK, Australia, the United States, and Canada [3,4]. In the UK, as in Poland, a pharmacist has discretionary power to dispense prescription-only medicine when a patient is unable to present the appropriate prescription and after interviewing the patient. This commonly occurs when a travelling patient forgot to pack their medication. Psychotropic medications and narcotics, except for phenobarbital (limited to a five-day course of treatment) for epilepsy sufferers, are excluded from these provisions. All such dispensing requires formal documentation [4] including a description of the exceptional circumstances. The pharmacist's discretion only extends to dispensing medicine and to the continuation of existing therapy, but does not authorize the pharmacist to initiate new therapy.

Beginning on 1 April 2020, during coronavirus epidemy, pharmacists were permitted to issue a prescription to any patient in any situation that posed a risk to health. Pharmacists may exceed the 180 days prescribing limit for consecutive pharmacist-prescribed renewals in circumstances where the patient is unable to be assessed by their primary care provider. This temporary provision allows pharmacists to exceed the 180 days prescribing limit for renewals during a public health emergency/crisis for patients who do not have a primary care provider or are unable to access them at this time. Pharmaceutical prescriptions may be issued for all medicines except for narcotics and psychiatric medications. The patient does not receive any reimbursement from the NHF. The pharmacist is not, however, authorized to carry out physical examinations, but must perform a diagnostic interview. Since 1 April 2020, the pharmacist was also authorized to self-prescribe. They are allowed to issue a reimbursed prescription for themselves or their family members. Initial statutory provisions (effective from 2002 to January 2020) required a pharmacist to issue a paper version of the prescription, but this was replaced by electronic documentation since January 2020. The record of each pharmaceutical prescription can identify the person who entered data and the date the prescription was filled. Table 1 summarizes Polish policies for issuing prescriptions by the pharmacist before and after the COVID-19 epidemic.

Pharmacists could prescribe in minor ailments. Enabling pharmacist prescribing for minor ailments to make easier access to health care in a more timely fashion, help improve health outcomes, and reduce costs-per-visit for a variety of non-critical medical conditions. This demonstrates that a significant number of patient visits to walk-in clinics, family doctors, and emergency departments would be prevented, as patients could receive care at the pharmacy. Minor ailments are considered health conditions that can typically be self-diagnosed by patients such as urinary tract infections, upper respiratory tract infections, contact dermatitis, conjunctivitis, and athlete's foot and can be managed with minimal treatment or straightforward self-care strategies [6]. Pharmacists could also prescribe in chronic conditions mainly renewals prescriptions. Chronic conditions are the largest cause of death and disability in the world. In ambulatory care settings, pharmacists assume responsibility for the management of chronic conditions such as hypertension, asthma, diabetes, hyperlipidaemia, and psychiatric disorders [7].

Table 1. Practice differences for issuing prescriptions in Poland before and after the COVID-19 epidemic was declared and law regulatory changes [5].

Pharmacist Prescribing Rules	Before 31st March 2020	After 1st April 2020
Prescription type	Only the paper version was technically possible	The electronic prescription is preferred and made available. The paper version only in exceptional cases
Reasons for issuing a prescription	Immediate health risk	Health risk
Amount of medicine	The smallest, single registered packet of the given medicine	In the case of electronic prescriptions, the amount of medicine required for 180 days of therapy for the given dose
Types of medicines	Prescription-only medicines except narcotics and psychotropic medication	Prescription-only medicines except narcotics and psychotropic medication
Information needed on the prescription	The same as on the prescription issued by a physician, and the reason for dispensing the medicine	The same as on the prescription issued by a physician and the reason for dispensing the medicine
Reimbursement	0%	0%, excluding prescriptions issued for the pharmacist himself/herself or his/her family members

To date, no study has been published that comprehensively describes pharmaceutical services associated with pharmacist prescribing in community pharmacies in Poland. The primary purpose of reviewing pharmacist prescribing practices, which is still evolving in Poland, is to help fill this knowledge gap. As of the 1 April 2020, Poland a country in Central Europe with a population of 37 million, has substantially expanded the pharmacists' competences by implementing the regulation that permits to issue a prescription to any patient in any situation posing a risk to health. This regulation and its consequences for the healthcare system may in the close future have significant impact on pharmaceutical regulation in other countries of the Central and Eastern Europe region, where Poland is the only one which permits pharmacists to prescribe [8,9].

The objective of this study was to analyze pharmacist prescribing practices in the Polish healthcare system and describe the evolution of that pharmacist service during 18 years. Comparison of prescribing practices including the most common therapeutic areas was made to find evidence for an expansion in the scope of pharmacists' practice in Poland. Findings may give an insight for future service planning in other European countries with no pharmacy prescribing service existing. Findings of this research add to the international literature on pharmacist prescribing and through identification of models of prescribing and medicines prescribed to inform future education and policy.

2. Materials and Methods
2.1. Study Designed and Settings

To understand and find the scope of pharmacist prescribing in Poland, the researchers conducted an analysis of the emergency prescription conditions and practice and then compared this data with an analysis of the actual patterns of prescribing by pharmacist prescribers. Data were obtained from two sources. A retrospective analysis of inspection reports from all community pharmacies in the study region (representative voivodeships in Poland) from the period 2002 to 2019 was carried out to assess emergency pharmacist prescribing practices in Poland (first phase of the study). During this time, all prescriptions were paper and not digitalized and could be filled only in an emergency situation. The scope of the study also assessed the preliminary effects of the new pharmaceutical law in Poland that was implemented in April 2020. In the second phase, a retrospective analysis of a database showing pharmacist prescribing habits in the study region from 1 April 2020 to 31 October 2020, when the pharmacy prescription was allowed not only in emergency situations was made. Digitalized data from 2020 was obtained from the e-Health Centre (Centrum e-Zdrowia [CeZ]), a governmental organization under the Ministry of Health responsible for the development of health care information systems in Poland.

The paper data, which were subjected to a first phase of the study were provided by the Regional Pharmaceutical Inspectorate in Bydgoszcz. The researcher, who was legally obliged to act under strict confidentiality terms and disclose only anonymized data, searched the inspectorate's archives. Every written inspection report from community pharmacies containing lists of issued pharmaceutical prescriptions was included in our study. Documentation from all community pharmacies that were in operation in this area during the study period was analyzed. There were 650 active pharmacies when the collection of the study's secondary dataset was completed. To obtain a complete picture, we also analyzed the paper records of pharmacies that were no longer in business, but that had operated at least for a short period following the introduction of the term "pharmaceutical prescription" in Polish legislation (i.e., following 1 October 2002). Consequently, data from a total of 842 community pharmacies were included in our analysis. Since the State Pharmaceutical Inspectorate neither collected nor stored data concerning pharmacies and inspections in electronic databases, we had to undertake a labor-intensive examination of paper-based reports stored in folders by pharmacies. The data were gathered from inspection reports issued following comprehensive elective controls conducted by pharmaceutical inspectors who inspected every operational aspect of each pharmacy. Occasionally, inspections' control of comply by legal regulations concerning pharmaceutical prescriptions was ad hoc. Audited area included a region of Poland with a population of over 2 million inhabitants.

The second stage of the study was based on an analysis of the data on all the pharmacist prescriptions from the public records held by the CeZ. This process involved writing to the CeZ with our research request, in which we were required to demonstrate that there was a significant public interest in the research findings that would result, before we were granted access to the data. We were also required to explain that ours was a scientific study that would generate neutral (objective) results showing trends and how implementation of pharmacist prescribing was working.

2.2. Ethical Considerations

The research project received approval from the Independent Bioethics Committee for Scientific Research at Nicolaus Copernicus University of Torun Collegium Medicum in Bydgoszcz (reference number 665/2015). The data acquired was anonymized by a suitable public administrator (Voivodeship Pharmaceutical Inspectorate in Bydgoszcz, CeZ) before sharing for researchers of the content and did not contain any personal data. Only information about the prescribed drugs and the patient's age was disclosed by both agencies (Voivodeship Pharmaceutical Inspectorate in Bydgoszcz, CeZ), without any possibility to identify a patient. Therefore, no informed consent from the patients was necessary. The study was designed to be a "non-invasive study". The study was conducted in accordance with the requirements of the Polish Data Protection Act, which implemented Regulation EU 2016/679 of the European Parliament and of the Council of 27 April 2016. According to this act and patients' rights act, anonymous data (with no possibility to identify the patient) do not need the informed consent from the patient. Data were stored on a Compact Disc (CD) secured with a login password and secured in a strongbox in a locked office.

2.3. Data Collection

Analysis of the data gathered from the paper reports allowed us to determine the number of pharmaceutical prescriptions issued, the reasons for dispensing each medicine, and the types of medicine dispensed. The Anatomical Therapeutic Chemical (ATC) Classification System was used to analyze the types of prescribed medicines. Prescriptions did not contain any information about the age of the patient, as this requirement was introduced in 2020. The location for each issuing pharmacy was recorded (i.e., village, city < 100,000, city > 100,000), their location within the town/city (e.g., in the vicinity of a hospital or outpatient clinic, in a shopping center, in a residential area, in the center of the town/city), and their operating hours (i.e., 24-h service, on Sundays and public and bank holidays).

Once we had received CeZ permission to get data from the public database, we were sent all the prescriptions on an encrypted CD. Because of the nature of the data contained in the file and the fact that they included prescriptions, the researchers were required to ensure that the data was kept secure. The data CD received was encrypted and the access code was provided to only one person from the research team. When not in use, the data CD was stored in a key-locked cabinet in a secure room with limited access to authorized personnel only.

2.4. Data Analysis

The data were manually digitized in a database using Microsoft Excel (Microsoft Corp., Redmond, WA, USA). Coding and data entry accuracy was checked by a second person from the research team. Statistical analysis was carried out to assess whether the pharmacies' operating schedule, location, or position within the town/city had any impact on the number of pharmaceutical prescriptions issued or filled. The following statistical tools were used: quantity and percent values, which were also presented as bar graphs; mean and standard deviation calculations; non-parametric Mann–Whitney U test to assess the differences between two populations; non-parametric Spearman's rank correlation coefficient to assess the relationship between two variables; non-parametric Kruskal–Wallis analysis of variance (ANOVA) rank test to assess the differences when multiple independent groups were compared; post hoc tests for multiple comparisons; and Fisher's least significant difference (LSD) test. In the second phase of the study, all analyzed variables were nominal using data from the CeZ. Frequency and contingency tables compiled on the basis of both raw data and percentages were used to assess the correlation between the aforementioned. Similar statistical tools were used, including quantity and percent values, which were also presented as bar graphs.

3. Results

The first phase of the study analyzed the records of pharmaceutical prescriptions from 842 pharmacies. One hundred and twelve (13.3%) were pharmacies operating in villages and towns with less than 1500 inhabitants, 375 (44.5%) were in towns and cities greater than 1500 and fewer than 100,000 inhabitants, and 355 (42.4%) were pharmacies in cities with a population greater than 100,000. A total of 569 pharmacies (67.6%) operated during standard opening hours Mondays to Saturdays, 17 (2.0%) were open 24 h and seven days a week, 143 pharmacies (17%) operated with extended opening hours, including Sundays, holidays and public holidays, and 113 pharmacies (13.4%) operated periodically on an on-duty basis at times stipulated by local authorities. The nature of the data enabled us to classify each according to their neighborhood characteristics. Three hundred (35.6%) were located in the vicinity of a hospital or an out-patient clinic, 74 (8.8%) operated in shopping centers, 281 (33.4%) were located in residential areas, and 187 (22.2%) were operated in town/city centers. Table 2 presents the quantitative distribution of pharmacies based on their position and the population size of where they were located.

Table 2. The distribution of the studied pharmacies based on their location and position within the town/city.

Location	Rural Area		City < 100,000		City > 100,000
Position	n	%	n	%	n
Neighborhood of out-patient clinic or hospital	59	52.7	134	35.7	107
Shopping center	2	1.8	35	9.3	37
Residential area	43	38.4	85	22.7	153
Town/city center	8	7.1	121	32.3	58
Total	112	100.0	375	100.0	355

Analysis of pharmacy inspection reports showed that 2189 pharmaceutical prescriptions were issued. The highest incidence rate of prescriptions issued was in cities with a population greater than 100,000. Our data showed that no pharmaceutical prescriptions were issued in pharmacies that were located in villages. With respect to operating hours, the highest rate of issued pharmaceutical prescriptions was in pharmacies open during standard hours from Monday to Saturday (3.04) and those operating periodically on an on-duty basis (1.98); the lowest number of prescriptions issued was in pharmacies open 24 h and seven days a week (0.76 prescriptions). In our data, only three prescriptions were issued at night in pharmacies operating on a 24-h basis. With respect to locations within their town/city, pharmacies in town/city centers and those in residential areas showed the highest index of prescriptions issued (4.14 and 3.48, respectively). The lowest index was observed in pharmacies situated near out-patient clinics or hospitals (1.11) (Table 3).

Table 3. Statistical analysis of the number of pharmaceutical prescriptions based on pharmacy location.

Pharmacy Location	n	Mean	SD	CI −95.0%	CI +95.0%	Minimum	Maximum
Neighborhood of out-patient clinic or hospital	300	1.11	13.421	−0.42	2.63	0.0	218.0
Shopping center	74	1.42	7.503	−0.32	3.16	0.0	53.0
Residential area	281	3.48	30.094	−0.05	7.01	0.0	431.0
Town/city center	187	4.14	30.816	−0.31	8.58	0.0	371.0

After the introduction of legislation in 2020 for pharmacist prescribing practices in the study region, a steady increase in the number of prescriptions issued by pharmacists was observed; over 1100 prescriptions were issued in April, which increased to almost 3900 in September and consisted of a total of over 18,500 pharmacist prescriptions at evaluated period. A detailed analysis of the number of pharmaceutical prescriptions is presented in Figure 1.

In Table 4, the percentage of medicines prescribed by pharmacist's including to the ATC Classification System from 1 April to 31 October 2020 is shown. Over a period of seven months, the highest percentage of prescriptions were related to those used for cardiovascular diseases (3436; 18.54%), alimentary tract diseases and metabolism disorders (2316; 12.50%), nervous system (2121; 11.45%), and those used in dermatological diseases (2057; 11.10%).

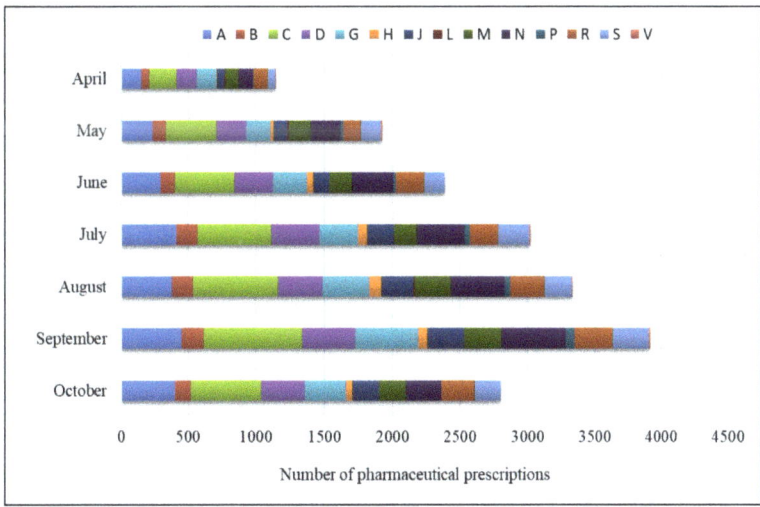

Figure 1. Pharmacist prescribing practices in the Kuyavian-Pomeranian and the types of prescribed medicines according to ATC Classification System from 1 April to 30 October 2020 (data provided by the CeZ); A—Alimentary tract and metabolism, B—Blood and blood forming organs, C—Cardiovascular system, D—Dermatologicals, G—Genito-urinary system and sex hormones, H—Systemic hormonal preparations, excluding sex hormones and insulins, J—Antiinfectives for systemic use, L—Antineoplastic and immunomodulating agents, M—Musculo-skeletal system, N—Nervous system, P—Antiparasitic products, insecticides and repellents, R—Respiratory system, S—Sensory organs, V—Various.

Table 4. Prescribed drugs by pharmacists according to the ATC Classification System in the analyzed region from 1st April to 30th October 2020.

ATC Code	Total Pharmacist Prescribing 1 April–30 October	Percentage of Pharmacist's Prescribing in the Month							Σ [%]
		April	May	June	July	August	September	October	
A	2316	0.80	1.27	1.59	2.23	2.03	2.43	2.16	12.50
B	859	0.32	0.51	0.58	0.83	0.86	0.87	0.65	4.64
C	3436	1.10	2.02	2.36	2.95	3.37	3.93	2.81	18.54
D	2057	0.82	1.21	1.55	1.93	1.77	2.09	1.73	11.10
G	1948	0.78	0.94	1.33	1.51	1.86	2.48	1.62	10.51
H	357	0.02	0.13	0.26	0.38	0.47	0.39	0.27	1.93
J	1151	0.30	0.54	0.62	1.02	1.25	1.46	1.03	6.21
L	22	0.02	0.05	0.00	0.00	0.04	0.00	0.00	0.12
M	1348	0.52	0.89	0.91	0.91	1.47	1.51	1.08	7.28
N	2121	0.60	1.16	1.62	1.93	2.16	2.57	1.40	11.45
P	193	0.02	0.11	0.13	0.23	0.22	0.34	0.00	1.04
R	1427	0.56	0.70	1.10	1.10	1.34	1.55	1.35	7.70
S	1256	0.30	0.78	0.84	1.25	1.12	1.46	1.03	6.78
V	38	0.02	0.05	0.00	0.04	0.04	0.05	0.00	0.21
Σ	18,529	6.20	10.39	12.89	16.28	18.00	21.13	15.11	100.00

A—Alimentary tract and metabolism, B—Blood and blood forming organs, C—Cardiovascular system, D—Dermatologicals, G—Genito-urinary system and sex hormones, H—Systemic hormonal preparations, excluding sex hormones and insulins, J—Antiinfectives for systemic use, L—Antineoplastic and immunomodulating agents, M—Musculo-skeletal system, N—Nervous system, P—Antiparasitic products, insecticides and repellents, R—Respiratory system, S—Sensory organs, V—Various.

Comparing the type of medicines prescribed by pharmacists from 2002–2019 and during 2020 indicated a difference in prescribing practices in ATC groups, including drugs use for systemic hormonal preparations (0.70% vs. 1.93% in 2020), medicines used to treat nervous system disorders (6.60% vs. 11.45% in 2020), anti-infectives medicines for systemic use (16.8% vs. 6.21% in 2020), medicines used in respiratory system diseases (15.20% vs. 7.70% in 2020), and medicines used in sensory organs diseases (13.50% vs. 6.78% in 2020), as shown in Figure 2. Important observations showed anti-infective drugs to have a reduced percentage level in pharmaceutical prescription in this therapeutic group. Additionally, drug prescription by pharmacists of new ATC groups: dermatological group (11.10%), genito-urinary system, and sex-hormones (10.51%) was observed, and no pharmaceutical prescription was found in the first part of the study.

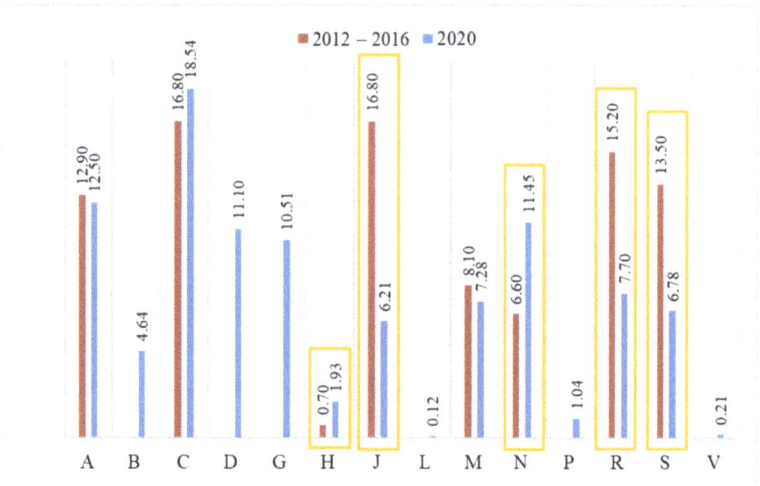

Figure 2. Medicines prescribed by pharmacists according to the ATC Classification System in the Kuyavian-Pomeranian Voivodeship from 2002 to 2016 and from 1 April to 30 October 2020.

4. Discussion

Twenty World Health Organization (WHO) member states (10% of member states) authorize pharmacists and nurses to prescribe medicines, which is widely accepted by both healthcare professionals and patients [10–12]. The evolution of pharmacist prescribing practices have differed among these countries. Sweden adopted the idea of "repeat prescribing" [13], while Canada and the United Kingdom (UK) adopted so-called "independent prescribing" [14–18]. One reason many developing and developed countries introduced pharmacist prescribing was to give patients better access to healthcare services, including access to medicines. Studies also indicate the importance pharmacist prescribing after-hours and in emergency situations [19,20]. Published studies on emergency prescribing practices are scarce. One UK study [4] analyzed the emergency dispensing processes of prescription-only medicines by pharmacists. The four-week, four-stage study took place in 22 community pharmacies with varying ownership arrangements, gathered data from patients, pharmacists, and general physicians. Eight pharmacies were in the vicinity of a healthcare facility, nine in shopping centers, three in town/city centers, and two in other parts of the town/city. Fourteen pharmacies operated Monday to Friday, five from Monday to Saturday, and three included Sunday trading. A total of 526 medicinal products were dispensed to 450 patients (in 90% of cases, the prescription was for a single preparation). The need for pharmacist intervention increased on weekends and public holidays was observed. Overall, most dispensing occurred on Mondays or Fridays. Fridays accounted for nearly 25% of all cases. Most dispensing was for elderly patients (137 events for patients aged 60–74, 116 for those aged 45–59, and 94 for those older than 75 years). Predominantly, patients sought medicines to continue their current therapy, a similar finding observed in our study. The medicines that were most commonly dispensed were for cardiovascular (32%), respiratory (13%), endocrine (12%), and gastrointestinal diseases (11%). The UK study indicates that demand for emergency and repeat prescribing emphasizes the important role of the pharmacist and community pharmacies in the healthcare system. An English study showed that patients commonly sought a recurrent need for medicines related to cardiovascular, endocrine, and gastrointestinal diseases [21]. The demand for medicines used to treat respiratory diseases was half of that found in the Morecroft et al. study [4]. In a study based on 401 pharmacists by George et al. that evaluated cases of supplementary prescribing, prescribed medicines were used mostly for cardiovascular diseases [17]. One American study indicated that 75% of pharmacists only fill emergency prescriptions several times a month and that they may dispense antibiotics, inhaled medications, antidiabetic medicines, and drugs used for nausea and vomiting [22]. Our own data analysis indicated that the most common prescriptions were for cardiovascular medicines and anti-infectives. Our study showed that most cases of pharmacist prescribing took place during normal business hours, similar to findings in Morecroft et al. [4].

Pharmacists who prescribe medicines for themselves or their family members when a long-term medicine was running low is a common practice and was granted legal status in the 2020 Law that included reimbursable and non-reimbursable medicines. Though providing healthcare services to oneself and/or family members is generally considered inappropriate and may be regarded as a conflict of interest, issuing a prescription to any person in an emergency situation, or when another appropriate health professional is not readily available, are both permitted.

In addition to peer-reviewed scientific studies, data on pharmacist prescribing practices may be gathered from official health sector reports such as the Prescription Analysis and Cost (PACT) reports in the UK. In the report summarizing the first period after the introduction of emergency prescribing in the UK (2004–2006), the data indicate that pharmacist prescribing practices initially remained low, but then increased from 2706 in 2004 to 31,052 by 2006; however, these values represent a small proportion (0.004%) of all medicines prescribed in UK healthcare facilities. The medicines most commonly prescribed by pharmacists were those used for chronic diseases, including cardiovascular (mainly acetylcholinesterase converting enzyme inhibitors, diuretics, nitrates, calcium channel blockers, antianginal medicines, and lipid level regulating drugs), nervous system therapy (pain medication, anxiolytics and hypnotics), respiratory conditions (bronchodilatators, mainly corticosteroids), endocrine disorders (for diabetes in more than 50% of cases), and gastrointestinal diseases. In monetary terms, emergency prescribing practices increased from GBP 25,348 in 2004 to GBP 278,634 in 2006 [23]. Studies have shown that oftentimes, when patients are unable to access emergency supply services, they stop taking their medication. In a UK study of 227 community pharmacies, a total of 2485 patients needed emergency dispensing and most went to the pharmacy on Saturdays and national holidays. The elderly were heavily represented in these data. Of 3226 dispensing cases, 439 were classified as high-risk events. Patients' easy access to the emergency services increased their willingness to contact the community pharmacy in the future for medication-related issues [24]. Studies have reported medication-related non-adherence as a frequent reason for hospital admissions [25]. Not having access to medications used in long-term therapy may pose a significant risk to the patient.

For the first time, data on pharmacist prescribing practices in study region after the introduction of legislation effecting pharmacist prescribing practices showed a steady increase in the number of prescriptions issued by pharmacists from April to October 2020. This confirms the impact of recent legislative changes and how pharmacists can help with the prescription of medicines to address health needs. Moreover its demonstrate the effective role of researchers (science advocacy) in helping preparation and validation of new regulatory solutions [26].

This study has a few limitations to note. Our study is a descriptive study, so the subject of the research was not an assessment of the adequacy of the prescriptions and economic evaluation of the costs of this practice. The identification of factors related to patient characteristics was not carried out by the investigators. Pre- and pending pandemic differences in the prescribed drugs was identified only according to ATC groups. The results presented in the figures illustrated the observing changes adequately to pharmacy law transformation and changes of pharmacist prescribing practices in Poland.

5. Conclusions

Polish pharmacists most commonly issue prescriptions for medicines used for cardiovascular diseases, alimentary tract and metabolism, nervous system, or for those used in respiratory system diseases. This indicates that patients regard pharmacies as important healthcare facilities. The observed decreased trend in the pharmaceutical prescription of anti-invectives drugs is an expected phenomena, especially in the case of increasing antibiotics resistance and the lack in pharmacies of rapid diagnostic tests to identification of infection cause. Our study shows that retaining pharmacist prescribing practices in the Polish healthcare system is justified. The application of these kind of results help advocate for science and help demonstrate the role that research has contributed to new legislation in Poland. This indicates that such studies are required in shaping policy and legislation regarding pharmacist dispensing practices, as evidenced by the analysis of pharmacist prescribing practices following the legislative amendment.

Author Contributions: Conceptualization, A.Z., J.P. and A.O.; Methodology, J.P., A.Z., N.W. and A.O.; Software, J.P. and A.O.; Validation, A.Z. and A.O.; Formal analysis, A.Z.; Investigation, J.P., A.Z., N.W. and A.O.; Writing—original draft preparation, A.Z. and J.P.; Writing—review and editing, A.Z. and A.O.; Visualization, J.P. and A.O.; Supervision, A.Z. and A.O. All authors have read and agreed to the published version of the manuscript.

Funding: This research received no external funding.

Institutional Review Board Statement: The research project received approval from the Independent Bioethics Committee for Scientific Research at Nicolaus Copernicus University of Torun Collegium Medicum in Bydgoszcz (reference number 665/2015). All complies with the Polish regulations for the protection of personal data. All information included in this study is anonymized.

Informed Consent Statement: Not applicable.

Data Availability Statement: There are legal restrictions on sharing a de-identified data set, as specified by the Medical University of Gdańsk's inner regulations dedicated to employees. However, all surveys data is available upon request to researchers who meet the criteria for access to confidential data. Requests may be sent to the corresponding author.

Conflicts of Interest: The authors declare no conflict of interest.

References

1. Zimmermann, A.; Cieplikiewicz, E.; Wąż, P.; Gaworska-Krzemińska, A.; Olczyk, P. The implementation process of nurse prescribing in Poland—A descriptive study. *Int. J. Env. Res. Public Health* **2020**, *17*, 2020–2417. [CrossRef] [PubMed]
2. Hibbert, D.; Rees, J.A.; Smith, I. Ethical awareness of community pharmacists. *Int. J. Pharm. Pract.* **2000**, *8*, 82–87. [CrossRef]
3. Yuksel, N.; Eberhart, G.; Bungard, T.J. Prescribing by pharmacists in Alberta. *Am. J. Health Syst. Pharm.* **2008**, *65*, 2126–2132. [CrossRef] [PubMed]
4. Morecroft, C.W.; Mackridge, A.J.; Stokes, E.C.; Gray, N.J.; Wilson, S.E.; Ashcroft, D.M.; Mensah, N.; Pickup, G.B. Emergency supply of prescription-only medicines to patients by community pharmacists: A mixed methods evaluation incorporating patient, pharmacist and GP perspectives. *BMJ Open* **2015**, *5*, e006934. [CrossRef]
5. Pharmaceutical Law of 6 September 2001 (JL No. 126, item 1381) Consolidated Text of 15 March 2019 (JL item 499) and Consolidated Text of 28 May 2021 (JL item 974). Available online: http://isap.sejm.gov.pl/isap.nsf/DocDetails.xsp?id=wdu20011 261381 (accessed on 7 July 2021).
6. Kim, J.J.; Tian, A.H.; Pham, L.; Nakhla, N.; Houle, S.K.; Wong, W.W.; Alsabbagh, M.W. Economic evaluation of pharmacists prescribing for minor ailments in Ontario, Canada: A cost-minimization analysis. *Int. J. Pharm. Prac.* **2021**, *29*, 228–234. [CrossRef]

7. Mossialos, E.; Courtin, E.; Naci, H.; Benrimoj, S.; Bouvy, M.; Farris, K.; Noyce, P.; Sketris, I. From "retailers" to health care providers: Transforming the role of community pharmacists in chronic disease management. *Health Policy* **2015**, *119*, 628–639. [CrossRef]
8. Nachtigal, P.; Šimůnek, T.; Atkinson, J. Pharmacy Practice and Education in the Czech Republic. *Pharmacy* **2017**, *9*, 54. [CrossRef]
9. Soares, I.B.; Imfeld-Isenegger, T.L.; Makovec, U.N.; Horvat, N.; Kos, M.; Arnet, I.; Hersberger, K.E.; Costa, F.A. A survey to assess the availability, implementation rate and remuneration of pharmacist-led cognitive services throughout Europe. *Res. Soc. Adm. Pharm.* **2020**, *16*, 41–47. [CrossRef]
10. Weiss, M.C.; Sutton, J. The changing nature of prescribing: Pharmacists as prescribers and challenges to medical dominance. *Sociol. Health Illness* **2009**, *31*, 406–421. [CrossRef]
11. Latter, S.; Blenkinsopp, A.; Smith, A.; Chapman, S.; Tinelli, M.; Gerard, K.; Little, P.; Celino, N.; Granby, T.; Nicholls, P.; et al. *Evaluation of Nurse and Pharmacist Independent Prescribing*; Keele University: Southampton, UK, 2011.
12. Bhanbro, S.; Drennan, V.M.; Grant, R.; Harris, R. Assessing the contribution of prescribing in primary care by nurses and professionals allied to medicine: A systematic review of literature. *BMC Health Serv. Res.* **2011**, *11*, 330. [CrossRef]
13. Andersson, K.; Melander, A.; Svensson, C.; Lind, O.; Nilsson, J.L.G. Repeat prescriptions: Refill adherence in relation to patient and prescriber characteristics, reimbursement level and type of medication. *Eur. J. Public Health* **2005**, *15*, 621–626. [CrossRef]
14. Riley, R.; Weiss, M.C.; Platt, J.; Taylor, G.; Horrocks, S.; Taylor, A. A comparison of GP, pharmacist and nurse prescriber responses to patients' emotional cues and concerns in primary care consultations. *Patient Educ. Couns.* **2013**, *91*, 65–71. [CrossRef]
15. Famiyeh, I.M.; MacKeigan, L.; Thompson, A.; Kuluski, K.; McCarthy, L.M. Exploring pharmacy service users' support for and willingness to use community pharmacist prescribing services. *Res. Soc. Adm. Pharm.* **2019**, *15*, 575–583. [CrossRef]
16. Hoti, K.; Hughes, J.; Sunderland, B. Expanded prescribing: A comparison of the views of Australian hospital and community pharmacists. *Int. J. Clin. Pharm.* **2013**, *35*, 469–475. [CrossRef]
17. George, J.; Pfleger, D.; McCaig, D.; Bond, C.; Stewart, D. Independent prescribing by pharmacists: A study of the awareness, views and attitudes of Scottish community pharmacists. *Pharm. World Sci.* **2006**, *28*, 45–53. [CrossRef]
18. Auta, A.; Strickland-Hodge, B.; Maz, J. Stakeholders' views on granting prescribing authority to pharmacists in Nigeria: A qualitative study. *Int. J. Clin. Pharm.* **2016**, *38*, 960–967. [CrossRef]
19. Smith, J.; Picton, C.; Dayan, M. Now or never: Shaping pharmacy for the future. In *The Report of the Commission on Future Models of Care Delivered through Pharmacy*; Royal Pharmaceutical Society of Great Britain: London, UK, 2013.
20. Law, M.R.; Morgan, S.G.; Majumdar, S.R.; Lynd, L.D.; Marra, C.A. Effects of prescription adaptation by pharmacists. *BMC Health Serv. Res.* **2010**, *10*, 313. [CrossRef]
21. O'Neill, R.; Rowley, E.; Smith, F. The emergency supply of prescription-only medicines: A survey of requests to community pharmacists and their views on the procedures. *Int. J. Pharm. Pract.* **2002**, *10*, 77–83. [CrossRef]
22. Shepherd, M.D. Examination of why some community pharmacists do not provide 72-hour emergency prescription drugs to Medicaid patients when prior authorization is not available. *J. Manag. Care Spec. Pharm.* **2013**, *19*, 527–533. [CrossRef]
23. Guillaume, L.; Cooper, R.; Avery, A.; Mitchell, S.; Ward, P.; Anderson, C.; Bissell, P.; Hutchinson, A.; James, V.; Lymn, J.; et al. Supplementary prescribing by community pharmacists: An analysis of PACT data, 2004–2006. *J. Clin. Pharm. Ther.* **2008**, *33*, 11–16. [CrossRef]
24. Nazar, H.; Nazar, Z.; Simpson, J.; Yeung, A.; Whittlesea, C. Summative service and stakeholder evaluation of an NHS-funded community Pharmacy Emergency Repeat Medication Supply Service (PERMSS). *BMJ Open* **2016**, *6*, e009736. [CrossRef] [PubMed]
25. Howard, R.L.; Avery, A.J.; Howard, P.D.; Partridge, M. Investigation into the reasons for preventable drug related admissions to a medical admissions unit: Observational study. *Qual. Saf. Health Care* **2003**, *12*, 280–285. [CrossRef] [PubMed]
26. Runkle, D. Advocacy in science. In *Summary of Workshop Convened by the American Association for the Advancement of Science*; Frankel, M.S., Ed.; American Association for the Advancement of Science: Washington, DC, USA, 2012.

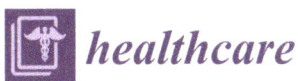

Article

Community Pharmacists' Practice, Awareness, and Beliefs about Drug Disposal in Saudi Arabia

Sultan Alghadeer [1,2,*] and Mohammed N. Al-Arifi [1]

[1] Department of Clinical Pharmacy, College of Pharmacy, King Saud University, Riyadh 11451, Saudi Arabia; malarifi@ksu.edu.sa
[2] Research Center, Basic Sciences Department, Prince Sultan College for EMS, King Saud University, Riyadh 11451, Saudi Arabia
* Correspondence: salghadeer@ksu.edu.sa

Abstract: The awareness among Saudi people regarding the good and safe practice of drug disposal is fairly low. Community pharmacists' potential toward drugs disposal directions and practice are not emphasized enough. Therefore, a cross sectional study was conducted in Riyadh, Saudi Arabia, to evaluate the practice, awareness and beliefs of community pharmacists about disposal of unused drugs. Out of 360 subjects who participated in the study, more than 70% returned the unused drugs to the pharmaceutical distributors. Around 80% of the participants confirmed the risk of environmental damage due to the inappropriate disposal of drugs, and 87.5% of them held themselves responsible for preventing such risk. Approximately 85% of surveyed pharmacists believed community pharmacies to be an appropriate location for the collection of unused drugs. There was no significant association between the community pharmacists' age group and years of practice as community pharmacists with either the awareness of unused medication disposal on environmental hazards, or the beliefs about the appropriate location for collecting unused drugs ($p > 0.05$). The awareness and proactive accountable responsibility, along with community pharmacists' belief of appointing pharmacies to collect unused drugs, strongly support the institution of drug take-back programs.

Keywords: community pharmacy; drug disposal; unused medication; environment; awareness; practice

Citation: Alghadeer, S.; Al-Arifi, M.N. Community Pharmacists' Practice, Awareness, and Beliefs about Drug Disposal in Saudi Arabia. *Healthcare* **2021**, *9*, 823. https://doi.org/10.3390/healthcare9070823

Academic Editor: Georges Adunlin

Received: 18 May 2021
Accepted: 25 June 2021
Published: 29 June 2021

Publisher's Note: MDPI stays neutral with regard to jurisdictional claims in published maps and institutional affiliations.

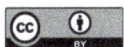

Copyright: © 2021 by the authors. Licensee MDPI, Basel, Switzerland. This article is an open access article distributed under the terms and conditions of the Creative Commons Attribution (CC BY) license (https://creativecommons.org/licenses/by/4.0/).

1. Introduction

In Saudi Arabia, the use of both prescribed and non-prescribed medications continues to increase. The concern for self-medication, regardless of whether they are prescribed items or over-the-counter drugs (OTC), seems to be a serious problem among the public in Saudi Arabia [1]. Such uncontrolled self-medication participates in avoidable excess of drug wastage, which has a negative impact financially and environmentally [2]. The mean drug waste was found to be 25.8% for Saudi families and 41.3% for families from other Gulf countries. A total of $150 million was the estimated expenditure on non-consumed drugs among people living in the Gulf countries [3].

Pharmaceuticals can go into the environment through human and animal excretion as well as through the disposal of unused medications [2,4]. Analgesics, anti-epileptics, beta-blockers and antidepressants were identified in 30 different locations in Sydney Harbor [5]. Additionally, the aforementioned pharmacological classes and other classes such as lipid-lowering agents, estrogens and others were identified on land and in the sea worldwide [6]. The most common sources for environmental contamination of pharmaceuticals included household disposal [7–9], industrial waste, hospital influent and effluent and human excreta [4,10]. Additionally, pharmaceuticals were found in low concentrations in surface water, ground water and treated drinking water [11–14]. Despite their availability in low concentrations in the environment, these pharmaceutical agents affect human health and water wildlife [15,16].

In Saudi Arabia, there is no authorized guideline for the disposal of unused drugs. A feasible option to deal with unused drugs is to return those drugs to the pharmacy [17]. However, this option seems to be seldom done in Saudi Arabia. Based on previous studies, the majority of the Saudi population dispose of their drugs in the household waste, while very few people return them to pharmacies [8,9]. These studies also showed that the awareness of Saudi people about the good and safe practice of drug disposal was fairly low.

Community pharmacists (CPs) have a great potential as accessible healthcare providers, who are approached by customers to recommend a pharmaceutical agent, dispense a prescription and counsel a patient regarding his/her medications. However, CPs' potential toward drugs disposal directions and practice are not emphasized enough. Therefore, the aim of this study was to evaluate the practice, awareness and beliefs of CPs about the disposal of unused drugs.

2. Materials and Methods

A cross sectional survey between July and August 2019 was conducted in the capital of the Kingdom of Saudi Arabia, Riyadh city. The self-administered survey was distributed in-person to investigate the CPs' practice, awareness and attitude about the disposal of drugs. Based on what about the community pharmacists' workforce in Saudi Arabia was determined by Alruthia et al. [18], the sample size (with 95% confidence interval and 5% margin of error) was calculated to be 368 participants. A convenient sample of community pharmacies from various areas was selected, based on the geographical areas of Riyadh city.

The questionnaire was adopted from previous studies and aimed to assess the practice and attitude of CPs towards drugs disposal in New Zealand and Kuwait [17,19]. The questionnaire consisted of four sections. The first section included questions about the demographic data of CPs. Three questions, aiming to assess the awareness of CPs towards environmental hazards, were available in the second section. All these questions were assessed utilizing a 5-point Likert scale of 1 to 5. However, the first two questions involved the terms 1 = do not know, 2 = no damage, 3 = no serious damage, 4 = some damage and 5 = serious damage, while the third question involved the terms 1 = strongly disagree, 2 = disagree, 3 = uncertain, 4 = agree and 5 = strongly agree. For suitability of statistical analysis, answers 'some damage' and 'serious damage' were compound to the response 'causes damage', and answers 'agree' and 'strongly agree' were compound to the answer 'agree'. The components of the third and fourth section were used to assess the beliefs of CPs associated to future procedures to control unused drugs, and to assess the practice of CPs towards the disposal of unused drugs, respectively. A pilot study was done among five CPs who have at least 5 years of experience working in community pharmacies in Saudi Arabia to assess the validity and reliability of the questionnaire. The content validity using the content validity index with a four-point Likert scale and the reliability using Cronbach's alpha coefficient were determined to be 0.8 and 0.7, respectively.

All collected data were entered into SPSS version 25, compatible with Windows for analysis. Fisher's exact test was conducted to find any significant association between respondents' demographic characteristics and items at a significance level of 0.05.

3. Results

The self-administered survey was distributed in-person to 400 CPs, and a total of 360 CPs (with 90% response rate) participated in the study. Table 1 shows the demographics of our participants.

Regardless of the various dosage forms, this survey found that the most common approaches for disposing unused medications were to send the medication back to the pharmaceutical distributor (between 73.3 and 75.3%), followed by putting medication in the medicines' bin (between 15.5 and 16.7%). Table 2 shows the disposal approaches of unused medications among CPs based on various dosage formulations.

Table 1. Demographics of participating pharmacists in the survey ($n = 360$ *).

Variables		N (%)
Age (years)	20–30	175 (48.6)
	31–40	134 (37.2)
	41–50	51 (14.2)
Qualification	B pharma	320 (88.9)
	Pharm D	15 (4.2)
	Master	17 (4.7)
	Diploma	3 (0.8)
Years of practice as community pharmacist	1–4	85 (23.6)
	5–9	156 (43.3)
	More than 10	118 (32.8.2)

* missing data; B pharm: Bachelor degree of pharmaceutical sciences; PharmD: Doctor of pharmacy degree.

Table 2. Disposal approaches of unused medications among community pharmacists based on various dosage formulations ($n = 360$ *).

Items	Answers	N (%)
SOLID dosage forms	In the rubbish bin	13 (3.6)
	In the sink	4 (1.1)
	In the toilet	7 (1.9)
	In a medicines' bin	58 (16.1)
	Sent back to pharmaceutical distributor	271 (75.3)
	Other	5 (1.4)
LIQUID dosage forms	In the rubbish bin	6 (1.7)
	In the sink	13 (3.6)
	In the toilet	16 (4.4)
	In a medicines' bin	55 (15.5)
	Sent back to pharmaceutical distributor	264 (73.3)
	Other	4 (1.1)
SEMI-SOLID preparations	In the rubbish bin	12 (3.3)
	In the sink	5 (1.4)
	In the toilet	10 (2.8)
	In a medicines' bin	60 (16.7)
	Sent back to pharmaceutical distributor	267 (74.2)
	Other	4 (1.1)

* missing data.

This study assessed the awareness of CPs regarding environmental hazards because of unused disposal drugs (Table 3). About 80% of CPs reported environmental damage as a result of unused medications being thrown in the sink or toilet. A very high percentage of CPs (87.5%) agreed that protecting the environment is one of their individual responsibilities. There was no significant association between the age group and years of practice as community pharmacy of CPs with any of the questions ($p > 0.05$).

Table 3. Awareness among community pharmacists of environmental hazards of unused medication disposal.

Items	Answers	N (%)
Effect of drug disposal on the environment	No damage	51 (14.7)
	Damage	284 (78.9)
	I don't know	23 (6.4)
Damage on the environment if you, as an individual, disposed of unused drugs by throwing them away in the sink or toilet	No damage	51 (14.2)
	Damage	287 (79.7)
	I don't know	22 (6.1)
Acknowledgment of personal responsibility	Disagree	25 (6.9)
	Uncertain	20 (5.612)
	Agree	315 (87.5)

For future reclaim programs in Saudi Arabia, the vast majority of the CPs believed that the most appropriate areas to place containers to collect unused medications were inside community pharmacies and pharmacies of public and private hospitals (Table 4). By assessing the impact of years of practice, no significant association was found between the age group of CPs and their years of practice in a community pharmacy with any of the beliefs ($p > 0.05$).

Table 4. Beliefs of community pharmacists about the appropriate location for collecting unused drugs.

Items	Answers	N (%)
Secure containers inside pharmacies within community pharmacies	Good idea	306 (85.0)
	Uncertain	30 (8.3)
	Not a good idea	23 (6.4)
Secure containers inside pharmacies within government hospitals	Good idea	309 (85.8)
	Uncertain	29 (8.1)
	Not a good idea	21 (5.8)
Secure containers inside pharmacies within private hospitals	Good idea	281 (78.1)
	Uncertain	37 (10.3)
	Not a good idea	41 (11.4)

4. Discussion

Inappropriate drug disposal can lead to potentially unfavorable consequences. Drug classes, such as antibiotics, analgesics and beta-blockers, have been identified in wastewater [20]. The uncontrolled presence of medications can negatively impact the natural living environment and health. The existence of antimicrobials in the environment may raise concern of antimicrobial resistance. Additionally, possible adverse effects and the unintended exposure risk of particular disposed medications were detected as affecting animals and humans, especially children [21–23]. Diclofenac (a non-steroidal anti-inflammatory medication) found in wastewater, for example, was shown to impair the renal function of brown trout [21]. The United States Food & Drug Administration (FDA) warned about fatalities among children due to accidental exposure to fentanyl patches, some of which were inappropriately wasted [22,23].

For this reason, many nations have established policies for the disposal of unused medications. The United States FDA developed governmental guidelines that encourage the availability of disposal instructions on drugs labels, establish a 'take-back' program for collecting and disposing unused medications in every city or county, and provide advice on disposing of unwanted drugs appropriately [23]. The integrated efforts of several agencies, such as the Department of Health and Social Care (DHSC), the National Health Services (NHS) of England and NHS Improvement, and the Pharmaceutical Services Negotiating Committee (PSNC) in the United Kingdom, resulted in formulating a policy necessitating community pharmacies to collect the unused medications from the public, and obligating the NHS to make a deal with a medical waste company to collect these medications from pharmacies frequently [24]. The Australian government conducted a similar program named 'Return Unwanted Medicine', where unused medications are collected by the community pharmacies [25]. In contrast, there are no policy guidelines for the disposal of unused medications in Saudi Arabia. Additionally, very few studies have been published about the knowledge and practice of appropriate disposal of drugs in the Middle East, particularly in Saudi Arabia [8].

In this study, the majority of CPs (between 73.3 and 75.3%) reported that the pharmaceutical supplier is the main route of disposing of solid or semi-solid as well as liquid unused medications. In contrast to a survey study conducted among pharmacists in Kuwait, about 73% of respondents disposed of unused medications in the trash and the toilet [19]. A similar survey study conducted among CPs in New Zealand revealed that the third-party contractors are a main route of disposal for solid (80%) and semi-solid (61%) unused medications [17]. However, the majority of surveyed CPs tends to dispose of the returned liquid (45%) and scheduled II controlled drugs (58%) into the sink inside the pharmacy. Such practice of disposing of the returned liquid and controlled drugs into sinks, and the practice of burning the unused medications by the third-party contractors, made 90% of community pharmacists in New Zealand call for the need of a destruction system by their health authority.

In Saudi Arabia, the current crucial need is for a policy to be formed by the Ministry of Health (MOH), which would permit community pharmacists to receive returned UMs from the general population and guide the pharmacists on their appropriate disposal [26]. The Saudi MOH published a general guideline for 'Implementing Regulations of Uniform Law for Medical Waste Management'. This guideline states that each health facility (including pharmacies) should have a contract with a company for waste removal. However, this guideline is general and does not focus on the return medication particularly. In addition, there is no guide or policy for community pharmacies to receive unused medications from the public.

Our CPs showed high awareness (79%) of the inappropriate disposal of medications, which may negatively impact the environment. Moreover, most of them (87.5%) held themselves responsible for protecting the environment from such risks. On the other hand, in another study, around 70% of Saudi drug consumers accounted themselves responsible for the proper way of disposing unused medications, and about 79% of them were willing to receive education or information on the proper way of disposing of unused medications [8]. About 85% of our surveyed pharmacists believe that community pharmacies are an appropriate location for the collection of unused medications. Additionally, the growing Saudi population requires the practice of the community pharmacy to be shifted more toward the paradigm of patient-centered care [27]. All these above-mentioned reasons may require immediate action to establish a drug-take program within community pharmacies in Saudi Arabia.

The study has some limitations. It was conducted only in one region, Riyadh. Saudi Arabia consists of thirteen regions. However, Riyadh is one of the largest regions in terms of population and area [28]. In addition, Riyadh has the highest number of pharmacists that comprise 35.64% of the total pharmacists in Saudi Arabia [18]. Our study was generalized, and doesn't specify the awareness and beliefs of disposing of 'hazardous medications' or 'controlled-drugs'. However, any drug could carry environmental or human risk if disposed inappropriately. Thus, our objective was to assess the practice, awareness and beliefs of drugs disposal in general regardless of any medications classifications.

5. Conclusions

The awareness and proactive accountable responsibility from both pharmacist and society, the beliefs of community pharmacists about the appropriate location for the collection of unused medications and the new practice of the community pharmacy strongly support the institution of drug take-back programs. To launch a national effective drug take-back program, the collaboration of different governmental sectors, along with national awareness on different levels, is necessary.

Author Contributions: Conceptualization, S.A. and M.N.A.-A.; methodology, M.N.A.-A.; validation, S.A.; formal analysis, M.N.A.-A.; investigation, S.A.; resources, M.N.A.-A.; data curation, M.N.A.-A.; writing—original draft preparation, M.N.A.-A. and S.A.; writing—review and editing, S.A.; visualization, S.A.; supervision, M.N.A.-A.; project administration, S.A.; funding acquisition, M.N.A.-A. All authors have read and agreed to the published version of the manuscript.

Funding: This research received no external funding.

Institutional Review Board Statement: This study was approved by the IRB at KSUMC as a part of project under the protocol number (E-19-3983).

Informed Consent Statement: Informed consent was obtained from all subjects involved in the study before conducting the survey.

Data Availability Statement: Data sharing not applicable.

Acknowledgments: The authors acknowledge the financial support from the Research Supporting Project (No. RSP-2021/81), King Saud University, Riyadh, Saudi Arabia.

Conflicts of Interest: The authors declare no conflict of interest.

References

1. AlKhamees, O.A.; AlNemer, K.A.; Maneea, M.W.B.; AlSugair, F.A.; AlEnizi, B.H.; Alharf, A.A. Top 10 most used drugs in the Kingdom of Saudi Arabia 2010–2015. *Saudi Pharm. J.* **2018**, *26*, 211–216. [CrossRef] [PubMed]
2. Glassmeyer, S.T.; Hinchey, E.K.; Boehme, S.E.; Daughton, C.G.; Ruhoy, I.S.; Conerly, O.; Daniels, R.L.; Lauer, L.; McCarthy, M.; Nettesheim, T.G.; et al. Disposal practices for unwanted residential medications in the United States. *Environ. Int.* **2009**, *35*, 566–572. [CrossRef]
3. Abou-Auda, H.S. An economic assessment of the extent of medication use and wastage among families in Saudi Arabia and Arabian Gulf countries. *Clin. Ther.* **2003**, *25*, 1276–1292. [CrossRef]
4. Kar, S.; Roy, K.; Leszczynski, J. Impact of Pharmaceuticals on the Environment: Risk Assessment Using QSAR Modeling Approach. *Methods Mol. Biol.* **2018**, *1800*, 395–443.
5. Scott, S.; Branley, A. Drugs Including Painkillers, Anti-Depressants Found in Tests on Sydney Harbour Water. *ABC News*. 6 July 2015. Available online: http://www.abc.net.au/news/2015-07-07/common-drugs-found-lurking-in-sydney-harbour-water/6599670 (accessed on 10 June 2021).
6. Murdoch, K. Pharmaceutical Pollution in the Environment: Issues for Australia, New Zealand and Pacific Island Countries. National Toxics Network. 2015. Available online: http://www.ntn.org.au/wp/wp-content/uploads/2015/05/NTN-Pharmaceutical-Pollution-in-the-Environment-2015-05.pdf (accessed on 10 June 2021).
7. Persson, M.; Sabelström, E.; Gunnarsson, B. Handling of unused prescription drugs—Knowledge, behaviour and attitude among Swedish people. *Environ. Int.* **2009**, *35*, 771–774. [CrossRef] [PubMed]
8. Al-Shareef, F.; El-Asrar, S.A.; Al-Bakr, L.; Al-Amro, M.; Alqahtani, F.; Aleanizy, F.; Al-Rashood, S. Investigating the disposal of expired and unused medication in Riyadh, Saudi Arabia: A cross-sectional study. *Int. J. Clin. Pharm.* **2016**, *38*, 822–828. [CrossRef] [PubMed]
9. Wajid, S.; Siddiqui, N.A.; Mothana, R.A.; Samreen, S. Prevalence and Practice of Unused and Expired Medicine—A Community-Based Study among Saudi Adults in Riyadh, Saudi Arabia. *BioMed Res. Int.* **2020**, *6539251*. [CrossRef]
10. Gómez, M.J.; Petrović, M.; Fernández-Alba, A.R.; Barceló, D. Determination of pharmaceuticals of various therapeutic classes by solid-phase extraction and liquid chromatography-tandem mass spectrometry analysis in hospital effluent wastewaters. *J. Chromatogr. A* **2006**, *1114*, 224–233. [CrossRef]
11. Celle-Jeanton, H.; Schemberg, D.; Mohammed, N.; Huneau, F.; Bertrand, G.; Lavastre, V.; Le Coustumer, P. Evaluation of pharmaceuticals in surface water: Reliability of PECs compared to MECs. *Environ. Int.* **2014**, *73*, 10–21. [CrossRef] [PubMed]
12. Sui, Q.; Cao, X.; Lu, S.; Zhao, W.; Qiu, Z.; Yu, G. Occurrence, sources and fate of pharmaceuticals and personal care products in the groundwater: A review. *Emerg. Contam.* **2015**, *1*, 14–24. [CrossRef]
13. Chander, V.; Sharma, B.; Negi, V.; Aswal, R.S.; Singh, P.; Singh, R.; Dobhal, R. Pharmaceutical Compounds in Drinking Water. *J. Xenobiot.* **2016**, *6*, 5774. [CrossRef] [PubMed]

14. Fick, J.; Söderström, H.; Lindberg, R.H.; Phan, C.; Tysklind, M.; Larsson, D.J. Contamination of surface, ground, and drinking water from pharmaceutical production. *Environ. Toxicol. Chem.* **2009**, *28*, 2522–2527. [CrossRef]
15. Schwab, B.W.; Hayes, E.P.; Fiori, J.M.; Mastrocco, F.J.; Roden, N.M.; Cragin, D.; Meyerhoff, R.D.; D'Aco, V.J.; Anderson, P.D. Human pharmaceuticals in US surface waters: A human health risk assessment. *Regul. Toxicol. Pharmacol.* **2005**, *42*, 296–312. [CrossRef]
16. Arnold, K.E.; Brown, A.R.; Ankley, G.T.; Sumpter, J.P. Medicating the environment: Assessing risks of pharmaceuticals to wildlife and ecosystems. *Philos. Trans. R. Soc. B* **2014**, *369*, 20130569. [CrossRef] [PubMed]
17. Tong, A.Y.; Peake, B.M.; Braund, R. Disposal practices for unused medications in New Zealand community pharmacies. *J. Prim. Health Care* **2011**, *3*, 197–203. [CrossRef] [PubMed]
18. AlRuthia, Y.; Alsenaidy, M.A.; Alrabiah, H.K.; AlMuhaisen, A.; Alshehri, M. The status of licensed pharmacy workforce in Saudi Arabia: A 2030 economic vision perspective. *Hum. Resour. Health* **2018**, *16*, 28. [CrossRef]
19. Abahussain, E.; Waheedi, M.; Koshy, S. Practice, awareness and opinion of pharmacists toward disposal of unwanted medications in Kuwait. *Saudi Pharm. J.* **2012**, *20*, 195–201. [CrossRef]
20. Sedlak, D.L.; Pinkston, K.E. Factors Affecting the Concentrations of Pharmaceuticals Released to the Aquatic Environment. *J. Contemp. Water Res. Educ.* **2001**, *120*, 56–64.
21. Hoeger, B.; Köllner, B.; Dietrich, D.R.; Hitzfeld, B. Water-borne diclofenac affects kidney and gill integrity and selected immune parameters in brown trout (Salmo trutta f. fario). *Aquat. Toxicol.* **2005**, *75*, 53–64. [CrossRef]
22. Saudi FDA. Updates on Safety Information of Fentanyl Patches: FDA Reminds the Public about the Potential for Life-Threatening Harm from Accidental Exposure to Fentanyl Transdermal Systems ("Patches"). 2012. Available online: https://www.sfda.gov.sa/sites/default/files/2019-06/1561839135%D8%AA%D8%B9%D9%85%D9%8A%D9%85%2014.pdf (accessed on 20 March 2021).
23. FDA Health Consumer Information. How to Dispose of Unused Medicines. 2013. Available online: https://www.fda.gov/files/about%20fda/published/How-to-Dispose-of-Unused-Medicines-(PDF).pdf (accessed on 20 March 2021).
24. Pharmaceutical Services Negotiating Committee (PSNC). NHS Community Pharmacy Contractual Framework Essential Service—Disposal of Unwanted Medicines. 2004. Available online: https://psnc.org.uk/wp-content/uploads/2013/07/Service-Spec-ES3-Waste-Disposal.pdf (accessed on 24 March 2021).
25. The National Return and Disposal of Unwanted Medicines Limited (by Australian Government-Department of Health). Return Unwanted Medicines (The RUM Project). Available online: https://returnmed.com.au/ (accessed on 25 March 2021).
26. Saudi Ministry of Health (MOH). Implementing Regulations of Uniform Law for Medical Waste Management (Modified 2019). Available online: https://www.moh.gov.sa/en/Ministry/Rules/Documents/Uniform-Law-for-Medical-Waste-Management.pdf (accessed on 20 April 2021).
27. Rasheed, M.K.; Alqasoumi, A.; Hasan, S.S.; Babar, Z.U. The community pharmacy practice change towards patient-centered care in Saudi Arabia: A qualitative perspective. *J. Pharm. Policy Pract.* **2020**, *13*, 59. [CrossRef] [PubMed]
28. General Authority for Statistics—Kingdom of Saudi Arabia. Chapter 01: Population & Demography. 2019. Available online: https://www.stats.gov.sa/en/1007-0 (accessed on 12 June 2021).

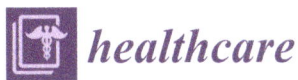

Article

Pharmacist Workforce at Primary Care Clinics: A Nationwide Survey in Taiwan

Wei-Ho Chen [1], Pei-Chen Lee [2,3], Shu-Chiung Chiang [4], Yuh-Lih Chang [2], Tzeng-Ji Chen [4,5,6,*], Li-Fang Chou [7] and Shinn-Jang Hwang [5]

1. Department of Medical Education, Taipei Veterans General Hospital, No. 201, Sec. 2, Shi-Pai Road, Taipei 11217, Taiwan; asdfg15995@gmail.com
2. Department of Pharmacy, Taipei Veterans General Hospital, No. 201, Sec. 2, Shi-Pai Road, Taipei 11217, Taiwan; kelseylee0612@gmail.com (P.-C.L.); ylchang@vghtpe.gov.tw (Y.-L.C.)
3. Graduate Institute of Clinical Pharmacy, College of Medicine, National Taiwan University, Taipei 10617, Taiwan
4. Institute of Hospital and Health Care Administration, National Yang Ming Chiao Tung University, No. 155, Sec. 2, Linong Street, Taipei 11217, Taiwan; scchiang0g@gmail.com
5. Department of Family Medicine, Taipei Veterans General Hospital, No. 201, Sec. 2, Shi-Pai Road, Taipei 11217, Taiwan; sjhwang@vghtpe.gov.tw
6. Big Data Center, Department of Medical Research, Taipei Veterans General Hospital, No. 201, Sec. 2, Shi-Pai Road, Taipei 11217, Taiwan
7. Department of Public Finance, National Chengchi University, Taipei 116, Taiwan; lifang@nccu.edu.tw
* Correspondence: tjchen@vghtpe.gov.tw; Tel.: +886-2-2875-7458; Fax: +886-2-2873-7901

Citation: Chen, W.-H.; Lee, P.-C.; Chiang, S.-C.; Chang, Y.-L.; Chen, T.-J.; Chou, L.-F.; Hwang, S.-J. Pharmacist Workforce at Primary Care Clinics: A Nationwide Survey in Taiwan. *Healthcare* 2021, 9, 863. https://doi.org/10.3390/healthcare9070863

Academic Editor: Georges Adunlin

Received: 25 May 2021
Accepted: 6 July 2021
Published: 8 July 2021

Publisher's Note: MDPI stays neutral with regard to jurisdictional claims in published maps and institutional affiliations.

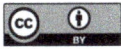

Copyright: © 2021 by the authors. Licensee MDPI, Basel, Switzerland. This article is an open access article distributed under the terms and conditions of the Creative Commons Attribution (CC BY) license (https://creativecommons.org/licenses/by/4.0/).

Abstract: Although dispensing is usually separated from prescribing in healthcare service delivery worldwide, primary care clinics in some countries can hire pharmacists to offer in-house dispensing or point-of-care dispensing for patients' convenience. This study aimed to provide a general overview of pharmacists working at primary care clinics in Taiwan. Special attention was paid to clarifying the relationship by location, scale, and specialty of clinics. The data source was the Government's open database in Taiwan. In our study, a total of 8688 pharmacists were hired in 6020 (52.1%) 11,546 clinics. The result revealed significant differences in the number of pharmacists at different specialty clinics among levels of urbanization. Group practices did not have a higher probability of hiring pharmacists than solo practices. There was a higher prevalence of pharmacists practicing in clinics of non surgery-related specialties than in surgery-related specialties. Although the strict separation policy of dispensing and prescribing has been implemented for 2 decades in Taiwan, most primary care clinics seem to circumvent the regulation by hiring pharmacists to maintain dominant roles in dispensing drugs and retaining the financial benefits from drugs. More in-depth analyses are required to study the impact on pharmacies and the quality of pharmaceutical care.

Keywords: ambulatory care facilities; health workforce; pharmacists; Taiwan

1. Introduction

Although the separation of prescribing and dispensing medication between physicians and pharmacists has been a common practice for a long time in North American and European countries, most Asian countries such as Korea, Malaysia, Japan, and Taiwan have only just begun to implement this separation system in recent decades [1]. Although the separation policy aimed to improve the quality of drug use, it could lead to patients' inconvenience. Physicians in these Asian countries continuously struggled for the right to dispense medication. In Korea, revenue from drugs had once accounted for more than 40% of the total revenue in many clinics. To settle the strike by physicians about the implementation of a strict separation policy, the Korean Government raised physician fees by as much as 44%, thus adding an extra financial burden on patients [2]. In Malaysia, because the separation system encountered vehement opposition from physicians, separation of prescribing and dispensing only occurred in governmental healthcare facilities [3]. In Japan, the Government adopted a slight reform by increasing the reimbursement of prescription fees for facilities without in-house dispensing and decreasing fees for in-house dispensing. Additionally, clinics were allowed to hire pharmacists [4].

In Taiwan, because physicians resisted the separation system and lobbied for dispensing rights, the Government followed the policy in Japan. In 1997, they implemented a so-called "dual track system", in which pharmacists could work either at independent pharmacies or at primary care clinics. The supporting argument was that since hospitals could hire pharmacists, clinics should be able to hire pharmacists in the same way [5]. According to the Pharmaceutical Affairs Act, any physician having dispensing facilities, could, for the purpose of medical treatment, dispense drugs by themselves based on their own prescriptions in remote areas where practicing pharmaceutical personnel was not available (as determined by the central or municipal competent health authorities) or in the case of urgent need of medical treatment services [6]. The strict separation policy restricted physicians from dispensing drugs independently in most cases. However, physicians could hire pharmacists to work for them at clinics. Therefore, the physician could still retain the benefits from dispensing fees and profit margins of medication. This may be contrary to the original goal of the separation policy, which expected the prescription given by the physician could be refilled at the community pharmacy. In Taiwan, the percentage of clinics hiring pharmacists in certain areas was more than 60% 1 year after the implementation of the new policy [7].

The retention of dispensing by clinics could be detrimental to the development of independent pharmacies. Although there was a wealth of literature on the introduction and influence of the separation system [1–3,8], there was a dearth of any published research on the pharmacist workforce at primary care clinics. The aim of this study was to conduct a nationwide survey of the pharmacist workforce at primary care clinics in Taiwan. Special attention was paid to geography, specialty, and scale of clinics. The unique phenomenon in Taiwan could offer valuable information for future discussion on healthcare policymaking.

2. Materials and Methods

2.1. Background

In Taiwan, the National Health Insurance program started in 1995 and covered almost all inhabitants [9]. There is no requirement for individuals to register with a primary care physician. Patients can freely consult with and switch between any kind of physician at local clinics and outpatient departments of hospitals without referral.

2.2. Data Source

Data were accessed through the website of Government's open data in Taiwan (https://data.gov.tw/) (accessed on 1 December 2020) [10]. The basic characteristics of 359 townships in 23 cities and counties in Taiwan were collected from the Monthly Bulletin of Interior Statistics [11]. The Ministry of Health and Welfare provided data, including the number of clinics, physicians, pharmacies, and pharmacists in Taiwan [12,13].

2.3. Study Design

A descriptive, cross-sectional study of the nationwide pharmacist workforce at primary care clinics in 2016 was performed. The variables in this study, such as geographical conditions, the number of physicians per clinic, and physician practice types, might influence the clinic hiring pharmacists. Information about these variables was available from the Government's open data. Therefore, we studied these factors to obtain deeper insight into current implementation of the policy for the separation of dispensing from prescribing in Taiwan.

To investigate the distribution of pharmacies and the pharmacist workforce in different regions, we adopted the urbanization stratification of Taiwan townships developed at Taiwan's National Health Research Institutes [14]. The degree of urbanization of townships in Taiwan was determined by demographic characteristics such as population density, degree of industrialization, distribution of medical resources, number of physicians per 100,000 people, population ratio of farmers, people over 65 years old, and people with higher educational levels [14]. The 359 townships in Taiwan were stratified into seven levels of urbanization [14], and clinics were grouped into seven levels of urbanization according to their location. The seven levels of urbanization were introduced as follows. Level 1 townships, so-called highly urbanized townships, had highest population density, with people of highest educational levels, and highest medical resource density. Level 2 townships, so-called moderately urbanized townships, were second to level 1 townships in terms of population density, people with educational levels, and medical resource density. Level 3 townships (so-called emerging townships), and level 4 townships (so-called general townships) had medium levels of development. Level 5 townships, so-called aging townships, had highest proportion of the elderly and the lowest number of physicians per 100,000 people. Level 6 townships, so-called agricultural townships, had highest population ratio of farmers, the lowest population density, and people of lowest educational levels. Level 7 townships, so-called remote townships, had second-least number of physicians per 100,000 people. We defined urban areas as levels 1 and 2, suburban areas as levels 3 and 4, and rural areas as levels 5, 6, and 7. The number of clinics, pharmacies, and pharmacists were investigated according to their location at different levels. The percentage of clinics hiring pharmacists was calculated on the basis of the collected data.

Besides geography, other key variables of interest to this study were the number of physicians in a clinic and physician practice types.

The number of physicians per clinic indicated the scale of the clinic. The total number of physicians in a clinic was grouped as one, two, three, and $\geq$four. Then, we put all the data into a mosaic plot, with the horizontal axis showing the percentage of clinics with different numbers of physicians per clinic and the vertical axis showing the percentage of clinics with different numbers of pharmacists per clinic. A solo practice in our study was defined as a clinic with one physician. A group practice in our study was defined as a clinic with more than one physician (>1).

Regarding physician specialty, although many physicians had more than one specialty certificate, they were categorized on the basis of the self-declared medical specialty as reported to the Government. In the present study, physician practice types were classified as a single-specialty practice or multi-specialty practice. We surveyed the pharmacist workforce in different single-specialty practices, including practices without specialist title, general medicine, family medicine, otolaryngology, pediatrics, ophthalmology, obstetrics and gynecology, dermatology, rehabilitation medicine, psychiatry, general surgery, plastic surgery, orthopedics, neurology, urology, neurosurgery, radiology, emergency, and anesthesiology. We grouped neurology, urology, neurosurgery, radiology, emergency, and anesthesiology as "others" because the number of clinics in these specialties was relatively small. We also analyzed multi-specialty practices, such as family medicine with pediatrics and family medicine with obstetrics and gynecology. The number of pharmacists hired by a clinic was classified into five groups: 0, 1, 2, 3, and $\geq$4. Then, we calculated the number of clinics in these groups. The percentage of clinics hiring pharmacists was calculated on the basis of the collected data. To perform additional statistical analysis by two-way ANOVA, we grouped specialty into six clusters according to their sample size and clinical pattern. We tried to keep the difference in sample size between groups as small as possible. In order to reduce intra-group variation, we performed grouping based on clinical practice patterns. The internal-medicine-related departments were grouped as group one. Surgery-related specialties were grouped as group two. Department of facial features (otolaryngology and ophthalmology) and pediatrics (patient's condition being similar to those in otolaryngology) were clustered as group three. The remaining specialties were classified as group four. Due to the highest percentage of pharmacists at clinics and their specific specialty attributes, dermatology and psychiatry were independently grouped into group five and six, respectively.

2.4. Statistical Analysis

The mean and standard deviation were reported by urbanization level and specialty for all continuous variables. The percentage of group or solo practices hiring pharmacists was examined through chi-square tests. We stratified the data by urbanization level and specialty to illustrate their impact on clinics hiring pharmacists. The number of pharmacists at clinics was analyzed by two-way analysis of variance (ANOVA) with levels of urbanization and specialty as factors. All analyses were performed using the Statistical Package for Social Science (SPSS, version 23.0) with the significance level set at $\alpha = 0.05$.

2.5. Ethical Approval

According to Taiwan's personal data privacy legislation and the regulations of the institutional review board (IRB) at Taipei Veterans General Hospital (Taipei, Taiwan), the use of publicly available data was exempted from the IRB approval procedure.

3. Results

As the first step, 480 hospitals (e.g., academic medical centers, regional hospitals, and local hospitals) were excluded from the total of 22,936 nationwide medical institutions. As Chinese medicine was not covered by the separation policy and there were different regulations for dental clinics, we excluded Chinese medicine clinics (3996 clinics) and dental clinics (6873 clinics). Clinics in isolated isles such as Kingmen and Lienchiang counties (41 clinics) were excluded. Finally, a total of 11,546 clinics were included in our study.

3.1. Distribution of Pharmacies and Pharmacists Workforce in Urban, Suburban, and Rural Areas

Among 11,546 clinics in 359 townships in Taiwan, the majority was situated in urban areas (65.2%) and suburban areas (28.2%) (see Table 1). Similarly, 4587 (55.8%) pharmacies and 2944 (35.8%) pharmacies were in urban and suburban, respectively. Most pharmacists worked in urban areas (66.7%) and suburban areas (28.4%). In addition, the overwhelming majority of pharmacists in clinics were found in urban areas (66.8%) and suburban areas (28.0%).

Table 1. Distribution of nationwide pharmacies and the pharmacist workforce at clinics in urban, suburban, and rural areas.

Urbanization Level	No. of Townships	No. of Pharmacists *	No. of Pharmacies	No. of Clinics	% of Clinics with Pharmacists	No. of Pharmacists in Clinics
Urban						
Level 1	27	10,872	1988	3526	50.5	2660
Level 2	43	12,659	2599	3998	53.4	3147
Suburban						
Level 3	56	5451	1696	1780	54.2	1424
Level 4	88	4561	1248	1478	51.0	1011
Rural						
Level 5	35	236	104	135	43.0	62
Level 6	61	661	266	295	51.9	162
Level 7	49	818	318	334	53.0	222
Total	359	35258	8219	11546	52.1	8688

* The total number of pharmacists included those working in hospital, clinics, pharmacies, and the pharmaceutical industry.

3.2. Distribution of the Nationwide Pharmacist Workforce at Clinics, Stratified by Number of Physicians Per Clinic

Figure 1 shows the distribution of the pharmacist workforce in 11,454 clinics after excluding clinics without any physicians (92 clinics), stratifying the number of physicians per clinic into four groups. As for the clinics with pharmacists (orange, yellow, green, and blue areas in Figure 1), the percentage of clinics hiring three (green areas) and four or more (blue areas) per clinic became more when the scale of the clinics became larger (more physicians per clinic in other words). Regarding the clinics without any pharmacists (gray areas in Figure 1), less than half of clinics with one, two, and three physicians hired no pharmacists (48.0%, 46.2%, and 45.2%, respectively). Interestingly, more than half of clinics (55.6%) with four or more physicians did not hire pharmacists.

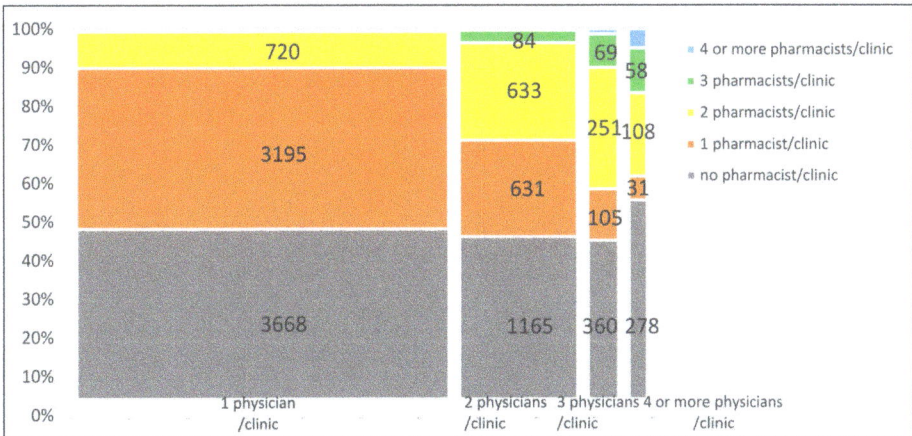

Figure 1. Distribution of the nationwide pharmacist workforce in clinics, stratified by the number of physicians per clinic. The numbers on the graph indicate the number of clinics.

3.3. Distribution of Pharmacist Workforce in Different Specialties Clinics

Of 11,546 clinics in Taiwan, more than four-fifths of clinics (87.1%; 10,053/11,546) were single-specialty (see Table 2). Practices without a specialist title, general medicine, family medicine, otolaryngology, pediatrics, and ophthalmology accounted for three-fourths of the single-specialty clinics (76.5%; 7694/10,053), and practices without a specialist title were the largest proportion of clinics (29.1%; 2932/10,053).

Table 2. Distribution of pharmacist workforce in clinics, stratified by specialty.

Specialty	Number of Clinics						% of Clinics with Pharmacists
	0 Pharmacist/Clinic	1 Pharmacists/Clinic	2 Pharmacists/Clinic	3 Pharmacists/Clinic	≥4 Pharmacists/Clinic	Total	
Single-specialty clinics	4857	3445	1504	212	35	10,053	51.7
Practices without specialist title	1558	1057	282	32	3	2932	46.9
General medicine	566	371	133	11	0	1081	47.6
Family medicine	493	391	158	27	3	1072	54.0
Otolaryngology	388	298	263	42	5	996	61.0
Pediatrics	317	344	211	31	5	908	65.1
Ophthalmology	232	286	164	20	3	705	67.1
Obstetrics and gynecology	251	218	62	2	2	535	53.1
Dermatology	150	133	126	26	12	447	66.4
Rehabilitation	278	31	3	0	0	312	10.9
Psychiatry	88	132	50	11	1	282	68.8
General surgery	160	74	13	0	1	248	35.5
Plastic surgery	209	11	0	0	0	220	5.0
Orthopedics	114	55	25	7	0	201	43.3
Others	53	44	14	3	0	114	53.5
Multi-specialty clinics	668	545	217	50	13	1493	55.3
All clinics	5525	3990	1721	262	48	11,546	52.1

The percentage of clinics with pharmacists varied by specialty. The average percentage of single-specialty clinics with pharmacists was around half (51.7%; 5196/10,053). Among most single-specialty clinics, about two-thirds of those specializing in psychiatry (68.8%), ophthalmology (67.1%), and dermatology (66.4%) hired at least one pharmacist. Other specialties in which over half of the clinics hired pharmacists included pediatrics (65.1%), otolaryngology (61.0%), family medicine (54.0%), obstetrics, and gynecology (53.1%), and others (53.5%). One-third of general surgery clinics (35.5%) hired pharmacists, and very few rehabilitation medicine and plastic surgery clinics hired pharmacists (10.9% and 5%, respectively).

On average, around half of multi-specialty clinics hired pharmacists (55.3%; 825/1496).

3.4. The Average Number of Pharmacists at Clinics by Urbanization Level and Specialty Group

To perform additional statistical analysis by two-way ANOVA, we grouped 15 specialties into six clusters according to their sample size and clinical pattern (see Table A1). Two-way ANOVA suggested that significant differences were observed in the number of pharmacists at different specialty clinics (F value of 5.8, degree of freedom = 5 and p value < 0.001) among levels of urbanization (F value of 2.3, degree of freedom = 6 and p value < 0.05). The results revealed an interaction between levels of urbanization and the specialty (F value of 2.2, and p value < 0.001). After we excluded group five and group six because of their smaller sample size, significant differences in the data still existed, along with the interaction between levels of urbanization and the specialty (F value of 2.8, and p value < 0.001).

The average number of pharmacists at clinics was put into a bar chart by urbanization level and specialty group (see Figure 2). Among specialty groups one to four, the average number of pharmacists at clinics in level 5 townships (red bar in Figure 2) was the lowest. Different colors of bars on the chart representing different levels of urbanization had a similar pattern, which revealed the lowest number of pharmacists at clinics in specialty group 2, and the highest one in specialty groups 5 and 6.

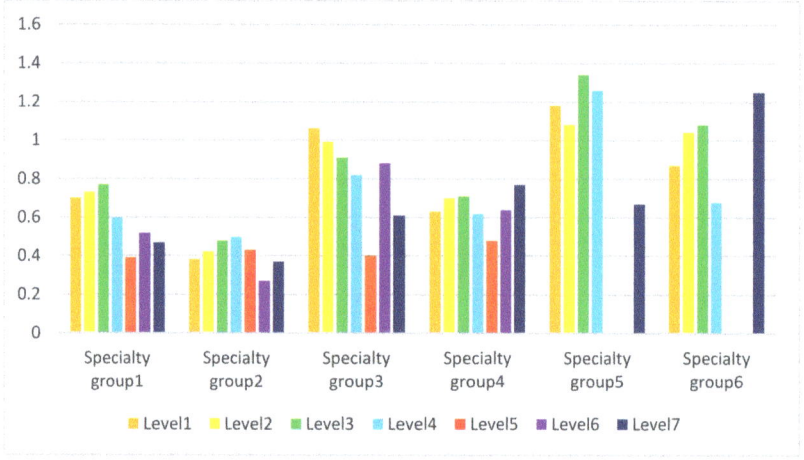

Figure 2. The average number of pharmacists at clinics by urbanization level and specialty group. We grouped specialty into six clusters according to their sample size and clinical pattern. The internal medicine-related departments were grouped as group one. Surgery-related specialties were grouped as group two. Department of facial features (otolaryngology and ophthalmology) and pediatrics (patient's condition being similar to those in otolaryngology) were clustered as group three. The remaining specialties were classified as group four. Due to the highest percentage of pharmacists at clinics and their specific specialty attributes, dermatology and psychiatry were independently grouped into groups five and six, respectively. There were almost no clinics of specialty groups 5 or 6 in level 5 or 6 townships, so data were not applicable there.

4. Discussion

To our knowledge, this was the first study to investigate the distribution of the pharmacist workforce at primary care clinics in Taiwan by location, scale, and specialty of the clinic.

It yielded several notable findings. First, there were significant differences in the number of pharmacists at different specialty clinics among levels of urbanization. Most clinics, pharmacies, and pharmacists were found in urban areas. Second, about half of clinics (52.1%) hired on-site pharmacists. We found that the larger the scale of the clinics, the higher the percentage of clinics that hired more than two pharmacists. The percentages of clinics hiring pharmacists were not obviously different between group practices versus solo practices. Finally, there was a lower probability of hiring pharmacists in surgery-related specialty clinics compared with non surgery-related clinics.

Globally, a lack of pharmacists in the workforce in rural areas has been reported in Australia, the United States, Canada, and Brazil [15–20]. Our study revealed an extremely low proportion of pharmacists working in rural areas (approximately 5%) in Taiwan. Based on our study, an uneven distribution of pharmacies was also found, with only 8.4% of pharmacies located in rural areas. The challenges for rural pharmacies' practices were mainly based on economic realities [21]. The lack of pharmacists may increase pharmacy-related medication errors and alter the operations of the pharmacy department [22]. Besides, more part-time staff has been recruited, and the expanded use of overtime pay was noted [22]. One previous report indicated that patient safety, even death, could be contributed to by a shortage of pharmacists [23].

According to a previous study, more than 60% of clinics hired pharmacists in certain areas just after the new policy was launched [7]. After the new policy had been in place for more than 2 decades, our nationwide results were consistent with those of an earlier study. Based on our study, around half of clinics (52.1%) hired pharmacists. Such a high probability of clinics hiring pharmacists may be related to an oversupply of pharmacists and the risk of operating a pharmacy business. The ratio of physicians to practicing pharmacists was 1.4 to 1 in Taiwan, and the ratio of those was 3.9 to 1 in Organization for Economic Cooperation and Development (OECD) countries [24,25], indicating an oversupply of pharmacists relative to the number of physicians. For pharmacists, running their own pharmacy business was harder than being hired in clinics [26–28], so fewer pharmacists were willing to participate in the labor force in pharmacies.

Our study showed that the percentage of clinics hiring more than two pharmacists increased when the scale of clinics became larger (see Figure 1). As group practices could better build local healthcare market power compared to solo practices [29], we assumed that more primary care physicians in the clinics translated into more daily patient visits. To ensure the quality of dispensing, a threshold had been set at 80 prescriptions per day for each pharmacist. If there were more than 80 prescriptions, the dispensing fee was reduced by half [30]. Therefore, as the daily number of outpatient visits grew, we assumed that clinics would hire more pharmacists to work in shifts to handle the increasing patient demand for medical health services.

Based on our study, the percentage of clinics hiring pharmacists was not significantly different (p value of 0.41) for group versus solo practices (see Figure 1). Moreover, clinics with four or more physicians were the most likely to not hire pharmacists (55.6%) among all groups. This may be related to next-door pharmacies. To encourage prescriptions from clinics to be refilled in community pharmacies, the Government provided financial incentives to both clinics (prescription releasing fee) and pharmacies [31]. According to laws in Taiwan, pharmacies must be managed by pharmacists, but they can be owned by non-pharmacists [32]. Some practitioners found this loophole in the law, so they established pharmacies nearby and hired pharmacists to manage the pharmacy as their employees. These next-door pharmacies were controlled by practitioners (often physicians) and were distinct from independent pharmacies controlled by pharmacists [31]. Under this loophole in the law, the physicians benefited from both the prescription releasing fee and the pharmacist dispensing fee [33]. Previous research showed that large-volume clinics tended to collaborate with next-door pharmacies or contracted pharmacies with long-standing relationships [34]. In 2006, about one-third of pharmacies were next-door pharmacies [31]. Next-door pharmacies were not unique to Taiwan. They also occurred in Japan (the so-called "second pharmacy ") and the United States, but they gradually disappeared after governmental intervention from 1990 to 2000 [4]. In Taiwan, although the Government amended the law, the number of next-door pharmacies remains unknown.

When the number of patient visits or medication needs became greater, clinics were more likely to hire pharmacists to retain the financial benefits from drugs [7,35]. In our research about the distribution of the pharmacist workforce among different specialties, the results revealed a lower percentage of clinics with a pharmacist (<50%) in surgery-related specialties (including plastic surgery, general surgery, and orthopedics) than in most non surgery-related counterparts. The major medical service from clinics of rehabilitation medicine and surgical-related specialties seemed to be various therapies and surgical intervention, respectively [36–38]. Regarding many non surgical-related specialties, polypharmacy had been noted worldwide for decades [39–41]. For example, almost one-third of patients visiting outpatient psychiatry departments are on three or more psychotropic drugs in the United States [42].

Analysis results of a two-way ANOVA (see Table A1) suggested that significant differences were observed in the number of pharmacists at different specialty clinics (p value < 0.001) among levels of urbanization (p value < 0.05). The results revealed an interaction between levels of urbanization and the specialty (p value < 0.001). Among specialty groups one to four, our result (see Figure 2) showed the average number of pharmacists at clinics in level 5 townships was the lowest. According to the previous study, Level 5 townships had the lowest number of physicians per 100,000 people [14]. There seemed to be the lowest medical resource density in level 5 townships, which needs more attention in medical care. In different urbanization level townships (see Figure 2), the specialty group 2 (primarily surgery-related specialty) had the lowest number of pharmacists at clinics, and the specialty groups 5 and 6 (dermatology and psychiatry) had the highest one. In addition to urbanization level and specialty, clinics hiring pharmacists could be influenced by multiple factors such as clinic business type, the competitiveness of the market, the number of prescriptions refilled at a community pharmacy, physician's trust in pharmacists, and practitioner's beliefs being consistent with the core value of the separation policy.

Our comprehensive analyses of the nationwide distribution of the primary care pharmacist workforce by geographic location, the scale of the clinics, and different specialty types have some limitations. First, part-time doctors and pharmacists may cause imprecision in the calculation and presentation of data. Second, although we presume that clinics with four or more physicians collaborate with next-door pharmacies or long-term contracted pharmacies, the number of next-door pharmacies remains unknown at present [31]. Third, specialty clinics cannot be accurately counted because some clinics with multiple specialties may be considered as a single-specialty if they register only one specialty. Moreover, when seeking care in community clinics, many patients with illnesses are treated similarly by otolaryngologists, pediatricians, and family physicians [43]. Thus, there is an overlap of patients' diseases among several specialties. Finally, we lacked information and could not consider the impact of potential confounding factors such as clinic business type, the competitiveness of the market, and the number of prescriptions refilled at a community pharmacy. We could obtain further information about the features of clinics with pharmacists if we implement a survey using a questionnaire. Hence, our study may not reflect a complete view of the pharmacist workforce in primary care clinics in Taiwan.

5. Conclusions

Our study shows significant differences in the number of pharmacists at different specialty clinics among levels of urbanization. Group practices do not have a higher probability of hiring pharmacists than solo practices. Clinics with non surgery-related specialties are more likely to hire pharmacists compared to surgery-related counterparts. In summary, a total of 8688 pharmacists have been hired to work in 6020 (52.1%) of 11,546 clinics, indicating that more than half of clinics hire on-site pharmacists. Although the strict separation between dispensing and prescribing has been implemented for 2 decades in Taiwan, most primary care clinics seem to circumvent the regulation by hiring pharmacists to maintain the dominant role in dispensing while maintaining control of the financial benefits from drugs. More in-depth analyses are required to further study the impact on pharmacies and the quality of pharmaceutical care.

Author Contributions: Conceptualization, W.-H.C. and T.-J.C.; methodology, W.-H.C., S.-C.C., and T.-J.C.; software, W.-H.C. and S.-C.C.; validation, W.-H.C., P.-C.L., S.-C.C., Y.-L.C., T.-J.C., L.-F.C., and S.-J.H.; writing—original draft preparation, W.-H.C.; writing—review and editing, W.-H.C., P.-C.L., T.-J.C., L.-F.C., and S.-J.H.; supervision, T.-J.C.; project administration, T.-J.C. All authors have read and agreed to the published version of the manuscript.

Funding: This research was funded by Taipei Veterans General Hospital, grant number V109E-002-1.

Institutional Review Board Statement: Not applicable.

Informed Consent Statement: Not applicable.

Data Availability Statement: Not applicable.

Conflicts of Interest: The authors declare no conflict of interest.

Appendix A

Table A1. The average number of pharmacists at clinics by urbanization level and specialty group, with their mean and standard error.

	Urbanization Level						
	Level 1	Level 2	Level 3	Level 4	Level 5	Level 6	Level 7
* Specialty group 1	0.70 ± 0.04	0.73 ± 0.03	0.77 ± 0.04	0.60 ± 0.05	0.39 ± 0.12	0.52 ± 0.09	0.47 ± 0.08
Specialty group 2	0.38 ± 0.03	0.42 ± 0.03	0.48 ± 0.06	0.50 ± 0.07	0.43 ± 0.31	0.27 ± 0.25	0.37 ± 0.19
Specialty group 3	1.06 ± 0.03	0.99 ± 0.03	0.91 ± 0.04	0.82 ± 0.05	0.40 ± 0.37	0.88 ± 0.17	0.61 ± 0.14
Specialty group 4	0.63 ± 0.02	0.70 ± 0.02	0.71 ± 0.03	0.62 ± 0.03	0.48 ± 0.09	0.64 ± 0.06	0.77 ± 0.06
Specialty group 5	1.18 ± 0.06	1.08 ± 0.06	1.34 ± 0.12	1.26 ± 0.13	N/A **	N/A	0.67 ± 0.48
Specialty group 6	0.87 ± 0.08	1.04 ± 0.08	1.08 ± 0.14	0.68 ± 0.18	N/A	N/A	1.25 ± 0.41

Values are expressed as mean ± standard error. * To perform additional statistical analysis by two-way ANOVA, we grouped specialty into six clusters according to their sample size and clinical pattern. The internal-medicine-related departments were grouped as group one. Surgery-related specialties were grouped as group two. Department of facial features (otolaryngology and ophthalmology) and pediatrics (patient's condition being similar to those in otolaryngology) were clustered as group three. The remaining specialties were classified as group four. Due to the highest percentage of pharmacists at clinics and their specific specialty attributes, dermatology and psychiatry were independently grouped into group five and six, respectively. ** There were almost no clinics of specialty group 5 or 6 in level 5 or 6 townships, so data were not applicable there.

References

1. Yokoi, M.; Tashiro, T. Influence of the separation of prescription and dispensation of medicine on its cost in Japanese prefectures. *Glob. J. Health Sci.* **2014**, *6*, 57–62. [CrossRef] [PubMed]
2. Kwon, S. Pharmaceutical reform and physician strikes in Korea: Separation of drug prescribing and dispensing. *Soc. Sci. Med.* **2003**, *57*, 529–538. [CrossRef]
3. Tiong, J.J.; Mai, C.W.; Gan, P.W.; Johnson, J.; Mak, V.S. Separation of prescribing and dispensing in Malaysia: The history and challenges. The International journal of pharmacy practice. *Int. J. Pharm. Pract.* **2016**, *24*, 302–305. [CrossRef] [PubMed]
4. Rodwin, M.A.; Okamoto, A. Physicians' conflicts of interest in Japan and the United States: Lessons for the United States. *J. Health Polit. Policy Law* **2000**, *25*, 343–375. [CrossRef] [PubMed]
5. Chen, M.-L. Discussion on the Restrictions and Possibilities of Social Practice of Separation Policy. Available online: https://www.rchss.sinica.edu.tw/app/ebook/journal/23-04-2011/4.pdf (accessed on 1 December 2020). (In Chinese)
6. Law and Regulation Database of The Republic of China. Available online: https://law.moj.gov.tw/LawClass/LawSingleRela.aspx?PCODE=L0030002&FLNO=50&ty=L (accessed on 1 December 2020). (In Chinese)

7. Chou, Y.J.; Yip, W.C.; Lee, C.H.; Huang, N.; Sun, Y.P.; Chang, H.J. Impact of separating drug prescribing and dispensing on provider behaviour: Taiwan's experience. *Health Policy Plan.* **2003**, *18*, 316–329. [CrossRef]
8. Yamamura, S.; Yamamoto, N.; Oide, S.; Kitazawa, S. Current state of community pharmacy in Japan: Practice, research, and future opportunities or challenges. *Ann. Pharmacother.* **2006**, *40*, 2008–2014. [CrossRef]
9. National Health Insurance Administration; Ministry of Health and Welfare. The Coverage Rate of National Health Insurance. 2019. Available online: https://www.nhi.gov.tw/Content_List.aspx?n=4DAAA0A111B2378D&topn=23C660CAACAA159D (accessed on 1 December 2020).
10. Taiwan Opening Data Government. Medical Institutions and Basic Information. Available online: https://data.gov.tw/ (accessed on 1 December 2020).
11. Taiwan Ministry of the Interior. Monthly Bulletin of Interior Statistics.1.7—Population for Township and District and by Urban Area. Available online: https://www.moi.gov.tw/files/site_stuff/321/1/month/month_en.html (accessed on 1 December 2020).
12. Taiwan Ministry of Health and Welfare. Annual Statistical Table. Available online: https://dep.mohw.gov.tw/DOS/lp-4934-113-1-20.html (accessed on 1 December 2020).
13. Taiwan Ministry of Health and Welfare. Pharmaceutical Administration-Number of Pharmaceutical Merchants in Each County and City-By Township and City. Available online: https://dep.mohw.gov.tw/DOS/cp-1729-2940-113.html (accessed on 1 December 2020).
14. Liu, C.Y.; Hung, Y.T.; Chuang, Y.L.; Chen, Y.J.; Weng, W.S.; Liu, J.S. Incorporating development stratification of Taiwan townships into sampling design of large scale health interview survey. *J. Health Manag.* **2006**, *4*, 1–22.
15. Taylor, S.M.; Lindsay, D.; Glass, B.D. Rural pharmacy workforce: Influence of curriculum and clinical placement on pharmacists' choice of rural practice. *Aust. J. Rural Health* **2019**, *27*, 132–138. [CrossRef]
16. Martin, S.L.; Baker, R.P.; Piper, B.J. Evaluation of urban-rural differences in pharmacy practice needs in Maine with the MaPPNA. *Pharm. Pract.* **2015**, *13*, 669. [CrossRef]
17. Soon, J.A.; Levine, M. Rural pharmacy in Canada: Pharmacist training, workforce capacity and research partnerships. *Int. J. Circumpolar Health* **2011**, *70*, 407–418. [CrossRef]
18. Faraco, E.B.; Guimarães, L.; Anderson, C.; Leite, S.N. The pharmacy workforce in public primary healthcare centers: Promoting access and information on medicines. *Pharm. Pract.* **2020**, *18*, 2048. [CrossRef]
19. Nattinger, M.; Ullrich, F.; Mueller, K.J. Characteristics of rural communities with a sole, independently owned pharmacy. *Rural Policy Brief* **2014**, *7*, 1–4.
20. Bono, J.D.; Crawford, S.Y. Impact of Medicare Part D on independent and chain community pharmacies in rural Illinois–A qualitative study. *Res. Soc. Adm. Pharm.* **2010**, *6*, 110–120. [CrossRef]
21. Stratton, T.P. The economic realities of rural pharmacy practice. *J. Rural Health* **2001**, *17*, 77–81. [CrossRef]
22. Walton, S.M. The pharmacist shortage and medication errors: Issues and evidence. *J. Med. Syst.* **2004**, *28*, 63–69. [CrossRef]
23. Young, D. Shortage of pharmacists may have contributed to patient's death. *Am. J. Health Syst. Pharm.* **2002**, *59*, 2042–2045. [CrossRef]
24. Health Care Resources: Pharmacists. Available online: https://stats.oecd.org/index.aspx?queryid=30178# (accessed on 26 January 2021).
25. Taiwan Ministry of Health and Welfare. Available online: https://dep.mohw.gov.tw/dos/cp-1735-3245-113.html (accessed on 26 January 2021). (In Chinese)
26. Rollins, B.L.; Gunturi, R.; Sullivan, D. A pharmacy business management simulation exercise as a practical application of business management material and principles. *Am. J. Pharm. Educ.* **2014**, *78*, 62. [CrossRef]
27. Davies, M.J.; Fleming, H.; Jones, R.; Menzie, K.; Smallwood, C.; Surendar, S. The inclusion of a business management module within the master of pharmacy degree: A route to asset enrichment? *Pharm. Pract.* **2013**, *11*, 109–117. [CrossRef]
28. Mattingly, T.J.; Mullins, C.D.; Melendez, D.R.; Boyden, K.; Eddington, N.D. A systematic review of entrepreneurship in pharmacy practice and education. *Am. J. Pharm. Educ.* **2019**, *83*, 7233. [CrossRef]
29. Lin, H.C.; Chen, C.S.; Liu, T.C.; Lee, H.C. Differences in practice income between solo and group practice physicians. *Health Policy* **2006**, *79*, 296–305. [CrossRef]
30. Bureau of National Health Insurance. Available online: https://www.nhi.gov.tw/Content_List.aspx?n=58ED9C8D8417D00B (accessed on 1 December 2020).
31. Investigation Bureau, Ministry of Justice in Taiwan. Available online: https://www.moj.gov.tw/2204/2795/2796/54190/ (accessed on 26 January 2021).
32. Chen, T.H.; Hsu, M.M. Disputes about the program of handling next-door pharmacies. *Taiwan Med. J.* **2005**, *48*, 549–550. (In Chinese)
33. Explanation of Law of Dispensing Medicine, Judicial Yuan in Taiwan. Available online: https://www.president.gov.tw/File/Doc/7b219027-bd5a-448c-9294-1de3c0036265 (accessed on 26 January 2021). (In Chinese)
34. Willing of Clinic Physicians to Approve Prescription Refills for Chronic Disease. Available online: https://www.asia.edu.tw/Main_pages/academics/teacher_research/pk_kung/10.pdf (accessed on 26 January 2021). (In Chinese)
35. Practicing Physicians' Views on the Implementation of Separation Policy in the Future. Available online: https://www.chimei.org.tw/main/cmh_department/57726/08/data/II-11.pdf (accessed on 26 January 2021). (In Chinese)

36. Brathwaite, D.; Aziz, F.; Eakins, C.; Charles, A.J.; Cristian, A. Safety precautions in the rehabilitation medicine prescription. *Phys. Med. Rehabil. Clin. N. Am.* **2012**, *23*, 231–239. [CrossRef] [PubMed]
37. What is Rehabilitation? Available online: https://www.who.int/news-room/fact-sheets/detail/rehabilitation (accessed on 26 January 2021).
38. Bicket, M.C.; Brat, G.A.; Hutfless, S.; Wu, C.L.; Nesbit, S.A.; Alexander, G.C. Optimizing opioid prescribing and pain treatment for surgery: Review and conceptual framework. *Am. J. Health Syst. Pharm.* **2019**, *76*, 1403–1412. [CrossRef] [PubMed]
39. Kukreja, S.; Kalra, G.; Shah, N.; Shrivastava, A. Polypharmacy in psychiatry: A review. *Mens Sana Monogr.* **2013**, *11*, 82–99. [CrossRef]
40. Tarn, D.M.; Schwartz, J.B. Polypharmacy: A five-step call to action for family physicians. *Fam. Med.* **2020**, *52*, 699–701. [CrossRef]
41. Masnoon, N.; Shakib, S.; Kalisch-Ellett, L.; Caughey, G.E. What is polypharmacy? A systematic review of definitions. *BMC Geriatr.* **2017**, *17*, 230. [CrossRef]
42. Mojtabai, R.; Olfson, M. National trends in psychotropic medication polypharmacy in office-based psychiatry. *Arch. Gen. Psychiatry* **2010**, *67*, 26–36. [CrossRef]
43. Chou, Y.C.; Lin, S.Y.; Chen, T.J.; Chiang, S.C.; Jeng, M.J.; Chou, L.F. Dosing variability in prescriptions of acetaminophen to children: Comparisons between pediatricians, family physicians and otolaryngologists. *BMC Pediatr.* **2013**, *13*, 64. [CrossRef]

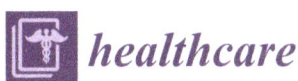

Article

Reproductive Health Services: Attitudes and Practice of Japanese Community Pharmacists

Shigeo Yamamura [1,*], Tomoko Terajima [1], Javiera Navarrete [2], Christine A. Hughes [2], Nese Yuksel [2], Theresa J. Schindel [2], Tatta Sriboonruang [3], Puree Anantachoti [3] and Chanthawat Patikorn [3]

1. Faculty of Pharmaceutical Sciences, Josai International University, Gumyo 1, Togane, Chiba 283-8555, Japan; terajima@jiu.ac.jp
2. Faculty of Pharmacy and Pharmaceutical Sciences, College of Health Sciences, University of Alberta, Edmonton, AB T6G 2H1, Canada; javiera@ualberta.ca (J.N.); cah1@ualberta.ca (C.A.H.); yuksel@ualberta.ca (N.Y.); terri.schindel@ualberta.ca (T.J.S.)
3. Faculty of Pharmaceutical Sciences, Chulalongkorn University, Bangkok 10330, Thailand; tatta.s@pharm.chula.ac.th (T.S.); puree.a@pharm.chula.ac.th (P.A.); Chanthawat.p@gmail.com (C.P.)
* Correspondence: s_yama@jiu.ac.jp; Tel.: +81-475-53-4583

Abstract: The provision of sexual and reproductive health (SRH) services is an important part of a community pharmacist's role in many countries. However, such services are not traditionally provided by pharmacists in Japan. We surveyed the practice and attitudes regarding the provision of SRH services among Japanese community pharmacists with a focus on reproductive health (RH) topics. The participants were asked about the provision of RH services, attitudes toward their role as SRH providers, and self-reported confidence in providing education to patients on RH topics. We obtained 534 effective responses. About half of the participants reported providing RH services, and only 21% were involved in dispensing emergency contraception pills. Although the proportion of pharmacists providing education on these topics was considerably lower, about 80% recognized the importance of their role as SRH advisors. Confidence in providing patient education about RH topics depended on their experience in providing such services. Most participants were interested in additional SRH training (80%). Our results suggest that training programs could help to expand Japanese community pharmacists' roles as SRH providers and increase their confidence in the education of patients. This study provides useful insights to expand pharmacists' roles in Japan as providers of comprehensive SRH services.

Keywords: reproductive health; contraception; emergency contraceptives; patient education; community pharmacists

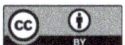

1. Introduction

The provision of sexual and reproductive health (SRH) services is an important part of public health and influences the development of a country; it is also a human rights concern [1]. SRH is defined as "a state of physical, emotional, mental, and social well-being in relation to all aspects of sexuality and reproduction" [2]. The World Health Organization (WHO) emphasizes that SRH is part of the global health goals, constituting a special team for promoting research in the SRH field [3]. The WHO vision is the attainment of the highest possible level of SRH for people worldwide.

In a statement issued in 2019, the International Pharmaceutical Federation (FIP) has indicated that pharmacists have the necessary perspective and interest in dealing with gender-related ethical or reproductive health issues [4]. Community pharmacists play an important role in the provision of SRH services, as they are the most accessible healthcare providers in the community. Some specific SRH services, such as chlamydia screening or hormonal contraception-dispensing are provided by community pharmacists in many countries; however, there are many other areas where pharmacists can expand their professional role [5].

One of the essential SRH services offered by community pharmacists is the provision of reproductive health services, such as pregnancy tests, contraception, including emergency contraception (EC), and strategies to prevent sexually transmitted infections. EC reduces the risk of pregnancy after unprotected sexual intercourse or missed or incorrect use of contraceptives [6,7]. In a number of countries, EC pills containing levonorgestrel EC (LNG-EC) are available without a prescription in pharmacies as over-the-counter (OTC) medication or as pharmacist-only access medicines [8–11].

Healthcare services offered in community pharmacies in Japan are undergoing reform to meet the needs of society [12]. However, in 2018, the ministry of health, labour and welfare decided that EC pills should not change to the OTC category because if a pharmacist sells the product, they need to have specialized knowledge about female reproduction, contraception, and emergency [13]. Japanese community pharmacists have also reported insufficient pharmacy training and a lack of appropriate knowledge and skills to provide enhanced pharmacy services, and therefore, they may feel unprepared to function as providers of SRH services [14]. To expand the role of pharmacists in SRH, it is necessary to assess the attitudes and practice of providing reproductive health services, including EC. In this study, we surveyed Japanese community pharmacists to answer the study question: what are community pharmacists' practices related to the provision of reproductive health services, attitudes toward these services, and self-reported confidence in providing reproductive health services (including EC) to patients?

This study is part of a broader study aimed at comparing community pharmacists' perspectives and attitudes regarding the provision of SRH services in Canada, Japan, and Thailand. The purpose of the broader study is to explore and compare the roles and attitudes toward the provision of SRH services by pharmacists in regions with different regulations around pharmacy practices. This report focuses on services related to reproductive health, including pregnancy tests, ovulation tests, contraception, and EC in the Japanese community pharmacy practice context.

Study Context

In Japan, the barrier contraceptive method, primarily condoms, is the most commonly used to reduce the probability of pregnancy, while the use of oral contraceptive pills is very low (3.0% in 2014) [15].

There are two business models for community pharmacies in Japan: pharmacies (chain or independent) and drugstores. Pharmacists working in settings that represent both models can dispense medicines with prescription. Pharmacies are usually located near clinics or hospitals and focus more on dispensing and compounding. On the other hand, drugstores can also dispense drugs, and focus on selling OTC medicines and miscellaneous products, such as cosmetics and food products.

In Japan, the 6-year Bachelor of Pharmacy program to educate pharmacists was initiated in 2006. The first cohort of graduates were certified as pharmacists based on passing the national examination of pharmacists conducted in 2012 [16,17]. Thus, about 10 years have passed since the introduction of the 6-year pharmacy education program. While the past 4-year Bachelor of Pharmacy program was focused on basic science, the 6-year program is more clinical [18]. Students in the 6-year program receive practical training at both hospital pharmacies and community pharmacies for 11 weeks each [19].

2. Materials and Methods

2.1. Study Design

This was a descriptive, cross-sectional, observational study. We used a web-based survey to answer the research question. A voluntary, anonymous online survey was distributed via Research Electronic Data Capture (REDCap) [20,21]. An information letter and a consent form were included at the beginning of the survey (Appendix A), completion of the survey and submission of responses implied participant consent. The survey was conducted between November 2020 and April 2021.

2.2. Participants

There was no sample size set a priori, a convenience sample of voluntary participants was recruited through email, list distribution, contact lists from pharmacy professional organizations (Ueda, Odawara, Japanese Association for Community Pharmacy), pharmacy chains (Pharcos, Medical system network group), drugstore chains (Welcia Yakkyoku, Aeon), and community pharmacists' group (Kyoto University SPH, Health informatics pharmacy group). The participants of continuing education programs conducted by the AEON Hapycom Comprehensive Training Organization [22] were also recruited. We also used Twitter and Facebook to recruit pharmacists. Any licensed Japanese pharmacist working in a community setting was able to participate. An initial screening question was used to capture eligible participants.

2.3. Data Collection Tool

The survey questions were first developed based on a literature review in English for an international audience. After, it was translated into Japanese. The translated version was refined further to ensure it represented the Japanese context and scope of practice. For face validity testing, the survey was reviewed by experts ($n = 2$, academic pharmacists) and pharmacists ($n = 5$), and then piloted with Canadian pharmacists working in community settings ($n = 10$) and Japanese pharmacists ($n = 5$) [23].

The survey focused on SRH and covered the following topics: pregnancy tests, ovulation tests, contraception (non-hormonal and hormonal), EC, sexually and blood-borne transmitted infections (STBBI), maternal and perinatal health, and general sexual health. However, the focus of this manuscript will be on results regarding reproductive health topics. The questionnaire included pharmacists' demographic information, educational background, practice regarding reproductive health, attitudes towards providing SRH services, and self-reported confidence in providing education to patients about reproductive health topics (Appendix B).

The primary outcomes were the proportion of pharmacists providing reproductive health, the proportion of pharmacists agreeing (or not) with a series of statements regarding the provision of SRH services, and self-reported confidence in providing reproductive health education to patients. Five-point Likert scales were used to explore attitudes towards providing SRH services and self-reported confidence in providing education on such topics. Additionally, we also assessed the differences in practice between pharmacists working in pharmacies versus drugstores, the influence of pharmacy education on attitudes towards the provision of SRH services, and the relationship between provision of patient education and self-reported confidence.

This study was approved by the research ethics review committee of Josai International (10M200001).

2.4. Statistical Analysis

The data were analyzed on JMP-pro version 15 (SAS Institute, Tokyo, Japan). Chi-square test and Fisher's exact test were used to analyze the association between categorical variables. The Cochran–Armitage test for trend or exact Cochran–Armitage test for trend were used to analyze the trends pertaining to categorical variables. The *p*-value for statistical significance was set at 0.05.

3. Results

3.1. Participant Characteristics

A total of 743 pharmacists attempted the survey. Of these, 534 (71.9%) were included in the final analysis. A total of 209 (28.1%) possible participants were excluded, 206 (27.7%) because they did not consent and 3 (0.4%) because they did not answer more than 80% of the questionnaire.

3.2. Reproductive Health Services Provided by Pharmacists

Most participants were women (55%), younger than 40 years in age (61%), and over half of the participants (51%) had less than 10 years of experience as practicing pharmacists. The majority of participants were employed at corporate chain pharmacies (60%), followed by at drugstores (25%), independent pharmacies (13%), and other types of pharmacies (2%) (Table 1).

Table 1. Background characteristics of participants.

Characteristics	n (%)
Gender	
Female	295 (55)
Age range	
20–30 years	208 (39)
31–40 years	116 (22)
41–50 years	97 (18)
51–60 years	81 (15)
61–70 years	29 (5)
71+ years	3 (1)
Professional Education	
Bachelor of Pharmacy (4 years)	245 (46)
Bachelor of Pharmacy (6 years)	257 (48)
Master (MSc or MPharm)	23 (4)
Doctor of Philosophy (PhD)	6 (1)
Years registered as a pharmacist	
<1 year	9 (2)
1–5 years	214 (40)
6–10 years	50 (9)
11–20 years	91 (17)
21–30 years	95 (18)
>31 years	74 (14)
Type of pharmacy	
Independent	68 (13)
Corporate/chain	323 (60)
Drugstore chain	134 (25)
Others	9 (2)

Table 2 summarizes the reproductive health services provided by Japanese pharmacists working in different settings. Most pharmacists working in drugstores reported selling pregnancy and ovulation tests (96% and 94%, respectively), but about one-third did not provide patient education on these topics (35% and 26%, respectively). Most participants reported working in a pharmacy which sold barrier contraceptives (95%), however most did not provide patient education on barrier contraceptives (87%). The availability of pregnancy tests and barrier contraceptives reported by pharmacists that worked in drugstores was higher than those working in pharmacy chains and independent pharmacies (96% vs. 42 and 38%, respectively). Almost half of the total samples of pharmacists filled prescriptions for combined hormonal contraceptives (47%). Approximately 20% of all community pharmacists participating in this study dispensed EC medication based on a prescription.

3.3. Pharmacists' Attitudes towards the Provision of SRH Services

About 80% of the participants strongly agreed or agreed with the statement "it is an important part of a community pharmacist's role to offer advice on sexual and reproductive health". More than 60% of the participants agreed with the following statements: "community pharmacists should be more involved in sexually transmitted infection prevention, screening, testing, and treatment.", "as a pharmacist, I have an ethical responsibility to provide SRH services", and "there is a need to expand the provision of SRH services in the community pharmacy where I work". The majority of the participants disagreed with the items regarding moral objections (63%), regular use by the community of SRH services offered (58%), and being adequately trained (57%) (Figure 1).

Table 2. Reproductive health services provided by Japanese community pharmacists.

Service	Total (n = 534) (%)	Drugstore (n = 134) (%)	Corporate/Chain (n = 323) (%)	Independent pharmacy (n = 68) (%)	Others (n = 9) (%)
Pregnancy Tests					
Does your pharmacy sell pregnancy tests?	293 (55)	127 (96)	134 (42)	26 (38)	6 (75)
Do you provide patient education on pregnancy tests?	192 (36)	87 (65)	90 (28)	9 (13)	6 (67)
Ovulation Tests					
Does your pharmacy sell ovulation tests?	297 (56)	127 (94)	147 (46)	18 (26)	5 (63)
Do you provide patient education on ovulation tests?	222 (42)	98 (74)	107 (33)	13 (25)	4 (44)
Contraception					
Does your pharmacy sell male non-hormonal (barrier) contraceptives? (e.g., condoms)	244 (46)	126 (95)	97 (31)	17 (26)	4 (57)
Do you provide patient education on male non-hormonal (barrier) contraceptives?	37 (7)	17 (13)	14 (4)	3 (4)	3 (33)
Do you dispense combined hormonal contraceptives? (with prescription)	250 (47)	80 (60)	141 (44)	24 (35)	5 (56)
Do you provide patient education on hormonal contraception?	207 (39)	77 (57)	109 (34)	16 (24)	5 (56)
Emergency contraception					
Do you dispense emergency contraception pills (ECPs)?	111 (21)	19 (16)	85 (27)	5 (7)	2 (25)
Do you provide patient education on ECPs?	81 (15)	20 (15)	51 (16)	6 (9)	4 (44)

Numbers of pharmacists who answered "yes" are presented, and the percentage is included in parentheses.

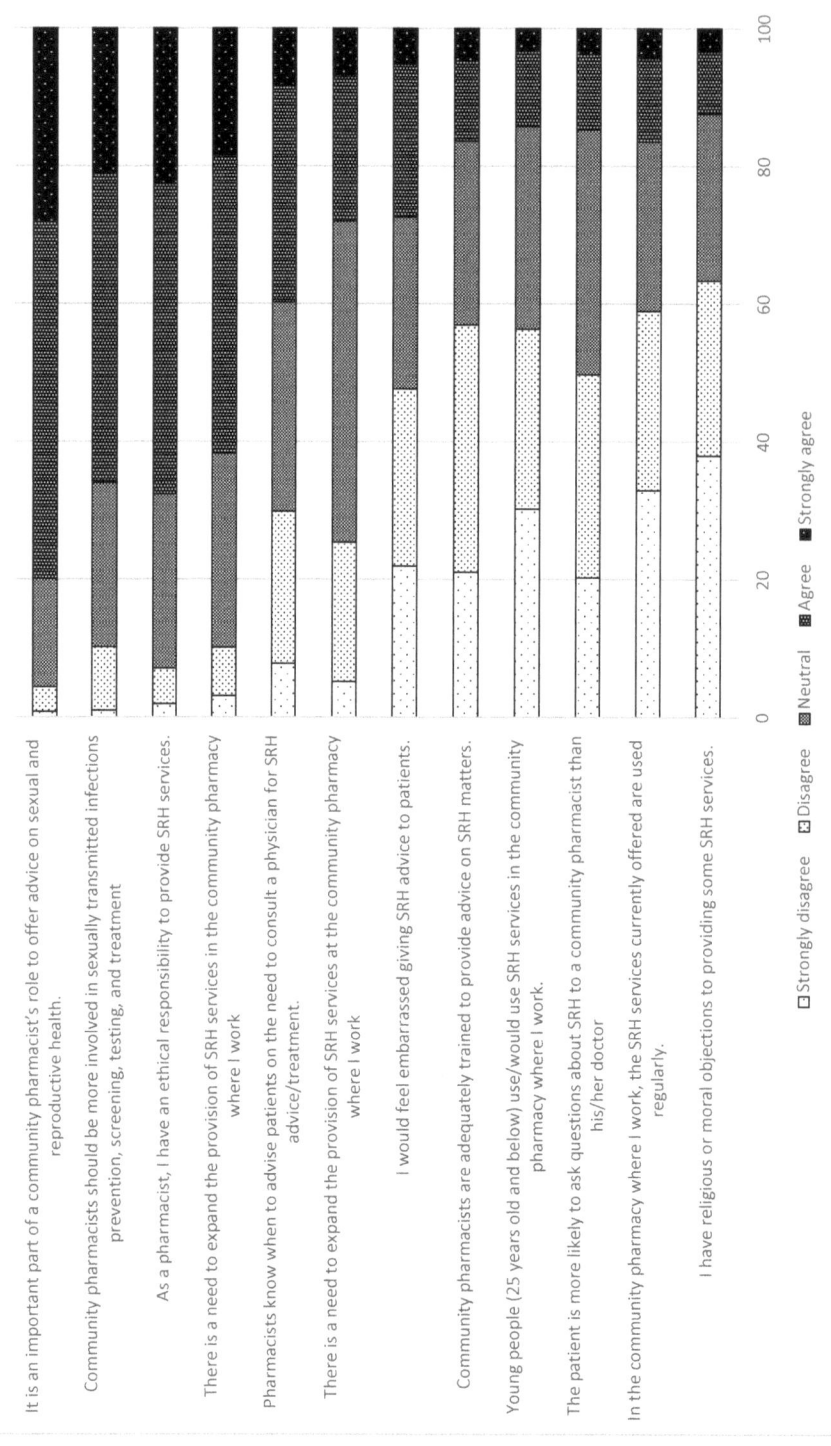

Figure 1. Attitudes toward the provision of sexual and reproductive health (SRH) services. SRH: sexual and reproductive health.

Table 3 summarizes the difference in attitudes towards the provision of SRH service based on the type of bachelor education program. Participants who graduated from the 6-year program tended to agree more with the expansion of the pharmacists' role in SRH (69% vs. 55%), but also agreed to feeling more embarrassed in giving SRH advice to people (34% vs. 21%). The influence of gender was also analyzed, but no statistical difference was found (data not shown).

Table 3. Statistically significant items regarding attitudes towards the provision of sexual and reproductive health (SRH) services (detailed in Figure 1), based on education programs.

There is a need to expand the provision of sexual and reproductive health services in this pharmacy ($p = 0.002$) *						
	Strongly disagree	Disagree	Neutral	Agree	Strongly agree	Total
Bachelor of Pharmacy (4 years)	9 (4)	25 (10)	74 (31)	100 (42)	31 (13)	239
Bachelor of Pharmacy (6 years)	6 (2)	10 (4)	64 (25)	116 (46)	58 (23)	254
There is a need for sexual health and reproductive services in the local area near this pharmacy ($p = 0.031$)						
	Strongly disagree	Disagree	Neutral	Agree	Strongly agree	Total
Bachelor of Pharmacy (4 years)	18 (7)	113 (46)	70 (29)	37 (15)	6 (2)	244
Bachelor of Pharmacy (6 years)	6 (2)	118 (47)	34 (13)	69 (27)	25 (10)	252
I would be embarrassed giving sexual and reproductive health advice to people ($p = 0.007$) *						
	Strongly disagree	Disagree	Neutral	Agree	Strongly agree	Total
Bachelor of Pharmacy (4 years)	59 (24)	58 (24)	73 (30)	44 (18)	8 (3)	242
Bachelor of Pharmacy (6 years)	51 (20)	66 (26)	51 (20)	69 (27)	18 (7)	255
Community pharmacists are adequately trained to provide advice on sexual and reproductive health matters ($p < 0.001$)						
	Strongly disagree	Disagree	Neutral	Agree	Strongly agree	Total
Bachelor of Pharmacy (4 years)	76 (31)	85 (35)	67 (27)	12 (5)	5 (2)	245
Bachelor of Pharmacy (6 years)	30 (12)	98 (38)	66 (26)	42 (16)	19 (7)	255
Young people (aged 25 years and below) would use sexual and reproductive health services at this pharmacy ($p < 0.001$)						
	Strongly disagree	Disagree	Neutral	Agree	Strongly agree	Total
Bachelor of Pharmacy (4 years)	114 (48)	10 (4)	57 (24)	58 (24)	1 (0)	240
Bachelor of Pharmacy (6 years)	39 (15)	44 (17)	88 (34)	70 (27)	15 (6)	256

Numbers and percentages in parentheses. p-values obtained using Fisher's exact test, except for * in the chi-square test.

3.4. Pharmacists' Self-Reported Confidence to Provide Education on Reproductive Health Topics to Patients

Figure 2 shows participants' confidence levels in providing education on various reproductive health topics. The reproductive health topics that participants reported more than moderate confidence were as follows: barrier contraception (27.7%), pregnancy tests (27.6%), ovulation tests (24.0%), hormonal contraceptives (22.3%), and EC (16.0%). However, more than half of the participants were only slightly confident or not at all confident when providing education on EC.

Table 4 shows the relationship between the provision of patient education on reproductive health topics and self-reported confidence. Participants who provided reproductive health education services tended to report higher self-confidence scores in educating patients about reproductive health topics ($p < 0.001$ for pregnancy tests, ovulation tests, hormonal contraception, and EC, and $p = 0.013$ for barrier contraceptives for men).

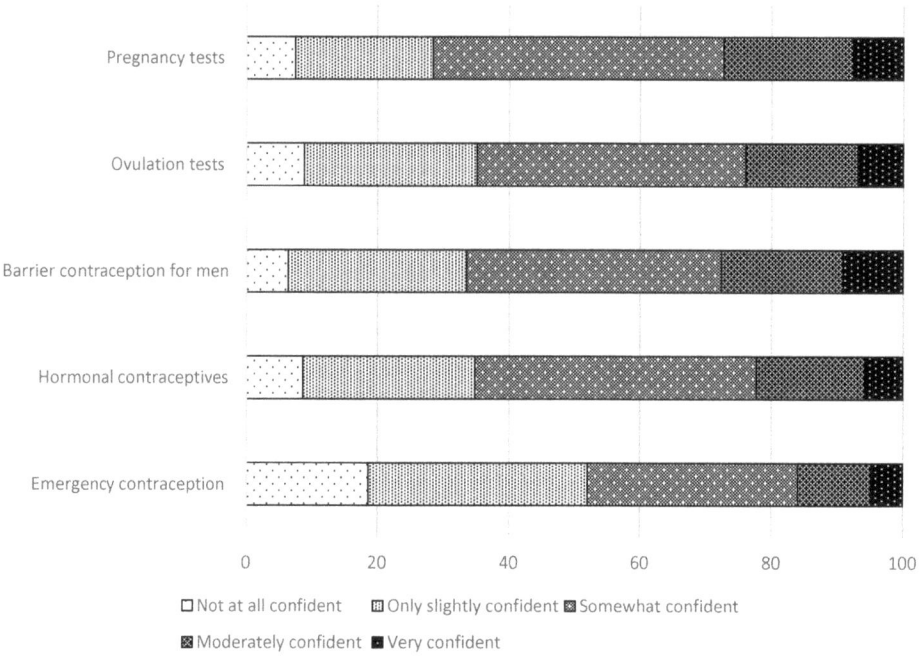

Figure 2. Confidence to provide education on topics related to reproductive health.

Table 4. Relationship between the provision of patient education with reference to sexual and reproductive health (SRH) services, and self-reported confidence.

Patient Education Service						
Pregnancy tests (p-value: chi-square test: <0.001, Cochran–Armitage test for trend: <0.001)						
Patient education	Very	Moderately	Confident Somewhat	Only slightly	Not at all	Total
Provided	25	45	92	25	3	190
Not provided	16	59	143	86	37	341
Ovulation tests (p-value: chi-square test: <0.001, Cochran–Armitage test for trend: <0.001)						
	Very	Moderately	Somewhat	Only slightly	Not at all	Total
Provided	22	56	104	32	6	220
Not provided	14	33	110	107	41	305
Barrier contraceptives for men (p-value: Fisher's exact e test: 0.0323, exact Cochran–Armitage test for trend: 0.013)						
	Very	Moderately	Somewhat	Only slightly	Not at all	Total
Provided	5	9	18	3	1	36
Not provided	44	88	185	140	33	490
Hormonal contraception (p-value: chi-square test: <0.001, Cochran–Armitage test for trend; <0.001)						
	Very	Moderately	Somewhat	Only slightly	Not at all	Total
Provided	18	45	96	40	6	205
Not provided	13	42	131	98	40	324
Emergency contraception (p-value: chi-square test: <0.001, Cochran–Armitage test for trend: <0.001)						
	Very	Moderately	Somewhat	Only slightly	Not at all	Total
Provided	7	19	30	18	7	81
Not provided	19	39	136	158	92	444

3.5. Pharmacists' Interest in Expanding Their SRH Role and Additional Training

Regarding pharmacists' role in SRH, two hundred and ninety participants (55%) reported that they would like to expand their role, while 13% indicated not being interested, and 33% did not know. In terms of SRH training, the majority of participants (80%) expressed interest in additional opportunities, and 6% of them would not like to have additional training. There were no statistically significant differences among participants based on educational background differences (data not shown).

4. Discussion

This study using a web-based survey revealed current practice and the willingness of Japanese community pharmacists to offer reproductive health services. The results also showed that their confidence to provide education to patients on reproductive health topics is not high, especially regarding EC. The pharmacists who participated in this survey reported that they were interested in expanding their role in SRH services. To achieve that, they need additional training in this regard. This is the first survey on the provision of SRH services and attitudes toward SRH services from Japanese community pharmacists' perspectives.

Most pharmacists working in drugstores currently sell pregnancy and ovulation test kits and barrier contraceptives, but only one-third of pharmacists working in pharmacies sell these items. This indicates that drugstores, as compared to pharmacies, are more likely to be locations where patients can access these test kits. This is because Japanese pharmacies are more focused on dispensing drugs based on prescriptions. Even among pharmacists working in drugstores, one third sell the test kits without patient education, and only 12% of pharmacists provide patient education for barrier contraceptives. This indicates the inadequacy of the reproductive health services provided by community pharmacists, regarding ensuring safety and proper use of contraceptives. This also implies that community pharmacists need to educate the patients on contraceptive methods because barrier contraception using condoms is the primary method of contraception in Japan [15].

Half of the participants provided the service of dispensing hormonal contraceptives with prescription, and about 20% dispensed EC pills. As a medical doctor's prescription is required to obtain EC pills in Japan, these pills are more commonly dispensed at clinics or hospitals than at pharmacies. Japanese women are reported to be uncomfortable with obtaining EC pills from pharmacists, or they may not be familiar with the fact that pharmacists dispense EC prescriptions because doctors have historically been permitted to both prescribe and dispense these pills to their patients [24,25]. Therefore, while pharmacists are willing to offer reproductive health services, it can involve a new process that requires adaptation. For example, they probably do not have enough experience dispensing EC pills (as it is commonly prescribed and dispensed by physicians) because they have not been involved with EC dispensing in the past due to national regulations and legislation. In line with these results, participants also reported the need for more training in EC medication. Our survey indicated that training and experience with EC would be expected to increase their confidence to provide reproductive health education to patients [26].

Most participants were willing to offer and expand their roles to provide SRH services, suggesting that Japanese community pharmacists may be attitudinally attuned to providing such services. As 160,000–180,000 abortions are reported per year in Japan [27], it is necessary to provide EC options and sex education for the younger generation. As community pharmacies constitute the most accessible healthcare facilities, the provision of accurate information on reproductive health to the community through such pharmacies would be desirable. Because participants of this study also reported a lack of confidence in providing such services, education and training related to SRH would enable them to expand their role in this field and provide the required services in their community.

Participants who had graduated from the 6-year program were more inclined to provide reproductive health services than those who graduated from the 4-year program. As 10 years have passed since the 6-year program was initiated, most participants who had graduated from the 6-year program were 34 years old or younger when the survey was conducted. Therefore, it is not clear whether this difference that was found was due to the type of pharmacy program undertaken and its curriculum, or the younger age of the participants who had graduated from the 6-year program. Sex education received in primary and secondary schools differs with age; therefore, the age of participants could affect the inclination to provide SRH services [28]. It is also important to consider that sex education provided in Japan may not be adequate and needs improvement [29]. Therefore, pharmacy education could be a stronger influence on whether the participants were willing to provide SRH services or not.

More than 80% of the participants who provided SRH services showed at least some confidence in providing education to patients about reproductive health topics. This suggested that prior experience raises their confidence in delivering such services. Most participants were interested in additional SRH training. Still, only 55% reported a desire to expand their role in SRH services, suggesting that they may not have enough confidence to provide SRH services or they may need additional support, for example, offered by pharmacy owners (such as installation of consulting rooms) or pharmacist organizations (additional training or education opportunities).

This study had some limitations. The generalizability of the results is limited because of voluntary response bias and non-response bias. The number of participants in the younger age group was higher than that of pharmacists in Japan. As the participants would have more interest in providing SRH services, this would imply a bias towards including more pharmacists who wanted to expand their role in SRH services.

Different strategies were used to distribute the survey, and participants were not identified in any way, so this makes it challenging to identify if pharmacists completed the questionnaire more than once. Furthermore, using Facebook and Twitter as recruitment platforms could lead to selection biases towards younger pharmacists. However, this could be mitigated by using other recruitment venues (pharmacists associations, pharmacy chains, and drugstores).

The characteristics of the Japanese cohort indicate that the survey represented a particular group of pharmacists, and the results may not be generalizable to all Japanese pharmacists. The sample of this study may not be representative of Japanese pharmacists because the proportion of women was slightly lower (55% vs. 61%), and the proportion of pharmacists aged <40 years old was higher (61% vs. 38%) [30]. However, it is relevant to mention that this survey aimed to target community pharmacists only, and there are no available national demographic statistics for the subgroup of Japanese pharmacists. Additionally, there was no sample size set a priori, and we approached this by using convenience sampling.

Despite these limitations, there are some strengths to this study. This is the first survey addressing the current situation and practice of reproductive health services from Japanese community pharmacists' perspectives. This study is also the first to reveal that most Japanese community pharmacists have a positive attitude toward providing SRH services and are interested in expanding their role and having additional training in SRH.

Differences in practices, attitudes towards sex or sexual health, and confidence on these topics might be partially influenced by experience and education as well as personal beliefs. It is necessary to expand pharmacists' roles beyond providing traditional product-focused services in several SRH areas. Further research could look into strategies to support the expansion of pharmacists' roles and the incorporation of comprehensive SRH pharmacy services into practice, as well as the impact of the SRH services that pharmacists provide to their communities.

5. Conclusions

To our knowledge, this is the first Japanese study to include several SRH topics and address them from a pharmacists' perspective lens. The findings of this study indicate that pharmacists are involved in the delivery of SRH pharmacy services to varying extents.

While Japanese community pharmacists are willing to offer reproductive health services, they do not feel confident enough to provide patient education on reproductive health topics, especially EC. Japanese community pharmacists are interested in expanding their role and receiving additional training on reproductive health topics. Education, experience, and training seem necessary to achieve that goal. The results of this survey can guide future studies to explore the reasons for disengagement of pharmacists in reproductive health services, and ways to support the incorporation of comprehensive SRH pharmacy services into practice.

Author Contributions: Conceptualization, S.Y., C.A.H., N.Y. and T.J.S.; methodology, C.A.H., J.N., N.Y. and T.J.S.; formal analysis, S.Y.; investigation, S.Y., T.T., J.N, C.A.H., N.Y., T.J.S., T.S., P.A. and C.P.; writing—original draft preparation, S.Y.; writing—review and editing, T.T., J.N, C.A.H., N.Y., T.J.S., T.S., P.A. and C.P.; supervision, C.A.H., N.Y. and T.J.S.; project administration, C.A.H. and J.N. All authors have read and agreed to the published version of the manuscript.

Funding: This work was supported by Faculty of Pharmacy and Pharmaceutical Sciences, University of Alberta (The Taiho Fund).

Institutional Review Board Statement: This study received approval from the research ethics review committee of Josai International (Approved Number: 10M200001).

Informed Consent Statement: An information letter and a consent form were included at the beginning of the survey; completion of the survey and submission of responses implied participants' consent.

Data Availability Statement: The data presented in this study are available on request from the corresponding author.

Acknowledgments: The authors wish to acknowledge the support of the EPICORE Center and the Alberta SPOR Support Unit Consultation and Research Services in the development and distribution of the online survey, and in data management.

Conflicts of Interest: The authors declare no conflict of interest directly relevant to the content of this article.

Appendix A

Appendix A.1. Informed Consent for Online Research

Your participation in this study is completely voluntary. Your consent to participate will be implied by completion of the survey. You can choose to not answer questions that you do not wish to and can withdraw from the survey with no adverse consequences at any time up until you press submit. Closing the window at any point prior to clicking the submit button will end your participation and will not submit your data. However, once you have clicked the "submit" button at the end of the survey, your data cannot be withdrawn.

All of the information that is collected will be kept confidential. Before results are released, any identifying data will be removed. If a publication or presentation results from this research, no names or identifying information will be used.

During the data collection and after, the information will be kept in a secure area (secure Canadian based database) by the principal investigators for a minimum of 5 years. We will not publish any information which could identify you in any way. By completing and submitting the survey, you give us permission to use your survey answers for the study.

There are no direct benefits or known risks from participation in this study. However, if any risks are discovered, you will be notified immediately.

If you have any questions, or would like a copy of this consent letter, you can contact Dr. Shigeo Yamamura – email: s_yama@jiu.ac.jp Tel: 0475-53-4583.

The plan for this study has been reviewed for its adherence to ethical guidelines and approved by the research ethics review committee of Josai International University (Approval Number: 10M200001)

Clicking the "Next" button indicates your willingness to complete the international comparison of community pharmacists' roles and attitudes in provision of sexual and reproductive health (SRH) services survey.

Thank you in advance for your participation

Questions used in this study. This is a part of survey questions in international comparison of community pharmacists' roles in provision of sexual and reproductive health (SRH) services

Appendix B

Appendix B.1. Provision of Sexual and Reproductive Health (SRH) Services

Please indicate whether the following products and services are currently provided at the pharmacy where you work.

1. Pregnancy tests.

    Does your pharmacy sell pregnancy tests?
    Do you provide patient education on pregnancy tests?

2. Ovulation Tests.

    Does your pharmacy sell ovulation tests?
    Do you provide patient education on ovulation tests?

3. Contraception.

    Does your pharmacy sell male non-hormonal (barrier) contraceptives? (e.g., condoms)
    Do you provide patient education on male non-hormonal (barrier) contraceptives?
    Do you dispense combined hormonal contraceptives (CHC)? (with prescription)
    Do you provide patient education on hormonal contraception?

4. Emergency contraception.

    Do you provide patient education on ECPs?
    Do you dispense emergency contraception pills (ECPs)?
    Do you dispense emergency contraception pills (ECPs)?

Appendix B.2. Attitudes toward Sexual and Reproductive Health (SRH) Services (We Used Five-Point Likert Scale for Following Questions)

Please indicate how strongly you agree or disagree with each of the following statements about SRH services:

1. It is an important part of a community pharmacist's role to offer advice on sexual and reproductive health.
2. Community pharmacists are adequately trained to provide advice on sexual and reproductive health matters.
3. There is a need for sexual health and reproductive services in the local area near this pharmacy.
4. Young people (25 years old and below) would use sexual and reproductive health services in this pharmacy.
5. Pharmacists know when to advise clients on the need to consult a physician for sexual and reproductive health advice/treatment.
6. Community pharmacists should be more involved in sexually transmitted infections prevention, screening, testing, and treatment.
7. The patient is more likely to ask questions about SRH to a community pharmacist than his/her doctor.
8. I would be embarrassed giving sexual and reproductive health advice to people.
9. I have religious or moral objections to providing sexual and reproductive health services.
10. In this community pharmacy, the sexual and reproductive health services currently offered are used regularly.
11. As a pharmacist, I have an ethical responsibility to provide SRH services.

12. There is a need to expand the provision of SRH services in the community pharmacy where I work.

Appendix B.3. Self-Reported Confidence in Providing Sexual and Reproductive Health (SRH) Services

Please indicate to what extent you feel confident about providing SRH education to patients in each of the following areas:
1. Pregnancy tests.
2. Ovulation tests.
3. Male barrier contraception (e.g., condoms).
4. Hormonal contraception.
5. Emergency contraception.

Appendix B.4. Sexual and Reproductive Health (SRH) Competencies and Training Preferences
1. Would you like to expand your role in SRH services?
2. Would additional training be beneficial in expanding your role in SRH services?

References

1. Fathalla, M.F.; Fathalla, M.M.F. Sexual and Reproductive Health: Overview: The International Encyclopedia of Public Health. In *Reference Module in Biomedical Sciences*, 2nd ed.; Associated Press: New York, NY, USA, 2017; pp. 481–490. [CrossRef]
2. Starrs, A.M.; Ezeh, A.C.; Barker, G.; Basu, A.; Bertrand, J.T.; Blum, R.; Coll-Seck, A.M.; Grover, A.; Laski, L.; Roa, M.; et al. Accelerate progress—Sexual and reproductive health and rights for all: Report of the Guttmacher–Lancet Commission. *Lancet* **2018**, *391*, 2642–2692. [CrossRef]
3. World Health Organization. Sexual and Reproductive Health and Research (SRH). Available online: https://www.who.int/teams/sexual-and-reproductive-health-and-research (accessed on 28 September 2021).
4. FIP STATEMENT OF POLICY. Pharmacists Supporting Women and Responsible Use of Medicines—Empowering Informal Careers. Available online: https://www.fip.org/file/4329 (accessed on 28 September 2021).
5. Navarrete, J.; Yuksel, N.; Schindel, T.J.; Hughes, C.A. Sexual and reproductive health services provided by community pharmacists: A scoping review. *BMJ Open.* **2021**, *11*, e047034. [CrossRef] [PubMed]
6. Emergency Contraception. Practice Bulletin No. 152 (2015), American College of Obstetricians and Gynecologists. Available online: https://www.acog.org/clinical/clinical-guidance/practice-bulletin/articles/2015/09/emergency-contraception (accessed on 28 September 2021).
7. Emergency Contraception. The Office on Women's Health in the U.S. Department of Health and Human Services. Available online: https://www.womenshealth.gov/a-z-topics/emergency-contraception (accessed on 28 September 2021).
8. Rafie, S.; Stone, R.H.; Wilkinson, T.A.; Borgelt, L.M.; El-Ibiary, S.Y.; Ragland, D. Role of the community pharmacist in emergency contraception counseling and delivery in the United States: Current trends and future prospects. *Integr. Pharm. Res. Pract.* **2017**, *23*, 99–108. [CrossRef] [PubMed]
9. Turnbull, G.; Scott, R.H.; Mann, S.; Wellings, K. Affiliations. Accessing emergency contraception pills from pharmacies: The experience of young women in London. *BMJ Sex Reprod. Health.* **2021**, *47*, 27–31. [CrossRef] [PubMed]
10. Stone, R.H.; Rafie, S.; Ernest, D.; Scutt, B. Emergency Contraception Access and Counseling in Urban Pharmacies: A Comparison between States with and without Pharmacist Prescribing. *Pharmacy* **2020**, *8*, 105. [CrossRef] [PubMed]
11. Collins, J.C.; Schneider, C.R.; Moles, R.J. Emergency contraception supply in Australian pharmacies after the introduction of ulipristal acetate: A mystery shopping mixed-methods study. *Contraception* **2018**, *98*, 243–246. [CrossRef] [PubMed]
12. Yamamura, S.; Yamamoto, N.; Oide, S.; Kitazawa, S. Current state of community pharmacy in Japan: Practice, research, and future opportunities or challenges. *Ann. Pharmacother.* **2006**, *40*, 2008–2014. [CrossRef] [PubMed]
13. The Results of the Review Meeting Regarding the Appropriateness of Switching Requested Ingredients to OTC, the Ministry of Health, Labour and Welfare. 2018. Available online: https://www.mhlw.go.jp/file/06-Seisakujouhou-11120000-Iyakushokuhinkyoku/0000193402.pdf (accessed on 28 September 2021).
14. Hasumoto, K.; Thomas, R.K.; Yokoi, M.; Arai, K. Comparison of community pharmacy practice in Japan and the US state of Illinois. *J. Pharm. Pract.* **2020**, *33*, 48–54. [CrossRef] [PubMed]
15. Yoshida, H.; Sakamoto, H.; Leslie, A.; Takahashi, O.; Tsuboi, S.; Kitamura, K. Contraception, Contraception in Japan: Current trends. *Contraception* **2016**, *93*, 475–477. [CrossRef]
16. Annual Report of JPA (2018–2019). Available online: https://www.nichiyaku.or.jp/assets/uploads/about/anuual_report2018j.pdf (accessed on 28 August 2021).
17. Home page of Japan Society for Pharmaceutical Education. Available online: http://www.jsphe.jp/en (accessed on 28 September 2021).

18. Model Core Curriculum for Pharmacy Education, The Pharmaceutical Society of Japan. Available online: https://www.pharm.or.jp/eng/curriculum.html (accessed on 28 September 2021).
19. Utsumi, M.; Hirano, S.; Fujii, Y.; Yamamoto, H. Evaluation of pharmacy practice program in the 6-year pharmaceutical education curriculum in Japan: Hospital pharmacy practice program. *J. Pharm. Health Care Sci.* **2015**, *1*, 18. [CrossRef]
20. Harris, P.A.; Taylor, R.; Thielke, R.; Payne, J.; Gonzalez, N.; Conde, J.G. Research electronic data capture (RED-Cap)—a metadata-driven methodology and workflow process for providing translational research informatics support. *J. Biomed. Inform.* **2009**, *42*, 377–381. [CrossRef]
21. Harris, P.A.; Taylor, R.; Minor, B.L.; Elliott, V.; Fernandez, M.; O'Neal, L.; McLeod, L.; Delacqua, G.; Delacqua, F.; Kirby, J.; et al. The REDCap consortium: Building an international community of software platform partners. *J. Biomed. Inform.* **2019**, *95*, 103208. [CrossRef] [PubMed]
22. AEON HAPYCOM. Comprehensive Personal Training Organization (Homepage). Available online: http://www.hapycom.or.jp (accessed on 28 September 2021).
23. Navarrete, J. Community Pharmacists' Roles in Sexual and Reproductive Health (A thesis for the degree of Master of Science in Pharmacy Practice, Faculty of Pharmacy and Pharmaceutical Sciences, University of Alberta). Available online: https://era.library.ualberta.ca/items/bd35cc3b-4cc8-4a67-8fbe-14ba05c54791/view/526f1df3-b158-4ac2-ac17-cb24c32f5fd2/Navarrete_Martinez_Javiera_Constanza_202101_MSc.pdf (accessed on 28 September 2021).
24. Article 19, in Pharmacists' Act in Japan. Available online: http://www.japaneselawtranslation.go.jp/law/detail/?id=2596&vm=04&re=01 (accessed on 28 September 2021).
25. Article 22 in Medical Practitioners' Act. Available online: http://www.japaneselawtranslation.go.jp/law/detail/?id=2074&vm=&re= (accessed on 9 September 2021).
26. Yuksel, N.; Schindel, T.J.; Eurich, D.; Tsuyuki, R.T. From prescription to behind the counter: Pharmacists views on providing emergency contraception. *J. Pharm. Res. Clin. Prac.* **2011**, *1*, 19–29. Available online: https://scholar.google.co.jp/citations?view_op=view_citation&hl=en&user=_nRWUOsAAAAJ&cstart=20&pagesize=80&citation_for_view=_nRWUOsAAAAJ:Zph67rFs4hoC (accessed on 28 September 2021).
27. Kamijo, K.; Kataoka, Y.; Shigemi, D. Challenges of accessing emergency contraceptive pills in Japan. *BMJ Sex Reprod. Health* **2021**, *47*, 232–233. [CrossRef] [PubMed]
28. Nishioka, E. Historical Transition of Sexuality Education in Japan and Outline of Reproductive Health/Rights [Article in Japanese]. *Nihon Eiseigaku Zasshi* **2018**, *73*, 178–184. [CrossRef] [PubMed]
29. Nishioka, E. Trends in Research on Adolescent Sexuality Education, Fertility Awareness, and the Possibility of Life Planning Based on Reproductive Health Education [Article in Japanese]. *Nihon Eiseigaku Zasshi.* **2018**, *73*, 185–199. [CrossRef] [PubMed]
30. Handbook of Health and Welfare Statistics 2019 Ministry of Health, Labour and Welfare. 2019. Available online: https://www.mhlw.go.jp/english/database/db-hh/xlsx/2-45.xlsx (accessed on 28 September 2021).

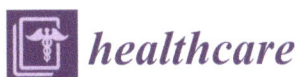

Article

Community Pharmacists' Perceptions towards the Misuse and Abuse of Pregabalin: A Cross-Sectional Study from Aseer Region, Saudi Arabia

Sultan M. Alshahrani [1,*], Khalid Orayj [1], Ali M. Alqahtani [2] and Mubarak A. Algahtany [3]

1 Clinical Pharmacy Department, College of Pharmacy, King Khalid University, Abha 61441, Saudi Arabia; korayg@kku.edu.sa
2 Pharmacology Department, College of Pharmacy, King Khalid University, Abha 62529, Saudi Arabia; amsfr@kku.edu.sa
3 Division of Neurosurgery, Department of Surgery, College of Medicine, King Khalid University, Abha 62512-2291, Saudi Arabia; mbalgahtany@kku.edu.sa
* Correspondence: shahrani@kku.edu.sa; Tel.: +96-650-874-7473

Abstract: Pregabalin is a first-line therapy for neuropathic pain and for chronic pain. It has abuse potential. This study was conducted to assess community pharmacists' perceptions towards pregabalin abuse and misuse in the Aseer region, Saudi Arabia, and identify predictors and associated factors. A cross-sectional survey using a structured questionnaire following a self-administrative study was conducted across community pharmacies in the Aseer region (Abha, Khamis Mushait, Mahayel, Sarat Abeeda, Ahad-Rufaida, and Bishah). A total of 206 respondents from community pharmacists participated in the study. Over the last six months, 136 respondents (66.0%) suspected pregabalin abuse in community pharmacies; male dominance in pregabalin abusers was also recorded (n = 165, 80.1%). Additionally, 40 (19.4%) respondents stated that a prescription was not issued for pregabalin demands. Over half (61.7%) of community pharmacists recorded an increased change in pregabalin abuse compared to the previous year. This is the first study to explore pharmacists' perceptions in the community of the Aseer region towards customers' misuse and abuse of pregabalin. Further monitoring and regulations on the prescribing and procurement of pregabalin are needed to avoid abuse.

Keywords: pregabalin; abuse; community pharmacists; Saudi Arabia; pain

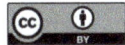

1. Introduction

Prescription drug misuse and abuse have been reported as a global issue [1]. The World Health Organization has clearly defined the rationale of drug use as when "patients receive medications appropriate to their clinical needs, in doses that meet their own individual requirements, for an adequate period of time, and at the lowest cost to them and their community" [2]. Drug misuse is when patients use medications in a way other than that prescribed by a physician [3]. However, the National Institute on Drug Abuse (NIDA) defines the misuse of prescription drugs as "taking a drug in a way or dosage that is not prescribed; taking somebody's prescription, even though it is for a valid medical reason like pain; or taking a drug to feel euphoric" [4,5]. On the other hand, drug abuse is the use of medications in a way that is inconsistent with legal and medical purposes. Both practices are considered inappropriate uses of medication [3]. Records state that the euphoria which appears as an adverse reaction in approximately 10% of patients is a leading cause of abuse [6]. As per statistics from the United Nations Office on Drugs and Crime, about 5% of adolescents who used drugs at least once in 2015 have reportedly suffered from drug use disorders, numbering 29.5 million in total [3,7]. Drug misuse is an increasing economic threat to public health. For problematic drug use in England and Wales, annual social costs have been assumed to be around GBP 11.961 million or GBP

35.455 per year/per user [8,9]. In Saudi Arabia, there is insufficient information on drug abuse; however, some studies have shown that opioids, alcohol, and cannabis are perhaps the most prevalent drugs abused in treatment centers [10].

Pregabalin is an analog of gamma-aminobutyric acid (GABA), the mammalian neurotransmitter. Pregabalin is structurally similar to gabapentin, which is known as an alpha 2 omega ligand [11]. For neuropathic pain, pregabalin is prescribed as the first-line therapy as well as for chronic pain [12,13]. Pregabalin inhibits the release of neurotransmitters (glutamate, noradrenaline, 5-hydroxytryptamine, dopamine, and substance P) at synapses by binding to the α2δ-subunits of presynaptic voltage-dependent calcium channels. The drug blocks the excitability of the neurons, particularly in the central nervous system (CNS) [14]. These neurons' blocking actions possibly account for the analgesic, anticonvulsant, anxiolytic, and sleep-modulating activities of pregabalin [14–16]. As per Pharma Marketing, net pregabalin (Lyrica®) sales worldwide in 2014 were ranked 12th (approximately USD 5.4 billion), with an annual growth rate of almost 12% [17].

Preclinical, clinical, and epidemiological observations have raised the issue of pregabalin abuse. In addition, case reports show that illegal pregabalin use is prevalent in opioid-addicted patients (68%) [17,18]. Pregabalin abuse and dependency were first recorded in 2006 in Italy, Germany, and Turkey [19]. Additionally, pregabalin is approved for use to treat neuropathic pain in Japan from fibromyalgia [20]. Pregabalin abuse has evolved from being a prescription drug to being mishandled, similarly to stimulants (methylphenidate), over the last ten years. Over time, it has become more widely available either through online outlets or on the illegal market [19,21]. To boost the overall psychogenic effect, pregabalin has often been mixed with alcohol, benzodiazepines (BZDs), zopiclone, gabapentin, cannabis, methamphetamine, morphine, amphetamines, LSD, and mephedrone [21]. The use of pregabalin and opiates at the same time has been linked to a substantially increased risk of mortality [19]. When combined with opioids or other CNS depressants, pregabalin's misuse potential raises concerns regarding greater risks of respiratory failure and death [22]. A study conducted in Jordan on community pharmacist's experiences of pregabalin misuse and abuse among their customers reveals that most participants (87.4%) reported cases of pregabalin abuse in their pharmacies [23]. Another study conducted in Lebanon reported that pharmacists might need to improve their knowledge concerning tramadol and gabapentinoids ($\alpha_2\delta$ ligands) [24]. Pregabalin was deemed a safe and effective medication for pain and helping with sleep in a Chinese study area at doses of 300–450 mg per day [25]. In Saudi Arabia, only a few studies have discussed pharmacists' awareness of the misuse and abuse of medications. They reported that pharmacy staff should have sufficient knowledge to identify medication abuse or misuse terminology. In addition, pharmacists' roles in Saudi Arabia should be clearly defined by drug legislators with policy and regulations toward the misuse and abuse of medication [3]. However, a previous study conducted in Saudi Arabia explored the prevalence of the misuse and abuse of pregabalin among healthcare workers [26].

Pregabalin was classified as a controlled substance in 2005 (USA, schedule V) and 2017 (Jordan, schedule III) [23]. Therefore, this study was designed to evaluate community pharmacists' perception in the Aseer region regarding pregabalin abuse and misuse by customers and determine its predictors and associated factors. The research will also focus on their practices regarding the dispensing of such drugs, especially with their high risk of misuse and abuse.

2. Materials and Methods

2.1. Study Design

This was a cross-sectional, questionnaire-based, self-administered study conducted across community pharmacies in the Aseer region.

2.2. Sample Size and Sampling Technique

The questionnaire was randomly distributed to 90 community pharmacies in six major cities in the Aseer region (Abha, Khamis Mushait, Mahayel, Sarat Abeeda, Ahad-Rufaida, and Bishah). Each community pharmacy had 2–3 pharmacists working over two shifts. As per the latest statistics, the number of registered community pharmacists in the Aseer region eligible to answer the study's survey was 747 pharmacists [27].

Using the sample size calculation website (http://www.raosoft.com/samplesize.html (accessed on 13 November 2020), the number of potential participants would be 252, implying a 95% confidence interval, 5% margin of error, and 50% response distribution. The data collection process was conducted by approaching community pharmacists in the designated cities and providing them with the survey. All survey-related questions and inquiries were answered. The pharmacists were asked to participate in the survey voluntarily. They were not asked about their ID or the location of their pharmacy. All data were kept confidential and treated with a minimal number of persons during data collection and analysis.

2.3. Measures

No previous study has been conducted on community pharmacists' perceptions towards pregabalin misuse and abuse in Saudi Arabia; therefore, the survey was adopted from four previous studies conducted elsewhere [3,23,24,28]. The questionnaire consisted of 21 questions on 2 domains; Domain I: 10 questions related to demographics; Domain II: 11 questions on perception with open and closed questions related to community pharmacists' perceptions towards pregabalin misuse and abuse. Initially, a pilot study was conducted on 14 faculty members in the College of Pharmacy at King Khalid University to evaluate the survey's reliability and validity. A self-administered questionnaire was created, and the pilot sample was then validated to ensure its quality and internal reliability. The Cronbach's alpha factor was determined as 0.81. In addition, three experts working within this field provided advice regarding the process. The pilot study results were not included in the final analysis.

2.4. Statistical Analyses

The questionnaires were reviewed for completeness and accuracy, and the data were cleaned, coded, and then entered into SPSS version 20 (IBM Corp., Armonk, NY, USA). The sociodemographic data were represented using descriptive analysis. Categorical variables were reported as frequencies and percentages, and continuous variables were described as means and standard deviations. Two multiple logistic regressions were conducted to investigate the factors that affected the following two dependent variables: (1) the perceived change in pregabalin abuse during the last year; and (2) the strategy used to limit suspected customers' access to pregabalin products of abuse. Regarding the second model (strategies used to limit the access to pregabalin), any effort to sell pregabalin without a prescription was considered as incorrect behavior, whereas refusing to sell the product was considered correct behavior. A particular independent variable was included in the final multiple logistic regression if it, upon conducting bivariate logistic regression with the previous two dependent factors, resulted in a p-value equal to or less than 0.20. Odds ratios and 95% confidence intervals were tabulated and analyzed.

3. Results

3.1. Demographics of the Respondents

A total of 206 respondents participated in the study. Community pharmacies completed questionnaires in the six major cities in the Aseer region (Abha, Khamis Mushait, Mahayel, Sarat Abeeda, Ahad-Rufaida, and Bishah). The majority of respondent pharmacists were male ($n = 157$, 76.2%), and the respondents' average age was between 20 and 30 years ($n = 125$, 60.7%). The most common educational backgrounds were found to be a Doctor of Pharmacy or PharmD ($n = 103$, 50%) and a Bachelor of Pharmacy ($n = 89$; 43.2%).

Almost half of the participating pharmacists had 1–4 years' experience ($n = 97$, 47.1%), whereas 30.1% had less than one year of experience ($n = 49$, 32.5%). Additionally, 90.8% of participants' pharmacies were located in an urban area ($n = 187$), and 88.3% were chain pharmacy types. Most of the pharmacies were located on a main road ($n = 130$, 63.1%). More than half of the pharmacists ($n = 114$, 535.3%) reported that they generally received an incentive for selling drugs. An overview of the respondents is given in Table 1.

Table 1. Demographics of the respondents.

Items	Sample ($n = 206$)	Percentage (%)
Gender		
Male	157	76.2
Female	49	23.8
Age		
20–30 years	125	60.7
31–40 years	61	29.6
41–50 years	18	8.7
Over 50 years	2	1.0
Education Level		
Pharmacy diploma	7	3.4
Bachelor in Pharmacy	89	43.2
Doctor of Pharmacy (PharmD)	103	50.0
Postgraduate	7	3.4
Years of Experience		
Less than one year	62	30.1
1–4 years	97	47.1
5–10 years	34	16.5
More than 10 years	13	6.3
Pharmacy Area		
Rural	19	9.2
Urban	187	90.8
Pharmacy Type		
Chain	182	88.3
Private	24	11.7
Pharmacy Location		
Main street	130	63.1
By street (village/district pharmacy)	52	25.2
Inside shopping center	24	11.7
Work-Shift Time		
Morning shift	74	35.9
Mid-day shift	80	38.8
Night shift	52	25.2
Do you receive incentives when you sell drugs in general? (Yes)	114	55.3

3.2. Community Pharmacists' Perceptions toward Customer's Misuse and Abuse of Pregabalin

Table 2 shows that 80.6% of the pharmacists sold pregabalin with the presentation of prescriptions, whereas 19.4% (n = 40) sold the drugs without prescriptions. The majority of respondents (n = 136, 66.0%) suspected pregabalin product abuse/misuse in community pharmacies in the last 6 months. Male dominance in the pregabalin-abusers was also reported (n = 165, 80.1%). Young adults aged 20–30 years (n = 128; 62.1%) were the majority of abusers, compared to those aged <20 years (9.7%) and >40 years (8.7%). The most commonly abused strengths were 75 mg (n = 72, 35%) and 150 mg (n = 73, 35.4%). It was reported that most abusers had indications of back pain (n = 60, 29.1%), followed by neuropathy (n = 44, 21.4%), epilepsy (n = 39, 18.9%), chronic pain (n = 33, 16%), and others (n = 30, 14.6%). The majority of those suspected of abusing or misusing pregabalin products were foreigners (non-usual customers of the pharmacy) (n = 152, 73.8%).

Table 2. Community pharmacists' perceptions towards customer's misuse and abuse of pregabalin.

Items	Subgroups	Sample (n = 206)	Percentage (%)
Do you receive requests to sell pregabalin with a prescription?	No, not at all	40	19.4
	Yes, sometimes	62	30.1
	Yes, usually	74	35.9
	Yes, always	30	14.6
In the last 6 months, have you received a request to sell pregabalin to someone who misused or abused them?	Yes	136	66.0
Most of the time, what is the gender of assumed pregabalin abusers who come to your pharmacy?	Male	165	80.1
Most of the time, what is the age of assumed pregabalin abusers who come to your pharmacy?	Less than 20 years	20	9.7
	20 to 30 years	128	62.1
	31 to 40 years	40	19.4
	More than 40 years	18	8.7
What is the most requested dose of pregabalin from assumed abusers who come to your pharmacy?	25 mg	6	2.9
	50 mg	23	11.2
	75 mg	72	35.0
	150 mg	73	35.4
	300 mg	32	15.5
What was indication that the assumed abusers of pregabalin claimed they had when they requested pregabalin?	Back pain	60	29.1
	Chronic pain (other than back pain)	33	16.0
	Neuropathy	44	21.4
	Epilepsy	39	18.9
	Other	30	14.6
Usually, who are the assumed abusers of pregabalin who come to your pharmacy?	Non-regular/foreign customers of the pharmacy	152	73.8
	Usual customers at the pharmacy	54	26.2

3.3. Perceived Change of Pregabalin Misuse and Abuse

The majority of the pharmacists who took part in the study noticed an increase (n = 127/206, or 61.7%) in the pattern of pregabalin abuse/misuse over last year, as shown in Figure 1. In contrast, a 38.7% decreased pattern was also observed for pregabalin abuse/misuse. The variables that calculated the logistic regression model for the perceived change in pregabalin abuse during the last year are presented in Table 3, and two of them were chosen to be included in the final multiple logistic regression (i.e., pharmacy type and the claimed indication of abusers). The final multiple logistic regression that examined the perceived change in pregabalin abuse during the last year is presented in Table 4. The "chain pharmacy" and "back pain" categories were considered reference or independent variables for pharmacy type and claimed indication of abusers, respectively. The multiple logistic regression indicated that the odds of increasing use of pregabalin in the last year was higher in private pharmacies compared to chain pharmacies (OR = 2.698). Furthermore, the abuser was more likely to have back pain compared to chronic pain (OR = 0.423), neuropathy (OR = 0.774), epilepsy (OR = 0.60), and others (OR = 0.406). However, none of these dependent variables reveal a significant p-value.

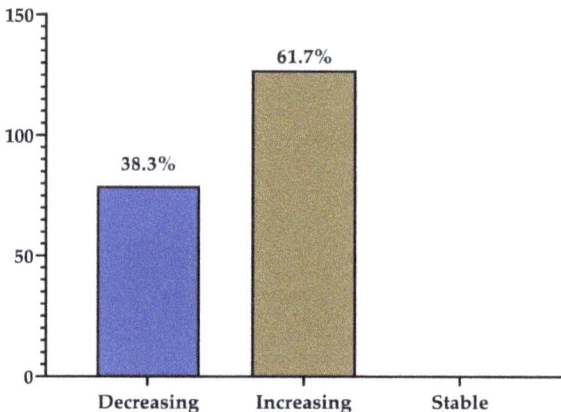

Figure 1. Perceived change of pregabalin misuse and abuse in the Aseer region (n = 206).

Table 3. Bivariate logistic regression analysis for the perceived change in pregabalin abuse during the last year.

Variable	Wald Test	p-Value
Gender	0.071	0.789
Age	0.275	0.675
Educational level	0.002	0.966
Work experience	6.408	0.421
Pharmacy area	0.125	0.724
Pharmacy type	3.325	0.068
Pharmacy location	0.916	0.339
Work shift	0.434	0.510
Incentives to sell drugs	0.007	0.935
Gender of abusers	0.949	0.330
Age of abusers	1.099	0.295
Claimed indication of abusers	2.176	0.140
Strategy used by you to limit suspected customers' access to pregabalin products of abuse	0.002	0.961

Table 4. Multiple logistic regression examining potential factors affecting the perceived change in pregabalin abuse during the last year (if OR is more than 1, this means that the misuse of pregabalin was increased in comparison to the last year).

Variable	OR (95% CI)	*p*-Value
Pharmacy type		
Chain Pharmacy	Reference	
Private pharmacy	2.698 (0.939–7.751)	0.651
Claimed indication of abusers		
Back pain	Reference	
Chronic pain (other than back pain)	0.423 (0.174–1.029)	0.058
Neuropathy	0.774 (0.326–1.834)	0.56
Epilepsy	0.6 (0.257–1.401)	0.237
Other	0.406 (0.163–1.011)	0.053

3.4. Strategy to Limit Suspected Customers' Access to Pregabalin Abuse

Pharmacists used various techniques to limit consumers' access to pregabalin abuse, with refusing to sell being the most mentioned in the present study (n = 177; 85.9%). However, 20 pharmacists (9.7%) reported that they did nothing about the issue and sold the demanded pregabalin (Table 5). All of these pharmacists were over the age of 30 (*p*-value $\leq$ 0.001). More than 115 pharmacists (55.8%) reported that the government's legal restrictions help reduce pregabalin use, although 57 pharmacists (27.7%) did not agree with this statement. Table 6 shows the variables chosen for inclusion in the final logistic regression model used to assess the strategy used to limit suspected customers' access to pregabalin products of abuse. The final multiple logistic regression is presented in Table 7. Younger pharmacists seemed to express the correct behaviors by not selling pregabalin without a prescription (i.e., pharmacists aged between 31 and 40 years were less likely to avoid selling pregabalin without a prescription (OR = 0.237) compared to pharmacists aged 20–30 years). Additionally, PharmD pharmacists were more likely to avoid selling pregabalin without a prescription (OR = 9.04) compared to pharmacists with a diploma degree.

Table 5. Strategy used to limit suspected abusers' access to pregabalin in the Aseer region (n = 206).

Items	Subgroups	Sample (n = 206)	Percentage (%)
What is the strategy used by you to limit suspected abusers' access to pregabalin products?	Do nothing. Just sell the product	20	9.7
	Selling smaller amount than requested	9	4.4
	Refusal of sale	177	85.9
Do you think that the legal restrictions applied by the government help in reducing pregabalin abuse?	No	57	27.7
	Yes	115	55.8
	I don't know	34	16.5

Table 6. Bivariate logistic regression analysis for the strategies used to limit suspected abusers' access to pregabalin products.

Variable	Wald Test	*p* Value
Gender	5.161	0.023
Age	11.47	<0.001
Educational level	3.080	0.079
Work experience	2.170	0.141

Table 6. *Cont.*

Variable	Wald Test	*p* Value
Pharmacy area	2.549	0.117
Pharmacy type	1.005	0.316
Pharmacy location	1.263	0.261
Work shift	0.638	0.424
Incentives to sell drugs	0.615	0.433
Gender of abusers	8.956	0.003
Age of abusers	5.656	0.017
Claimed indication of abusers	1.035	0.905
Usually, the assumed abusers of pregabalin who come to your pharmacy are usual or foreigner customers	22.158	<0.001

Table 7. Multiple logistic regression examining potential factors affecting the strategy used to limit suspected abusers' access to pregabalin products (if OR is more than 1, this means that the odds of correct behavior, i.e., not selling pregabalin, was higher in this group compared to the reference).

Variable	OR (95% CI)	*p*-Value
Gender		
Female	Reference	
Male	0.123 (0.015–1.005)	0.051
Age of the Pharmacist		
20–30 years	Reference	
31–40 years	0.237 (0.079–0.712)	0.01
41–50 years	0.224 (0.057–0.874)	0.031
Over 50 years	0.175 (0.003–10.281)	0.401
Education level		
Pharmacy diploma	Reference	
Bachelor in Pharmacy	5.322 (0.926–30.583)	0.061
Doctor of pharmacy (PharmD)	9.04 (1.513–53.999)	0.016
Postgraduate	1.19 (0.116–12.169)	0.884
Work Experience		
Less than one year	Reference	
1–4 years	2.901 (0.886–9.497)	0.078
5–10 years	1.629 (0.436–6.091)	0.468
More than 10 years	6.002 (0.708–50.904)	0.1
Pharmacy Area		
Rural	Reference	
Urban	1.526 (0.406–5.738)	0.532
Gender of Abusers		
Female	Reference	
Male	2.319 (0.829–6.486)	0.109

Table 7. *Cont.*

Variable	OR (95% CI)	*p*-Value
Age of Abusers		
Under 20 years	Reference	
20 to 30 years	3.85 (0.799–18.551)	0.093
31 to 40 years	9.625 (2.828–32.761)	<0.001
Over 40 years	21.962 (3.545–136.042) 0.001	<0.001
Types of Customers		
Non-usual/Foreigner customers of the pharmacy	Reference	
Usual customers at the pharmacy	5.394 (1.967–14.794)	0.001

4. Discussion

This study underlined community pharmacists' perceptions towards the misuse and abuse of pregabalin in the Aseer region of Saudi Arabia. The area studied included six cities: Abha, Khamis Mushait, Mahayel, Sarat Abeeda, Ahad-Rufaida, and Bishah. There has been no such type of study of community pharmacists regarding pregabalin misuse in the Aseer region of Saudi Arabia. However, a study was conducted from July 2017 to July 2018 in the Aseer region among healthcare professionals (physicians, pharmacists, nurses, and paramedical staff) regarding the prevalence of pregabalin abuse. This study among healthcare professionals reported that 42.9% of abusers used pregabalin for stress management, whereas 52% of abusers used it with more than one other drug [26]. In a cross-sectional study in the Eastern Region of Saudi Arabia, 48.9% (*n* = 44) of the respondents stated that the misuse and abuse of drugs in Saudi Arabia was at an alarming level [3]. Pregabalin was listed as a controlled drug in the United States in 2005 (schedule V) and 2017 in Jordan (schedule III) [23]. As for Saudi Arabia, selling pregabalin without prescriptions is restricted, although some reports have found that this still occurs. We also believe that there have been more confirmed cases of pregabalin abuse in community pharmacies.

According to some reports, pharmacists receive inadequate instruction or training in the area of drug abuse. Pharmacy students and pharmacists, in particular, are under-prepared to identify, interact with, or manage patients and co-workers who have drug abuse issues [29]. The pharmacy profession's licensing laws and ethics are designed to protect the public and maintain professional boundaries [30]. Community pharmacists are by far the most responsive healthcare professionals and the first line of support against prescription and non-prescription drug abuse; therefore, it is considered that scheduling the drug and the subsequent strengthening of inspections on its sale in community pharmacies would help minimize this issue [23,31]. In one study, 89.5% of community pharmacists distributed antipsychotic medications based on co-worker's requests without reviewing the prescriptions [32]. In this study, 19.4% of community pharmacists received a request to sell pregabalin without a prescription. However, according to the survey, 36.4% of the community pharmacists agreed that dispensing drugs without a prescription is vital for the pharmacy's profits [29]. In this study, 55.3% of community pharmacists reported receiving incentives while selling drugs in general.

More than half of the community pharmacists in our study indicated that they had received suspicious demands for pregabalin in the previous six months, most of which were for strengths of 75 mg or 150 mg and with indications of back pain (29.1%), followed by neuropathy (21.4%), epilepsy (18.9%), and chronic pain (16%). According to a previous survey, pregabalin abusers used the drug for euphoria (28.6%), whereas 42.9% used it for stress management [26]. Furthermore, in this study, males were suspected of abusing pregabalin in 80.1% of cases. This study is similar to a previous study conducted in the Aseer area for healthcare professionals [26]. Several other studies in the literature look at the male gender as a possible cause for addictive behavior [23,33,34]. It also observed that foreign (i.e., non-regular) customers are more likely to be pregabalin product abusers compared to local or usual customers.

The majority of pharmacists reported a growth (61.7%) in pregabalin abuse/misuse patterns over the previous year, although a decrease (38.7%) was noted by some. This increase in pregabalin abuse might be due to the incentives offered by customers for sales, which is also mentioned by Al-Husseini and colleagues [23]. The perceived change in pregabalin abuse during the last year was also associated with the work experience, where it was reported that pharmacists with less than one year of experience were mostly involved. A study showed that only 71% of community pharmacists had received comprehensive instruction on drug misuse/abuse since Pharmacy School graduation [35]. In another survey from the Center on Addiction and Substance Abuse in 2005, only 48% had received training to prevent drug addiction [36]. However, one study showed that most community pharmacists were taught or trained to detect abuse or dependency during a pharmacy bachelor's degree. However, approximately 85.8% of community pharmacists indicated a desire to receive advanced educational programs in drug abuse [29,30]. Pharmacist participation in community service and substance addiction management studies should be facilitated as well as the inclusion of training or specialization in pharmacy residency programs [30].

Prescription-only medication does not authorize pharmacists to dispense medicine without a prescription written by a doctor, and this is where a pharmacist's professional and ethical judgment is essential. Some pharmacists might respond by selling large quantities of the products that have been requested [37]. In this study, 9.7% of community pharmacists agreed to sell the requested pregabalin, despite it being an unethical practice to do so. The community pharmacists in the Aseer area studied in this study limited pregabalin product abuse by applying the legal restrictions from the government; 55.8% of the community pharmacists agreed with the above statement. Traditionally, pharmacists have used different strategies, such as refusing to sell such drugs, placing them out of sight, or demanding a medical prescription [38,39]. Therefore, our study results suggested that 85.9% of community pharmacists agreed to refuse the sale to limit suspected customers' access. However, these techniques are of little use because patients can obtain supplies from other pharmacies [40]. This issue can be reduced if pharmacists network with each other more often; if a suspected abuser is identified to other local pharmacies, they can be notified systematically by linking all pharmacies on a national level by an electronic system. This form of model requires community pharmacist training as well as increased collaboration with healthcare professionals [40,41].

This study has a few limitations, which are: (1) Saudi Arabia's health authorities have restricted the sale of pregabalin without a prescription [42], but some people can still obtain the drug; (2) The data presented in this study were focused on community pharmacists' perceptions towards day-to-day events, which are utterly personal and only represented single perspectives. As a result, a critical reflection in the pharmacy-based analysis is more reliable in this context; (3) The questionnaire was answered by community pharmacists in Saudi Arabia's Aseer area, which is not representative of Saudi Arabia overall; and (4) The sample size was relatively small. As a result, the current study's findings can only reflect the situation in the Aseer area. Future research should include a higher proportion of community pharmacies from various regions across Saudi Arabia.

5. Conclusions

This study provides a basic representation of community pharmacists' attitudes, awareness, and opinions in the Aseer region of Saudi Arabia, addressing pregabalin abuse. According to participating pharmacists, pregabalin could be abused, with young males being the most likely pregabalin abusers. A substantial number of pregabalin demands were not followed by a prescription. There was a perceived change in pregabalin misuse and abuse in the Aseer region over the previous year. These results highlight the importance of developing better pharmacy-based programs to increase drug prescribers' (e.g., physicians, neurosurgeons, and pharmacists) awareness regarding the potential misuse of pregabalin. Further monitoring and regulations on the prescribing and procurement of pregabalin are needed to avoid the abuse, and a strict policy for pharmacists regarding drug misuse and abuse is also needed in Saudi Arabia.

Author Contributions: Conceptualization, S.M.A. and K.O.; methodology, K.O.; A.M.A. software, K.O.; validation, S.M.A., M.A.A., A.M.A. and K.O.; formal analysis, K.O.; investigation, M.A.A., K.O.; resources, M.A.A., A.M.A.; data curation, K.O., S.M.A.; writing—original draft preparation, S.M.A., A.M.A., K.O., M.A.A.; writing—review and editing, S.M.A., A.M.A.; visualization, K.O.; supervision, S.M.A.; project administration, S.M.A. All authors have read and agreed to the published version of the manuscript.

Funding: This research received no external funding.

Institutional Review Board Statement: The Research Ethics Committee at King Khalid University (HAPO-06-B-001) has reviewed and agreed to the conducting of this project: Approval No. ECM#2020-3211; Approval date 24 December 2020.

Informed Consent Statement: Informed consent was obtained from all subjects involved in the study.

Data Availability Statement: Data are available upon request.

Acknowledgments: The authors would like to acknowledge King Khalid University for administrative and technical support.

Conflicts of Interest: The authors declare no conflict of interest.

References

1. Lessenger, J.E.; Feinberg, S.D. Abuse of Prescription and Over-the-Counter Medications. *J. Am. Board Fam. Med.* **2008**, *21*, 45. [CrossRef] [PubMed]
2. World Health, O. *Promoting Rational Use of Medicines: Core Components*; World Health Organization: Geneva, Switzerland, 2002.
3. Alshayban, D.M.; Chacko, R.J.; Aljishi, F.; Lucca, J.M. Knowledge, perception, and practice of pharmacy professionals on drug misuse and abuse in eastern region of Saudi Arabia. *J. Rep. Pharm. Sci.* **2020**, *9*, 86. [CrossRef]
4. Hughes, G.F.; McElnay, J.C.; Hughes, C.M.; McKenna, P. Abuse/misuse of non-prescription drugs. *Pharm. World Sci.* **1999**, *21*, 251–255. [CrossRef] [PubMed]
5. Wazaify, M.; Hughes, C.M.; McElnay, J.C. The implementation of a harm minimisation model for the identification and treatment of over-the-counter drug misuse and abuse in community pharmacies in Northern Ireland. *Patient Educ. Couns.* **2006**, *64*, 136–141. [CrossRef]
6. Schwan, S.; Sundström, A.; Stjernberg, E.; Hallberg, E.; Hallberg, P. A signal for an abuse liability for pregabalin—results from the Swedish spontaneous adverse drug reaction reporting system. *Eur. J. Clin. Pharmacol.* **2010**, *66*, 947–953. [CrossRef] [PubMed]
7. Ali, S.F.; Onaivi, E.S.; Dodd, P.R.; Cadet, J.L.; Schenk, S.; Kuhar, M.J.; Koob, G.F. Understanding the Global Problem of Drug Addiction is a Challenge for IDARS Scientists. *Curr. Neuropharmacol.* **2011**, *9*, 2–7. [CrossRef] [PubMed]
8. Petry, N.M.; Tedford, J.; Austin, M.; Nich, C.; Carroll, K.M.; Rounsaville, B.J. Prize reinforcement contingency management for treating cocaine users: How low can we go, and with whom? *Addiction* **2004**, *99*, 349–360. [CrossRef]
9. Godfrey, C.; Eaton, G.; McDougall, C.; Culyer, A. *The Economic and Social Costs of Class A Drug Use in England and Wales, 2000*; Home Office Research, Development and Statistics Directorate: London, UK, 2002.
10. Bassiony, M. Substance use disorders in Saudi Arabia: Review article. *J. Subst. Use* **2013**, *18*, 450–466. [CrossRef]
11. Papazisis, G.; Tzachanis, D. Pregabalin's abuse potential: A mini review focusing on the pharmacological profile. *Int. J. Clin. Pharmacol. Ther.* **2014**, *52*, 709–716. [CrossRef]
12. Wiffen, P.J.; Derry, S.; Moore, R.A.; Aldington, D.; Cole, P.; Rice, A.S.C.; Lunn, M.P.T.; Hamunen, K.; Haanpaa, M.; Kalso, E.A. Antiepileptic drugs for neuropathic pain and fibromyalgia—An overview of Cochrane reviews. *Cochrane Database Syst. Rev.* **2013**, *2013*, CD010567. [CrossRef]
13. Shmagel, A.; Ngo, L.; Ensrud, K.; Foley, R. Prescription Medication Use Among Community-Based U.S. Adults With Chronic Low Back Pain: A Cross-Sectional Population Based Study. *J. Pain* **2018**, *19*, 1104–1112. [CrossRef]
14. Zhang, Y.; Wang, X.; Dong, G. The analgesic efficiency of pregabalin for the treatment of postoperative pain in total hip arthroplasty: A randomized controlled study protocol. *Medicine* **2020**, *99*, e21071. [CrossRef]
15. Wong, L.; Turner, L. Treatment of post-burn neuropathic pain: Evaluation of pregabalin. *Burn. J. Int. Soc. Burn Inj.* **2010**, *36*, 769–772. [CrossRef]
16. Schifano, F.; D'Offizi, S.; Piccione, M.; Corazza, O.; Deluca, P.; Davey, Z.; Di Melchiorre, G.; Di Furia, L.; Farré, M.; Flesland, L. Is there a recreational misuse potential for pregabalin? Analysis of anecdotal online reports in comparison with related gabapentin and clonazepam data. *Psychother. Psychosom.* **2011**, *80*, 118–122. [CrossRef]

17. Schjerning, O.; Rosenzweig, M.; Pottegård, A.; Damkier, P.; Nielsen, J. Abuse Potential of Pregabalin. *CNS Drugs* **2016**, *30*, 9–25. [CrossRef]
18. Pergolizzi, J.V.; Taylor, R.A.; Bisney, J.F.; LeQuang, J.A.; Coluzzi, F.; Gharibo, C.G. Gabapentinoid use disorder: Update for clinicians. *EC Anaesth* **2018**, *4*, 303–317.
19. Lancia, M.; Gambelunghe, A.; Gili, A.; Bacci, M.; Aroni, K.; Gambelunghe, C. Pregabalin Abuse in Combination With Other Drugs: Monitoring Among Methadone Patients. *Front Psychiatry* **2020**, *10*, 1022. [CrossRef] [PubMed]
20. Taguchi, T.; Nakano, S.; Nozawa, K. Effectiveness of Pregabalin Treatment for Neuropathic Pain in Patients with Spine Diseases: A Pooled Analysis of Two Multicenter Observational Studies in Japan. *J. Pain Res.* **2021**, *14*, 757. [CrossRef] [PubMed]
21. Lapeyre-Mestre, M.; Dupui, M. Drug abuse monitoring: Which pharmacoepidemiological resources at the European level? *Therapie* **2015**, *70*, 147–165. [CrossRef]
22. Bonnet, U.; Scherbaum, N. How addictive are gabapentin and pregabalin? A systematic review. *Eur. Neuropsychopharmacol. J. Eur. Coll. Neuropsychopharmacol.* **2017**, *27*, 1185–1215. [CrossRef]
23. Al-Husseini, A.; Abu-Farha, R.; Van Hout, M.C.; Wazaify, M. Community pharmacists experience of pregabalin abuse and misuse: A quantitative study from Jordan. *J. Subst. Use* **2019**, *24*, 273–279. [CrossRef]
24. Tarhini, F.; Taky, R.; Jaffal, L.H.; Kresht, J.; El-Chaer, G.; Awada, S.; Lahoud, N.; Khachman, D. Awareness of Lebanese Pharmacists towards the Use and Misuse of Gabapentinoids and Tramadol: A Cross-sectional Survey. *Dr. Sulaiman Al Habib Med. J.* **2020**, *2*, 24–30. [CrossRef]
25. Zhang, X.; Xu, H.; Zhang, Z.; Li, Y.; Pauer, L.; Liao, S.; Zhang, F. Efficacy and Safety of Pregabalin for Fibromyalgia in aPopulation of Chinese Subjects. *J. Pain Res.* **2021**, *14*, 537. [CrossRef]
26. Alsubaie, S.; Zarbah, A.; Alqahtani, A.; Abdullah, A.S.; Aledrees, N.S. Prevalence of pregabalin (Lyrica) abuse among healthcare professionals in Asser Province Saudi Arabia. *Int. J. Ment. Health Psychiatry* **2020**, *6*, 2.
27. Alshahrani, S.M. Assessment of Knowledge, Attitudes, and Practice of Community Pharmacists Regarding Weight Reduction Agents and Supplements in Aseer Region, Saudi Arabia. *Risk Manag. Healthc. Policy* **2020**, *13*, 347–353. [CrossRef]
28. Al-Husseini, A.; Wazaify, M.; Van Hout, M.C. Pregabalin misuse and abuse in Jordan: A qualitative study of user experiences. *Int. J. Ment. Health Addict.* **2018**, *16*, 642–654. [CrossRef]
29. Mobrad, A.M.; Alghadeer, S.; Syed, W.; Al-Arifi, M.N.; Azher, A.; Almetawazi, M.S.; Babelghaith, S.D. Knowledge, Attitudes, and Beliefs Regarding Drug Abuse and Misuse among Community Pharmacists in Saudi Arabia. *Int. J. Environ. Res. Public Health* **2020**, *17*, 1334. [CrossRef] [PubMed]
30. Kenna, G.A.; Erickson, C.; Tommasello, A. Understanding substance abuse and dependence by the pharmacy profession. *US Pharm* **2006**, *31*, HS-21–HS-33.
31. Dole, E.J.; Tommasello, A. Recommendations for implementing effective substance abuse education in pharmacy practice. *Subst. Abus.* **2002**, *23* (Suppl. 3), 263–271. [CrossRef] [PubMed]
32. Al-Mohamadi, A.; Badr, A.; Bin Mahfouz, L.; Samargandi, D.; Al Ahdal, A. Dispensing medications without prescription at Saudi community pharmacy: Extent and perception. *Saudi Pharm. J.* **2013**, *21*, 13–18. [CrossRef] [PubMed]
33. Gahr, M.; Freudenmann, R.W.; Hiemke, C.; Kölle, M.A.; Schönfeldt-Lecuona, C. Pregabalin abuse and dependence in Germany: Results from a database query. *Eur. J. Clin. Pharmacol.* **2013**, *69*, 1335–1342. [CrossRef]
34. Gahr, M.; Freudenmann, R.W.; Kölle, M.A.; Schönfeldt-Lecuona, C. Pregabalin and addiction: Lessons from published cases. *J. Subst. Use* **2014**, *19*, 448–449. [CrossRef]
35. Wagner, G.A.; Andrade, A.G.D. Pharmacist professionals in the prevention of drug abuse: Updating roles, and opportunities. *Braz. J. Pharm. Sci.* **2010**, *46*, 19–27. [CrossRef]
36. Merriman, A.; Harding, R. Pain control in the African context: The Ugandan introduction of affordable morphine to relieve suffering at the end of life. *Philos. Ethics Humanit. Med.* **2010**, *5*, 1–6. [CrossRef] [PubMed]
37. Jaber, D.; Bulatova, N.; Suyagh, M.; Yousef, A.-M.; Wazaify, M. Knowledge, attitude and opinion of drug misuse and abuse by pharmacy students: A cross-sectional study in Jordan. *Trop. J. Pharm. Res.* **2015**, *14*, 1501–1508. [CrossRef]
38. Albsoul-Younes, A.; Wazaify, M.; Yousef, A.-M.; Tahaineh, L. Abuse and Misuse of Prescription and Nonprescription Drugs Sold in Community Pharmacies in Jordan. *Subst. Use Misuse* **2010**, *45*, 1319–1329. [CrossRef] [PubMed]
39. Wazaify, M.; Abood, E.; Tahaineh, L.; Albsoul-Younes, A. Jordanian community pharmacists' experience regarding prescription and non-prescription drug abuse and misuse in Jordan–An update. *J. Subst. Use* **2017**, *22*, 463–468. [CrossRef]
40. Van Hout, M.C. "Doctor shopping and pharmacy hopping": Practice innovations relating to codeine. *Drugs Alcohol Today* **2014**, *14*, 219–234. [CrossRef]
41. Manchikanti, L.; Whitfield, E.; Pallone, F. Evolution of the National All Schedules Prescription Electronic Reporting Act (NASPER): A public law for balancing treatment of pain and drug abuse and diversion. *Pain Physician* **2005**, *8*, 335. [CrossRef]
42. Saudi Food and Drug Authority. *Guidance for Classifying the Prescription & Distribution Status of Medicinal Products*; Saudi Food and Drug Authority: Riyadh, Saudi Arabia, 2018.

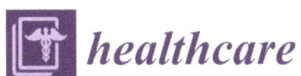

Article

Assessing the Impact of a Global Health Fellowship on Pharmacists' Leadership Skills and Consideration of Benefits to the National Health Service (NHS) in the United Kingdom

Claire Brandish [1], Frances Garraghan [2], Bee Yean Ng [1], Kate Russell-Hobbs [1], Omotayo Olaoye [3] and Diane Ashiru-Oredope [3,*]

[1] Pharmacy, Buckinghamshire Healthcare NHS Trust, Aylesbury HP21 8AL, UK; claire.brandish@nhs.net (C.B.); beeyean.ng@nhs.net (B.Y.N.); kate.russellhobbs@nhs.net (K.R.-H.)
[2] Pharmacy, Manchester University NHS Foundation Trust, Manchester M13 9PL, UK; frances.garraghan@mft.nhs.uk
[3] The Commonwealth Pharmacists Association (CPA), London E1W 1AW, UK; omotayo.olaoye@commonwealthpharmacy.org
* Correspondence: diane.ashiru-oredope@commonwealthpharmacy.org

Abstract: Antimicrobial resistance (AMR) poses a global, public health concern that affects humans, animals and the environment. The UK Fleming Fund's Commonwealth Partnerships for Antimicrobial Stewardship (CwPAMS) scheme aimed to support antimicrobial stewardship initiatives to tackle AMR through a health partnership model that utilises volunteers. There is evidence to indicate that NHS staff participating in international health projects develop leadership skills. Running in parallel with the CwPAMS scheme was the first Chief Pharmaceutical Officer's Global Health (CPhOGH) Fellowship for pharmacists in the UK. In this manuscript, we evaluate the impact, if any, of participation in the CwPAMS scheme and the CPhOGH Fellowship, particularly in relation to leadership skills, and consider if there are demonstrable benefits for the NHS. The 16 CPhOGH Fellows were invited to complete anonymised baseline and post-Fellowship self-assessment. This considered the impact of the Fellowship on personal, professional and leadership development. Senior colleagues were invited to provide insights into how the Fellows had performed over the course of the Fellowship. All Fellows responded to both the pre- and post-Fellowship questionnaires with a return of 100% (16/16) response rate. There was a significant improvement in Fellows' perception of their confidence, teaching abilities, understanding of behaviour change, management and communication skills. However, there was no change in the Fellows' attitude to work. Feedback was received from 26 senior colleagues for 14 of the CPhOGH Fellows. Overall, senior colleagues considered CPhOGH Fellows to progress from proficient/established competencies to strong/excellent when using the national pharmacy Peer Assessment Tool and NHS Healthcare Leadership Model. The majority (88%) of senior colleagues would recommend the Fellowship to other pharmacists. The analysis of the data provided suggests that this CPhOGH Fellowship led to the upskilling of more confident, motivated pharmacist leaders with a passion for global health. This supports the NHS's long-term plan "to strengthen and support good compassionate and diverse leadership at all levels". Constructive feedback was received for improvements to the Fellowship. Job satisfaction and motivation improved, with seven CPhOGH Fellows reporting a change in job role and five receiving a promotion.

Keywords: Commonwealth Partnerships for Antimicrobial Stewardship (CwPAMS); National Health Service (NHS); Chief Pharmaceutical Officer's Global Health Fellowship; CPhOGH Fellows; CwPAMS; pharmacy; fellowship; health partnerships; antimicrobial resistance (AMR); global health; leadership

Citation: Brandish, C.; Garraghan, F.; Ng, B.Y.; Russell-Hobbs, K.; Olaoye, O.; Ashiru-Oredope, D. Assessing the Impact of a Global Health Fellowship on Pharmacists' Leadership Skills and Consideration of Benefits to the National Health Service (NHS) in the United Kingdom. *Healthcare* **2021**, *9*, 890. https://doi.org/10.3390/healthcare9070890

Academic Editor: Georges Adunlin

Received: 30 May 2021
Accepted: 29 June 2021
Published: 15 July 2021

Publisher's Note: MDPI stays neutral with regard to jurisdictional claims in published maps and institutional affiliations.

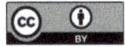

Copyright: © 2021 by the authors. Licensee MDPI, Basel, Switzerland. This article is an open access article distributed under the terms and conditions of the Creative Commons Attribution (CC BY) license (https://creativecommons.org/licenses/by/4.0/).

1. Introduction

1.1. A Health Partnerships Approach to Supporting Antimicrobial Stewardship in Four African Countries: The Commonwealth Partnerships for Antimicrobial Stewardship (CwPAMS)

Antimicrobial resistance (AMR) poses a global, public health concern that affects humans, animals and the environment [1]. In 2015, the World Health Assembly endorsed a global action plan to tackle the worldwide problem of AMR [1]. This plan encourages the use of a One Health, multi-sectoral approach, and calls for collaboration and coordination locally, and globally. The UK 5-year AMR Action Plan [2], the 20-year Vision for AMR [3] and the NHS Long-Term Plan [4], align with these intentions and build on existing achievements. Engagement and leadership are required at all levels to support progress internationally and to achieve the ambitions for containment and control of AMR globally. Sustained and focused efforts are required to minimise infections, provide safe and effective care to patients and raise awareness of AMR. Pharmacists have been at the forefront of successful antimicrobial stewardship (AMS) programmes across the NHS and, as such, are well placed to support further developments [5,6].

In recognition of the need to create leaders within this field, the Commonwealth Pharmacists Association (CPA) and the Tropical Health and Education Trust (THET) received UK Aid funds through the Department of Health and Social Care's Fleming Fund, for the pioneering Commonwealth Partnerships for Antimicrobial Stewardship scheme (CwPAMS) in 2019 [7]. A total of 12 health partnerships were formed between multidisciplinary teams from institutions in the UK, including NHS Trusts, together with institutions in Ghana, Tanzania, Uganda, and Zambia. These partnerships were created to allow ideas and knowledge exchange to further develop innovative ways to tackle the problem of AMR and raise awareness, which will mutually benefit the UK and low-to-middle-income countries (LMICs) [8,9]. Success of the CwPAMS projects was dependent on strong leadership and project management within each partnership. Similar qualities are required to facilitate effective approaches for systemwide working in the UK as transitions are made towards Integrated Care Partnership models of care [10].

1.2. Pharmacy Leaders and the NHS

Strong and influential leaders across a wide range of healthcare disciplines are essential in undertaking the WHO global AMR action plan [1]. There is evidence to indicate that NHS staff participating in international health projects develop leadership skills essential for influencing change and develop ways of working in the UK [9]. All NHS staff need inclusive leadership skills, which reinforce values and standards of care to drive improvement, leading to the highest quality of patient care [11–16]. Accessible leadership development programmes are fundamental to ensure that the NHS workforce is competent in the core leadership domains outlined in the NHS Healthcare Leadership Model [17]. Leadership should be integrated into the training and development offered to NHS staff to ensure good engagement and representation systemwide alongside clinical competencies [11,12].

The national professional body for pharmacists—the Royal Pharmaceutical Society (RPS)—has identified leadership as a key skill required of a pharmacist and has developed frameworks to support this [18]. In addition, the RPS has developed a policy on 'The pharmacy contribution to antimicrobial stewardship' and has identified the role that pharmacy leadership has in effective antimicrobial stewardship [19]. Internationally, leadership development and antimicrobial stewardship feature as 2 of the 21 development goals of the International Pharmaceutical Federation (FIP) [20]. Despite the existence of these frameworks and recognition of leadership as a desirable attribute, there are few opportunities available for pharmacists specifically to develop and demonstrate these skills.

1.3. Chief Pharmaceutical Officer's Global Health (CPhOGH) Fellowship Programme

Health Education England (which exists to provide national leadership and coordination for education and training within the health and public health workforce in England) offer an Improving Global Health (IGH) Fellowship to support the delivery of sustainable improvements in LMICs, whilst developing the transferrable leadership skills of the IGH Fellows to apply on return to the UK [21]. Historically, global health fellowship participants have mainly been doctors and nurses, despite being open to all NHS cadres. The CwPAMS scheme was the first of its kind to mandate that NHS pharmacists be included as essential members of each global health partnership.

Running in parallel with the CwPAMS scheme was the first Chief Pharmaceutical Officer's Global Health (CPhOGH) Fellowship programme. The CPhOGH scheme was a unique leadership development programme with the aim of cultivating pharmacists as clinical leaders of the future [22]. The development of the fellowship followed a request from Dr Keith Ridge, England's Chief Pharmaceutical Officer, recognising the positive impact the scheme could have for NHS staff [7]. In addition, the fellowship supported the participants by broadening their knowledge and understanding of global health. The Fellowship was led by CPA and funded by Health Education England (HEE).

The yearlong CPhOGH Fellowship required attendance at an inception workshop, to develop an awareness of skills and behaviours related to the Myers–Briggs Type Indicator (MBTI) questionnaire [23] and NHS Healthcare Leadership Model [17]. The Fellowship also involved completion of the Edward Jenner Professional Leadership Programme [24], a project management module, attendance and engagement in global pharmacy webinars, online action learning sets and responsibility for at least one deliverable within their respective CwPAMS partnership project. Each Fellow was assigned a leadership mentor through HEE's IGH International Health Fellowship programme [25] for the duration of the Fellowship to discuss the MBTI, reflect on the NHS Healthcare Leadership Model [17] and to provide support and challenge.

In this manuscript, we evaluate the impact, if any, of participation in the CwPAMS scheme and the CPhOGH Fellowship, particularly in relation to leadership skills, and consider if there are demonstrable benefits for the NHS. This will allow understanding of the value of the fellowship and potential future as a personal and professional development opportunity for NHS pharmacists.

2. Materials and Methods

Following a selection process, sixteen pharmacists that were involved in CwPAMS partnerships were appointed to join the CPhOGH Fellowship year. These pharmacists were all included in the evaluation of the Fellowship and are referred to as CPhOGH Fellows.

2.1. Pre- and Post-Fellowship Self-Assessment by Fellows

The 16 CPhOGH Fellows were invited to complete an online baseline questionnaire (see Supplementary Table S1) designed to capture demographic data and motivations for applying to the CPhOGH Fellowship. Leadership and global health experience was ascertained using a combination of open and closed questions. The questionnaire incorporated the Measuring the Outcomes of Volunteering for Education-Tool (MOVE-iT), a validated tool used to understand the impact of international placements [25]. This questionnaire was reviewed by members of Health Education England and the CPA. For the post-Fellowship evaluation, the baseline questionnaire was reviewed to consider which questions were most relevant and should be repeated in the post-Fellowship questionnaire (see Supplementary Table S2). Additional questions were included to elicit further information on the participants' leadership skills, development, project management skills and to understand if there were any benefits for the NHS. The pre-CPhOGH Fellows questionnaire consisted of 39 questions and the post-CPhOGH Fellows questionnaire consisted of 45 questions. These comprised free-text responses and statements to be answered according to a 7-pointed Likert scale ranging from "strongly agree" to "strongly disagree" [26]. The survey allowed for qualitative and quantitative analysis of the results.

2.2. Assessment by Senior Colleagues

Since this was a programme of leadership and development, the CPhOGH Fellows were invited to seek feedback from at least two senior colleagues who had worked with them prior to starting the Fellowship and for at least a year thereafter. This was in the form of an anonymous online questionnaire to comment on the CPhOGH Fellows' development and leadership skills (see Supplementary Table S3). A 16-item questionnaire was constructed to gain an understanding of how the CPhOGH Fellows had developed or changed, and how performance was perceived according to their senior peers over the course of the CPhOGH Fellowship. It was based on the NHS Healthcare Leadership Model [17] and the RPS Peer Assessment Tool, adapted and used with permission from the RPS [27]. These were chosen as they are validated, evidence-based models currently used to assess leadership skills in healthcare settings [17,27]. The questionnaire assessed the CPhOGH Fellows on the following dimensions:

- Teamwork;
- Influencing for results;
- Vision, Motivation and capability;
- Inspiring shared purpose;
- Managing change;
- Innovative working and practice.

Within each dimension, senior colleagues were invited to answer a series of questions using a scoring system to indicate their perception of the CPhOGH Fellow's level of competence before and after the CPhOGH Fellowship [17,27]. The scoring system adopted, ranged from 0 (Unable to comment), 1 (Essential); 2 (Proficient); 3 (Strong) to 4 (Exceptional), which aligns with the RPS Tool [27]. There was a free-text section for each dimension to capture additional feedback and examples (see Supplementary Table S3).

2.3. Distribution of Questionnaires

All three questionnaires were hosted on Survey Monkey©. The pre-Fellowship survey was open in June 2019 and CPhOGH Fellows were invited to complete this prior to attending the inception workshop 4–6 July 2019. The post-Fellowship survey and assessment by senior colleagues were open between 9 and 14 August 2020.

2.4. Data about Contributions, Achievements, and Communications of CPhOGH Fellows

Using the Fellow's network, the sixteen CPhOGH Fellows were invited to provide examples of achievements, contributions, and work undertaken to demonstrate the depth and breadth of the experiences gained since being inducted onto the Fellowship. Twitter© and self-reported activities were utilised to capture events and communications using the hashtags #CwPAMS and #CPhOGHFellows to monitor activity. A list of activities was collated and grouped into themes (see Supplementary Tables S4 and S5).

2.5. Data Analysis

Some of the data captured in the CPhOGH Fellows' self-assessment questionnaires were not analysed as they were not considered relevant to this leadership peer review; see Supplementary Tables S1 and S2 for the list of included and excluded questions as well as the rationale for exclusion. All data from the assessment of CPhOGH Fellows' leadership skills by senior colleagues were included in analysis.

Data were exported to Microsoft Excel© and anonymised before analysis and interpretation. Likert scale responses for components of the MOVE-iT tool, and reflective statements for professional activities and skills undertaken and developed over the CPhOGH Fellowship year were assigned values (7 = Strongly agree to 1 = Strongly disagree) resulting in an aggregate score for each assessed section. The higher the score, the more positive the Fellow's perception of the assessed components of the MOVE-iT tool and professional development during the Fellowship, respectively.

The Wilcoxon signed rank test was used to evaluate if there was any evidence of differences in average aggregated scores for components of the MOVE-iT tool before and after the Fellowship. Spearman's correlation test was also used to investigate the evidence of a relationship between Fellows' previous global health experience and reflective statements for professional activities and skills undertaken and developed over the CPhOGH Fellowship year. Both analyses were conducted using R software. Statistical significance was set at $p < 0.05$. Non-parametric tests (Wilcoxon signed rank test and Spearman's correlation) were conducted because of the population size and relatively skewed distribution of Fellows' responses.

Two CPhOGH Fellows reviewed the anonymised, qualitative data independently using thematic analysis to determine the key themes. Non-specific or duplicated quotes were removed, for example "leadership skills ". Where names were used or "he" or "she", these were changed to "the Fellow" to maintain anonymity.

Ethical approval was not required as per NHS Health Research Authority guidance and the NHS health research decision tool because this was a service evaluation of CPA's programme of activities to lead the CPhOGH Fellowship [28]. Data were anonymized and participants provided informed consent prior to each survey, including the peer feedback, and understood that the data would be used for the purposes of evaluation. They also had the opportunity to review and retract the data used in the production of this paper.

3. Results

3.1. CPhOGH Fellows

All sixteen CPhOGH Fellows responded to both the pre- and post-Fellowship questionnaires with a return of 100% (16/16) response rate. However, not all questions were answered by all. The demographics of the 16 CPhOGH Fellows that participated in the baseline and post-fellowship questionnaires are presented in Supplementary Table S6. The greatest number of respondents were aged 31–40 years (7 respondents) followed by those aged 41–50 years (5 respondents), reflecting the mid-career nature of the majority of the CPhOGH Fellows.

3.2. Self-Assessment

3.2.1. Expected Goals of the Fellowship Year

In the baseline questionnaire, CPhOGH Fellows were asked to select three statements from eight, to reflect what they hoped to gain from the Fellowship year. The responses were then compared with the responses to the post-fellowship questionnaire. Understanding of AMS in a low- and middle-income context and a greater understanding of international development and health partnership principles were both the most popular answers reported after the Fellowship. The responses varied and were different to the outcomes predicted by the CPhOGH Fellows at the start of the Fellowship, as shown in Figure 1. A total of 53 responses were received pre-Fellowship and 52 responses were received post-Fellowship against a request of 48, but one participant qualified this by adding in the comments section that "I could have honestly ticked every box here as I feel that I have been exposed to so many of these opportunities".

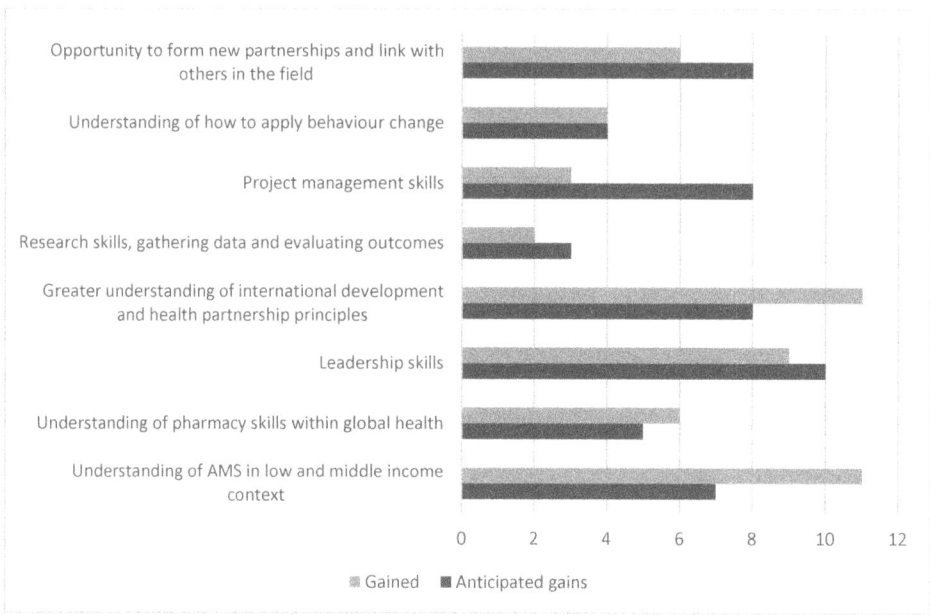

Figure 1. Values represent number of responses to the questions "What do you hope to gain?" and "what have you gained most from the Fellowship year?".

Many CPhOGH Fellows reported that they gained more from the Fellowship than they anticipated:

"Vastly useful and applicable. I feel I learned more than I taught during my visit! Although I do believe we made a difference for our partnership as well."

"I have gained more skills and knowledge than I anticipated through the Fellowship".

"Will enable me to confidently apply for funding for future projects."

3.2.2. Measuring the Outcomes of Volunteering for Education Tool (MOVE-iT)

Summary statistics of Fellows' feedback on components of the MOVE-iT tool before and post Fellowship are presented in Table 1 (see Supplementary Table S7 for raw data). Overall, there was an increase in the mean and median values of all assessed components and a lower variability in the responses post-Fellowship. The Wilcoxon signed rank test revealed that post-Fellowship, there was a statistically significant increase in Fellows' perception of their confidence ($v = 91$, $p = 0.001$), teaching abilities ($v = 61$, $p = 0.012$), behaviour change ($v = 136$, $p = < 0.001$), management ($v = 66$, $p = 0.003$) and communication skills ($v = 108$, $p = 0.006$). However, the improvement in Fellows' attitude to work was not statistically significant ($v = 92.5$, $p = 0.064$).

Table 1. Summary statistics for cumulative Likert-rated responses for the components of MOVE-iT.

	Pre-Fellowship			Post-Fellowship			p-Values
	Mean	Median	Standard Deviation	Mean	Median	Standard Deviation	
Confidence	53.31	52	6.23	58.69	61	4.81	0.001
Teaching	17.31	18.5	2.75	19.13	19	1.89	0.012
Behaviour change	19.31	19	5.50	22.88	24.5	5.56	<0.001
Management	17.50	18	3.39	19.81	21	1.83	0.003
Attitude to work	35.81	36	3.56	38.00	37	3.41	0.064
Difficult communication	15.00	15	4.07	18.44	18.5	2.99	0.006

3.2.3. Leadership Development, Experience, and Knowledge

When baseline and post-Fellowship questionnaires were compared, more leadership and project management activities were reported after the Fellowship compared to before (Table 2). Additionally, new professional development experiences were reported over the Fellowship year (Table 3).

Table 2. Leadership and project management activities experienced by the CPhOGH Fellows pre- and post-CPhOGH Fellowship programme.

Activities	Pre CPhOGH (n = 15)		Post CPhOGH (n = 16)			
	Yes	No	Yes (through Fellowship)	Yes (Alternative Route)	No	Not Answered
360 Assessment Questionnaire	4	11	7	3	6	
NHS Healthcare Leadership Model Self-Assessment	2	13	15	1		
Other leadership self-assessment	5	10	7	1	5	3
Project Management Course	6	9	10		6	
Myers–Briggs Type Indicator questionnaire	8	7	15			1
Other personality type indicator questionnaire	5	10	2	3	11	
A formal/semi-formal discussion with a mentor for your professional activities	5	10	16			
Written a project plan	10	5	15	1		
Formally led a project or project deliverable	11	4	15	1		
Led a quality improvement project	10	5	7	4	5	

Table 3. Professional activities undertaken by CPhOGH Fellows during the Fellowship year, including new experiences.

Activities Undertaken for the Last 12 Months (June 2019–June 2020)	N = 16 (New Experience)
Publication/presentation of work at a conference	12 (3)
Publication of work for a journal	9 (3)
Publication/presentation of work within Trust setting	13 (3)
Promotion of work on social media	11 (6)
Collaboration on work within Trust	13 (2)
Collaboration on work at a regional/local level (outside Trust)	12 (3)
Collaboration on work at a national level	13 (7)
Collaboration on work at an international level	13 (7)

Table 3. *Cont.*

Activities Undertaken for the Last 12 Months (June 2019–June 2020)	N = 16 (New Experience)
Utilised a mentor	15 (8)
Become a mentor	6 (4)
Changed job role	7
Had a promotion	5
Undertaken Faculty assessment	4 (1)
Written a business case	7 (1)
Undertaken an audit	14
Undertaken a project with a focus on quality improvement	12 (1)
Undertaken teaching	16
Enrolled or undertaken a leadership course	14 (9)

All 16 CPhOGH Fellows agreed that the skills and knowledge they gained during the Fellowship year were useful for the current stage in their careers and were applicable to their positions in the UK. Examples of application of improved leadership skills to everyday work situations were given by several CPhOGH Fellows:

"I have been able to apply aspects of the leadership skills and knowledge I gained through undertaking the Fellowship to facilitate antimicrobial stewardship work streams which are important to my organisation."

"I have definitely applied the leadership skills learnt through the facilitator study days . . . . I have also learnt the importance of reflection when things do not always go to plan. I have learnt new ways to deal with conflict which has helped my personal development and ensure that I am able to work effectively."

"I have adapted the flow of work in our team, I am more able to delegate tasks and together we regularly discuss our roles and responsibilities, which has made us more productive as a team."

"I felt the Fellowship has been worthwhile because it introduced me to the leadership course and a tool for me to assess my own leadership skills, identify my gap and act on it."

Some CPhOGH Fellows also reported enhanced research involvement and academic teaching opportunities.

"I have become involved in a research project with health psychologists teaching AMS and behaviour change. I never would have imagined doing this prior to the Fellowship!"

"Engagement of the NHS with higher education institutions and improved understanding and participation in research."

Additional reflective statements on professional activities and application of skills are shown in Table 4.

Table 4. Reflective statements for professional activities and skills undertaken and developed over the CPhOGH Fellowship year.

Reflecting between June 2019–June 2020 State How Much You Agree with the Following Statement (n = 16)	Strongly Agree/Agree	Somewhat Agree	Neutral	Somewhat Disagree	Strongly Disagree/Disagree
I undertake more MDT work compared to a year ago.	7	2	4	1	2
I am more likely to work with other disciplines on a regular basis	8	3	3		2
I have worked across disciplines in delivering AMS/IPC	14		1		1
I find myself working more with different professional groups	11	2	1		2
I am more confident to approach people I have never worked with before compared to a year ago	14		1		1
I am happy to work with/approach people who work outside the NHS in order to collaborate compared to a year ago.	14	1			1
I have started managing a new aspect of service.	10	2	2		2
I recognise the need to review/manage/introduce a new aspect of service.	12	2	1		1
I have become more involved in research.	7	3	2	1	3
I have made changes to the way in which I work as a team	12	3	1		
I have made changes to the way in which I engage with others in the work environment.	13	3			
I have made changes to the way in which I teach	13	2			1
I have made changes to the way in which I engage with the wider Trust/organisation.	10	1	2		3
I have made changes to the way I practice.	13	1	1		1
I have made changes to the way in which I engage with others outside a work environment.	12	2	1		1

A Spearman's correlation coefficient $\varrho = 0.23$ ($p = 0.3983$) was obtained from the comparison of previous global health experience (Supplementary Table S6) to reflective statements for professional activities and skills undertaken and developed over the CPhOGH Fellowship year (Table 4).

The themes identified from the free text in the post-Fellowship questionnaires were career development, job satisfaction and motivation, communication skills, networking, Global Health and frugal innovation/working with limited resources, education and training (improvements in confidence and adaptation of teaching methods, including the use of behaviour change techniques were reported by the majority of CPhOGH Fellows) and resilience. Table 5 contains the themes that have been identified from the open questions asked in the post-CPhOGH Fellows survey and the corresponding quotes.

3.3. Assessment by Senior Colleagues

Results of the leadership questionnaire by colleagues more senior than the CPhOGH Fellows are reported in Table 6. These findings represent the feedback of 26 senior colleagues and responses were received for 14 CPhOGH Fellows by the end of the data collection period; four responses were excluded due to incomplete data sets. One respondent only completed the post-CPhOGH Fellowship section. Two CPhOGH Fellows received feedback from three colleagues; eight CPhOGH Fellows received feedback from two colleagues; and five CPhOGH Fellows received feedback from one senior colleague. Respondents consisted of a wide range of healthcare professionals with six medical consultants, six more senior pharmacy colleagues, five more senior non-pharmacy colleagues, four line managers, three chief pharmacists and two medical colleagues.

There was a shift in responses when the pre- was compared to the post-CPhOGH Fellowship performance for all dimensions. On average, the CPhOGH Fellows progressed from proficient/established score of 2.5 pre-CPhOGH Fellowship to strong/excellent score of 3.3 post-CPhOGH Fellowship. Only one CPhOGH Fellow was considered to have the same overall score (2.9) for the pre-and post-Fellowship questionnaire. This performance was rated proficient/strong overall, across all dimensions. The respondent did not provide any narrative for this individual (see supplementary Figure S1).

3.4. Impact of the CPhOGH Fellowship on the Performance of Participating Pharmacists from a Senior Perspective

The one theme that constantly featured among all the dimensions was confidence. This was often regarded as a result of a change in the perception of self-efficacy, referring to an individual's belief in their capabilities to perform a task. The respondents felt that the Fellowship had empowered the CPhOGH Fellows to be more confident in striving for things that the CPhOGH Fellows perceived outside their reach. These included confidence to voice their opinions, integrating outside their comfort zone, accepting new challenges, and volunteering to lead a working group or project. The following feedback reflects this:

"Professionally the Fellow is more confident, able to allow their voice to be heard. The Fellow has developed their ability to manage change and people skills and works confidently within wider teams."

"Professionally the Fellow is more confident, more strategic in their thoughts and planning, ambitious and excited for improvement. The Fellow has developed their networks extensively, working across networks globally with ease."

"Increased confidence in ability to adapt to new situations and different environments. Ability to manage stressful situations and turn them to an advantage."

"Confidence, ability to think outside the box and use successful techniques in a different context."

A total of 96% ($n = 25$) of the seniors thought the CPhOGH Fellows were ready for more senior roles and 88% ($n = 23$) of them would recommend the CPhOGH Fellowship to others pharmacy colleagues.

"It has been a pleasure to watch the Fellow grow during the year and overall, this programme has been a positive influence on the department as a whole."

3.5. Contributions, Achievements and Communications

Feedback from the CPhOGH Fellows on the scope of the work published/presented was wide ranging, with national and international representation at conferences, webinars, blogs, podcasts and community engagement events (see Supplementary Tables S4 and S5).

Table 5. Themes from Open questions in the post-CPhoGH Fellows survey.

Themes from Open Questions	Selected Quotes
Career development In addition to the seven CPhOGH Fellows who reported a change in job role and the five CPhOGH Fellows who reported a promotion (Table 3), the written feedback supports improved development and professional progression through the experiences of the Fellowship programme.	*"It has also given me the confidence to apply for a managerial role, I wouldn't have considered only months before."* *"I have had opportunities e.g. projects with significant budgets which I believe I may not have been offered if it weren't for the Fellowship"* *"The Fellowship has empowered me to push myself further and broaden my horizons."* *"It has provided me with the tools for the next stage of my pharmacy career."* *"Lots of experiences during the last year motivated me to change role. Fellowship was one of them."*
Job satisfaction/motivation The results of the MOVE-iT tool, shown in Table 1, do not indicate a significant change in attitude to work. However, the following statements suggest improved job satisfaction, pro-active working and motivation.	*"Improvements in staff happiness and retention."* *"Increased confidence. Increased motivation"* *"The Fellowship has given me another focus, and has improved my motivation and job satisfaction in my role."* *"I've expanded my goals and through the support of my peers and Fellows I have achieved things I would never have dreamed of 18 months ago."* *"The CaPAMs projects and CPhOGH Fellowship has offered unique opportunities for us which have been very enjoyable. They have encouraged me to work hard and with more enthusiasm than before and I feel very happy and proud to work within the pharmacy profession."*
Communication skills Improvements in managing challenging conversations and difficult people were reported in the post-CPhOGH Fellows MOVE-iT survey when compared to the baseline (Table 1). This is further substantiated by the following:	*"My improved negotiation and communication skills, especially in tricky circumstances"* *"The coaching on the Fellowship weekend really allowed me to explore this in a safe environment and practice difficult conversations"* *"Coaching course delivered on the Fellowship weekend. This was amazing and has really improved my confidence and communication style."* *"I have learnt new ways to deal with conflict which has helped my personal development and ensure that I am able to work effectively."*
Networking Collaboration within Trusts, at a regional, national and international level, was reported by the majority of CPhOGH Fellows (Table 3). Stronger and more cohesive networks were developed locally as illustrated. Collaborations across sectors and specialties and outside the NHS were also fostered as described in Table 4 and by these CPhOGH Fellows:	*"The networks I have made also were useful in other areas of healthcare. Such as project plans for in house service development."* *"Wider network which I can call on to enhance what we are doing at work."* *"felt more empowered to work differently and innovatively within and outside our organisation."* *"It has connected me to inspiring and like-minded colleagues who all have a passion for improving global health in particular focusing on AMR."* *"I feel more confident to network now and have learnt a huge amount from positive role models outside of healthcare."* *"Greater collaboration. I have paired up the Uganda researchers with colleagues in South Africa to write a grant proposal."* *"Improved ability of staff involved to work beyond the traditional boundaries and to consider how collaborative efforts can provide further benefits to all."*

Table 5. Cont.

Themes from Open Questions	Selected Quotes
Global Health and Frugal Innovation/Working with limited resources The CPhOGH Fellows demonstrated a greater ability to work within the confines of limited resources as indicated by the greater agreement with the statements in the MOVE-iT (Table 1). Examples of benefits of this in the UK setting are illustrated here:	"In addition, having increased understanding of the global health context has helped me believe that anything is achieveable with the resources in the UK, you just need the will to make change." "Ability to produce outcomes and results in a very resource limited setting" "Greater awareness of how LMIC institutions are run and how cohesive relations are built. This is something that can benefit NHS organisations" "More appreciation of what the NHS has to offer (as a patient and an employee) and how improvements do not always require money and more often, a better understanding of how things actually work in practice." "The opportunity to participate in the CwPAMS project and the CPhOGH Fellowship has been eye opening. I have learnt how to improvise and find solution despite limited resources. I also learnt to be more adaptive to the environment and change way of working depending on the local context. This has been very useful given the COVID-19 pandemic." "It has been worthwhile, as it has given me greater exposure to the way in which a pharmacists role can be done even with great lack of resource. It has shown me how when undertaking the role of a leader you are able to accomplish a lot, despite any challenges."
Education and training All CPhOGH Fellows considered education and training to be part of their job roles prior to the Fellowship and CwPAMS experiences (Table 3). However, improvements in confidence and adaptation of teaching methods, including the use of behaviour change techniques, were reported by the majority of CPhOGH Fellows (Tables 1 and 4). Delivery and provision of education and training was also reported to be further reaching. This is highlighted here:	"The key benefits to my trust is the Fellowship has changed the way we conduct education and training through the introduction of behaviour change." "…. link with partnership and UK local university school of pharmacy to support overseas opportunities for undergraduate programme" "Far greater understanding of requirements to deliver high quality education at scale" "Together with colleagues in Uganda we developed a MOOC that has been accessed in 50 countries by over 2000 learners on AMS." "education strategies have changed to move away from didactic teaching to more workshop type training and in addition our work has made the team more visible in the trust. It also has embedded AMS into the long-term strategy of all areas."
Resilience When the CPhOGH Fellows were asked how they believed they had coped with the COVID-19 pandemic in April and May 2020, five answered extremely well, seven answered very well and three answered somewhat well. One CPhOGH Fellow did not respond. For some CPhOGH Fellows, they reported that they used their CwPAMS placements to be helpful:	"a better sense of self-awareness (after a lot of reading/research into this area, borne from the Fellowship study days)" "I built upon my experience in my new role and also the increased leadership skills I have been building on during the Fellowship which helped me to cope when I was redeployed to a clinical role during COVID." Others considered perspective of the situation to be important and utilised the leadership and educational skills they had developed: "I think the experiences of the past year have helped in dealing with the COVID19 emergency response and this has put into context what is important in life." "Positive outlook. Good communication. Open teamwork. Task delegation. Feeling prepared by having additional teaching." "I was re-deployed to support a clinical research team and having international experience … during the Fellowship and working with and managing international teams helped me cope with being in a new environment and responding to new and as yet unknown research needs and questions." "Leadership demonstrated by caring for my colleagues and my team's mental health and wellbeing. I take the time to listen and be there for colleagues, despite my very busy schedule."

Table 6. Leadership questionnaire adapted from RPS Peer Assessment Tool and Healthcare Leadership Model.

Statement	Pre CPhOGH (n = 25)					Post CPhOGH (n = 26)				
	Essential	Proficient	Strong	Exceptional	U/C*	Essential	Proficient	Strong	Exceptional	U/C*
Teamwork										
The pharmacist listens attentively to other team members and values their suggestions		3	17	5			1	10	15	
The pharmacist is an established and effective member of a multidisciplinary team	2	4	15	4			1	10	15	
The pharmacist is consulted for advice which requires their in-depth professional expertise	1	6	12	6				10	16	
The pharmacist consistently works effectively across boundaries to build relationships and share information, plans and resources.	2	6	9	7	1		1	5	19	1

U/C* Unable to comment

Supporting quotes

"... ability to network and be collegiate widens the scope and impact of Fellow work, and the Fellow is fundamental in keeping our team connected and on task."

"Their positive, "can-do" attitude and unrelenting support for ALL members of the team means you can face any challenge with them!"

"The Fellow is a core member of and contributor to the Antimicrobial Stewardship Committee ... developed strong working relationships with clinicians, pharmacists and specialist nurses in both hospital and community settings ... taken an active leadership role in the Trust response to COVID-19 working across site and specialities."

"The Fellow has always been strong team player and has developed strong networks ... sought for expert clinical advice at a National level"

	Influencing for Results									
The pharmacist is able to share issues and information to help others understand his/her point of view	1	11	8	5			3	11	12	
The pharmacist tailors his/her communication group or presentation according to the audience or stakeholder.	4	8	9	3	1		2	14	10	
The pharmacist directly or indirectly links different working groups across the organisation to achieve a common goal.	3	7	9	5	1		6	9	11	
The pharmacist gains reputational influence by sharing experience and best practice nationally	3	5	10	4	3		5	6	14	1

U/C* Unable to comment

Supporting quotes

"The Fellow is able to communicate and build relationships with anyone, irrespective of position or background. They have been proactive in sharing theirs and the team's work both locally and at conferences."

"The Fellow has worked hard to establish their place in the team with confidence, they now have a much stronger voice in our QI huddles and across the department"

"As Lead Antimicrobial Pharmacist the Fellow has to communicate with a variety of professionals in a number of different settings, all of whom may have differing agendas e.g. harmonisation of antimicrobial guidelines following the merger of two large hospital Trusts ... has spoken at national conferences and set up a professional Twitter account for dissemination and sharing of information and networking."

Table 6. Cont.

Statement	Pre CPhOGH (n = 25)					Post CPhOGH (n = 26)				
	Essential	Proficient	Strong	Exceptional	U/C*	Essential	Proficient	Strong	Exceptional	U/C*
Vision, Motivation and Developing Capability										
The pharmacist creates a clear vision of the future for his/her team in accordance with the organisations vision.	3	12	7	3			1	3	11	11	
The pharmacist often looks for opportunities to develop him/herself and learn things outside his/her comfort zone.	2	11	9	3				3	9	14	
The pharmacist often provides constructive feedback to his/her team to help them focus on the right area in order to develop professionally	4	6	6	3	6		1	6	8	6	5
The pharmacist is involved in strategy planning	4	7	9	2	3		2	4	11	8	1

U/C* Unable to comment

Supporting quotes

"The Fellow sees the bigger picture but is also able to home in on the key steps required to implement change and is detail-orientated when it is appropriate."

"very sensible and objective in discussions, also very good at providing feedback, identifying colleagues who need support and providing help to the best of their abilities."

"The Fellow has taken on the responsibility of being a diploma tutor . . . . . . and also actively engages with other diploma students and gives constructive and positive development suggestions."

"Lead role in development of Antimicrobial Stewardship strategy . . . . . involvement in Trust Infection Service strategy working group"

"The Fellow has been pivotal in planning the next steps of the project and disseminating the links work at a national level"

Inspiring shared purpose										
The pharmacist demonstrates the characteristics of a role model of the Pharmacy profession.	1	4	12	6	2			3	9	16	1
The pharmacist inspires others, even when they are under pressure, by helping them to focus on the value of their contribution	1	10	8	6				3	10	13	
The pharmacist supports his/her colleagues to keep challenging others cohesively to achieve a shared purpose.	1	10	9	5				3	12	11	

U/C* Unable to comment

Supporting quotes

"The Fellow is supportive, encouraging and inspiring in their enthusiasm, drive and outlook."

"The Fellow responded positively to the COVID crisis, showing calm yet strong leadership for the staff delivering clinical services to ward areas."

"The Fellow has managed the recent changes in working due to COVID-19 with grace and understanding . . . been a role model to their colleagues. Fellow has forged strong links with psychology colleagues at the university to provide behaviour change education to Stewardship Committee members and regularly demonstrates what they has learned from these sessions in leadership role."

Table 6. Cont.

Statement	Pre CPhOGH (n = 25)					Post CPhOGH (n = 26)				
	Essential	Proficient	Strong	Exceptional	U/C*	Essential	Proficient	Strong	Exceptional	U/C*
Managing Change										
The pharmacist is able to adapt to different way of working especially in times of crisis	1	8	11	3	2			10	15	1
The pharmacist consistently reflects on his/her service and manages processes of change or service improvement	4	4	11	3	3		1	16	7	2
The pharmacist applies a behaviour change approach in change management or education and training	3	12	2	3	5		3	12	8	3
U/C* Unable to comment										
Supporting quotes										

"The Fellow is very good at identifying the context for change and making on-going assessment of the potential impact of change."
"The Fellow has embraced new concepts of behaviour change in terms of education and training and has applied this new learning into practice."
"The Fellow worked hard to develop their confidence and her voice in the team, now confidently able to establish their ideas into change." "Use of QI methodology to understand problems, adapt processes and work differently."
"…. can take on a variety of challenges, whether that involves service improvement, additional clinical responsibilities or education and training."
"Working in a LMIC has provided an opportunity to apply skills in a new context and learning can be applied in future roles."

Statement	Pre CPhOGH					Post CPhOGH				
Innovative working and practice										
The pharmacist strives to improve his/her service within the limitation of resources.	3	8	9	3	2		2	16	8	
The pharmacist is able to analyse essential data and utilise the results to improve services.	2	8	8	4	3		3	13	8	2
The pharmacist is able to identify the key stakeholders and understand their agenda.	4	12	4	5			4	12	10	
The applicant takes the lead to ensure innovation produces demonstrable improvement	2	11	6	2	4	1	3	13	8	1
The Fellow effectively strives to improve quality within limitations of service	3	9	7	5	1		3	13	10	
The pharmacist recognises and implements innovation from the external environment.	3	12	4	3	3		3	13	8	2

U/C* Unable to comment

Supporting quotes

"The Fellow has an open mind to new ideas/innovation and change, i.e., not afraid of trying new ways of working. The Fellow has an increased awareness of stakeholder engagement and project work and in mindful of influences."
"Pushed forward with new prescribing models to address deficiencies brought about by staffing issues"
"Recognises areas for improvement using resources such as audit and incident reporting, makes an action plan and delivers on these plans"
"… interested in research and finding innovative ways of doing things … also good at giving due consideration to new and innovative ideas, as observed during our partnership project. I was impressed by … enthusiasm and dedication"

4. Discussion

This evaluation aimed to consider the impact, if any, of participation in the CPhOGH Fellowship, particularly in relation to leadership skills. It also deliberates whether this programme offers a development opportunity to provide demonstrable benefits to pharmacists as individuals and the wider NHS. The overall impression from the responses provided in the questionnaires indicates that all CPhOGH Fellows underwent a great deal of personal and professional development over the one-year Global Health Fellowship.

The responses indicate the significance of the Fellowship in honing vital traits beneficial to individual pharmacists and the NHS. Research in the UK has highlighted that the best performing hospitals were those in which staff demonstrated high levels of engagement in decision making and where there was evidence of distributed leadership in the organisation [29]. Increasing the confidence and leadership skills of pharmacists not employed in traditional leadership roles provides additional benefit to their organisations (evidenced by 10 fellows managing new aspects of service since commencing on the fellowship) and the NHS. This aligns with participants' most anticipated gain from the Fellowship from the pre-Fellowship survey—development of leadership skills. Although the impact of the Fellowship on pharmacists' 'Attitude to work' was not statistically significant, descriptive statistics show an increase in the mean and median values of respondents' perceptions of their abilities after the Fellowship. Improvements in confidence were mirrored in the feedback from senior colleagues when asked to assess the Fellow's performance. The use of feedback from senior colleagues is similar to the recommendation to use 360° assessments to move beyond the weaknesses of self-reported changes. [29–31].

The majority of CPhOGH Fellows reported that they gained the most from understanding AMS in an LMIC context, understanding international development and health partnership principles and leadership skills. This supports the intention of CwPAMS—to strengthen AMS capacity in LMIC health institutions as part of collaborative, partnership efforts, whilst providing leadership training as part of the CPhOGH Fellowship. In retrospect, this question was too restrictive as it allowed only three options to be selected from a pre-set of eight. There were more responses than requested and there was a spread of responses for all statements. The narrative provided allowed additional and more extensive insights to be captured.

Nearly a third of the CPhOGH Fellows had previous experience in global health. The results indicate insufficient evidence of a correlation between Fellows' previous global health experience and reflective statements for professional activities and skills undertaken and developed over the CPhOGH Fellowship year. Hence, factors other than previous global health experience could be responsible for the professional activities and skills undertaken and developed during the Fellowship year.

In some instances, it was difficult to unpick the developments and progression of the CPhOGH Fellowship experience from their routine job roles, as many CPhOGH Fellows reported that they practiced many of the professional activities and utilised the leadership skills regularly. Despite 74% of CPhOGH Fellows having 11 or more years' experience as a pharmacist, undertaking some of the professional activities routinely, most Fellows reported improvements or changes to the way in which they undertake the activities they were asked to self-reflect on. For example, CPhOGH Fellows reported more structured knowledge of tools and application of these in practice, resulting in a more holistic approach when undertaking quality improvement and project management tasks.

This fellowship has facilitated increased opportunities and new experiences for the Fellows with extended networks and visibility on a national and international level. This is evidenced by feedback from senior colleagues who credited the positive influence that the CPhOGH Fellows exhibited within their own departments to motivate others and act as role models. Workplace-based leadership training has been shown to increase willingness to lead [32]. These qualities and skills were challenged during the COVID-19 pandemic and it was acknowledged that the CPhOGH Fellows responded positively and were able to adapt to new ways of working.

The follow-up questionnaire revealed that job satisfaction and motivation improved, with seven CPhOGH Fellows reporting a change in job role and five receiving a promotion. This is similar to reports from MacPhail et al. (2015), where 'The clinical leadership programme significantly increased willingness to take on leadership roles' (93%), and participants reported that they were more willing to take on a leadership role within their team [32]. Progress was noted across all domains by senior colleagues when considering the NHS Healthcare Leadership Model and the RPS peer assessment tool.

Despite a small initial cohort of participants, the evaluation and feedback indicate that the CPhOGH Fellowship is beneficial as a development opportunity for pharmacists. However, future programmes should be offered to a wider number of pharmacy staff, including technicians, to allow for more representative analysis. Feedback should also be sought from LMIC partners to facilitate a more holistic review of performance and support bidirectional learning.

5. Limitations

The benefits of the CPhOGH Fellowship are intertwined with the benefits of participating in a global health project and therefore, it is difficult to identify the independent benefits of each. In hindsight, the leadership skills questionnaire for senior colleagues should have been completed at baseline and after the Fellowship to reflect answers more accurately. In comparison with other global health Fellowships [8], the number of participants included was small and the time spent in the partnership country was limited. Tools that elicit self-reported attainment and behaviour changes are considered to provide weak evaluation evidence, are of variable accuracy [33] and most studies use unvalidated tools. In this study, however, we combined a validated tool (MOVE-iT) for self-reporting [25] pre- and post-fellowship, [34] alongside independent peer assessment using nationally recognised leadership framework tools [18,28]. The use of a non-random population could also impact the results of our findings. Hence, the inference from this study should be treated with caution. Whilst this paper focusses on the impact of a Global Health Fellowship on UK-based pharmacists, it does not account for the leadership skills and development of pharmacists from LMICs involved in the CwPAMS projects.

Due to the impact of the COVID-19 pandemic, there was limited opportunity to obtain feedback from the Fellows' LMIC partners on the progress of the Fellows during the CwPAMS project.

6. Conclusions

This was the first global health fellowship for pharmacists in the UK. Overall, the Fellowship was a valuable experience for all those that took part in it. The engagement in the questionnaires and the extensive narrative provided by the Fellows showed their commitment to the Fellowship and the many outputs derived from it. The analysis of the data provided suggests that this CPhOGH Fellowship led to the upskilling of more confident, motivated pharmacist leaders with a passion for global health. This supports the NHS's long-term plan "to strengthen and support good compassionate and diverse leadership at all levels" [4]. There was some constructive feedback for how the Fellowship could be improved in anticipation of the offer of another CPhOGH Fellowship, as benefits can clearly be seen by CPhOGH Fellows and senior colleagues alike.

Supplementary Materials: The following are available at https://www.mdpi.com/article/10.3390/healthcare9070890/s1, Table S1: Self-assessment questionnaire (baseline), Table S2: Post-CPhOGH Fellowship Self-assessment questionnaire, Table S3: Assessment of CPhOGH Fellows Leadership skills by Senior Leaders, Table S4: Additional activities of the CPhOGH Fellows during the Fellowship year Table S5: Themes from the additional activities of the CPhOGH Fellows, Table S6: Demographic of the CPhOGH Fellows Table S7: Statements for the components of MOVE-iT, Figure S1: Average Leadership Dimension Score per CPhOGH Fellows.

Author Contributions: Conceptualization, C.B., F.G., B.Y.N., K.R.-H. and D.A.-O.; Data curation, C.B., F.G., B.Y.N. and K.R.-H.; Formal analysis, C.B., F.G., B.Y.N., K.R.-H. and O.O.; Funding acquisition, D.A.-O.; Methodology, C.B., F.G., B.Y.N., K.R.-H. and D.A.-O.; Project administration, C.B. and D.A.-O.; Supervision, D.A.-O.; Validation, D.A.-O.; Writing—Original draft, C.B., F.G., B.Y.N., K.R.-H. and O.O.; Writing—Review and editing, C.B., F.G., B.Y.N., K.R.-H., O.O. and D.A.-O. All authors have read and agreed to the published version of the manuscript.

Funding: CwPAMS was funded by the Department of Health and Social Care using UK aid funding and is managed by the Fleming Fund. The Fleming Fund is a GBP 265 million UK aid investment to tackle antimicrobial resistance by supporting low- and middle-income countries to generate, use and share data on AMR. The Fleming Fund programme is managed by the UK Department of Health and Social Care. The CwPAMS programme is managed by the Commonwealth Pharmacists Association and the Tropical Health Education Trust (THET). The views expressed in this publication are those of the authors and not necessarily those of the Department of Health and Social Care, the NHS, the represented NHS Trusts, CPA or THET. The CPhOGH Fellowship was funded by Health Education England.

Institutional Review Board Statement: Ethical approval was not required as per NHS Health Research Authority guidance because this was a service evaluation of CPA's programme of activities to lead the CPhOGH Fellowship [28]. Data were anonymised and informed consent was obtained as part of the data collection.

Informed Consent Statement: Informed consent was obtained from all participants involved in the study.

Data Availability Statement: Data is contained within the article or supplementary material.

Acknowledgments: The authors acknowledge: Keith Ridge, Chief Pharmaceutical Officer for initiating the CPhOGH Fellowship; the Commonwealth Pharmacists Association and Tropical Health Education Trust (THET) for co-leading the CwPAMS programme. The CPhOGH Fellows for their participation in this evaluation: Amritpal Atwal, Esmita Charani, Kate Russell-Hobbs, Scott Barrett, Claire Brandish, Joseph Brayson, Frances Garraghan, Fiona Rees, Bee Yean Ng, Joyce Mahungu, Preet Panesar, Misha Ladva, Edwin Panford-Quainoo, Reem Santos, Frances Kerr, Alison Cockburn. Global Pharmacy support from the Commonwealth Pharmacists Association: Emma Foreman, Sarah Marshall, Sarah Cavanagh and Victoria Rutter. The Health Education England team who supported the fellowship: Fleur Kitsell, Peter Morgan, Chris Cutts, Mohamed Sadak. Change Exchange, University of Manchester, for advice on how to incorporate the MOVE-iT tool: Lucie Byrne Davies and Joanne Hart. Statistical support and advice: Michael Fleming and Margaret Dennis. The following people who reviewed the article: Fleur Kitsell, Lucie Byrne Davies, Sarah Marshall, Esmita Charani, Edwin Pandord-Quainoo, Richard Skone-Jones and William Townsend.

Conflicts of Interest: Diane Ashiru-Oredope was technical programme lead for CwPAMS and lead for the CPhOGH Fellowship. C.B., F.G., B.Y.N. and K.R.-H. were all CPhOGH Fellows. O.O.—None.

References

1. World Health Organization. Global Action Plan on Antimicrobial Resistance. Available online: https://apps.who.int/iris/bitstream/handle/10665/193736/9789241509763_eng.pdf?sequence=1 (accessed on 21 August 2020).
2. Department of Health and Social Care. Tackling Antimicrobial Resistance 2019–2024. The UK's Five-Year National Action Plan, HM Government. 24 January 2019. Available online: https://assets.publishing.service.gov.uk/government/uploads/system/uploads/attachment_data/file/784894/UK_AMR_5_year_national_action_plan.pdf (accessed on 21 August 2020).
3. Department of Health and Social Care. Contained and Controlled. The UK's 20-Year Vision for Antimicrobial Resistance, HM Government. 24 January 2019. Available online: https://assets.publishing.service.gov.uk/government/uploads/system/uploads/attachment_data/file/773065/uk-20-year-vision-for-antimicrobial-resistance.pdf (accessed on 21 August 2020).
4. National Health Service. Long Term Plan, Updated 21 August 2019. Available online: https://www.longtermplan.nhs.uk/wp-content/uploads/2019/08/nhs-long-term-plan-version-1.2.pdf (accessed on 21 August 2020).
5. Hand, K. Antibiotic pharmacists in the ascendancy. *J. Antimicrob. Chemother.* **2007**, *60*, i73–i76. [CrossRef] [PubMed]
6. Gilchrist, M.; Wade, P.; Ashiru-Oredope, D.; Howard, P.; Sneddon, J.; Whitney, L.; Wickens, H. Antimicrobial Stewardship from Policy to Practice: Experiences from UK Antimicrobial Pharmacists. *Infect. Dis. Ther.* **2015**, *4*, 51–64. [CrossRef]
7. Commonwealth Partnerships for Antimicrobial Stewardship. Available online: https://commonwealthpharmacy.org/commonwealth-partnerships-for-antimicrobial-stewardship/ (accessed on 22 August 2020).
8. Monkhouse, A.; Sadler, L.; Boyd, A.; Kitsell, F. The Improving Global Health Fellowship: A qualitative analysis of innovative leadership development for NHS healthcare professionals. *Glob. Health* **2018**, *14*, 69. [CrossRef]

9. Tropical Health and Education Trust. Health Partnership Scheme Impact Report 2011–2019. Available online: https://www.thet.org/wp-content/uploads/2017/09/20443_HPS_Impact_Report-2019-8.pdf (accessed on 20 August 2020).
10. Care Quality Commission; Public Health England; National Health Service. *Five Year Forward View*; NHS: England, UIK, 2015. Available online: https://www.england.nhs.uk/wp-content/uploads/2014/10/5yfv-web.pdf (accessed on 27 May 2021).
11. Francis, R. Report of the Mid Staffordshire NHS Foundation Trust Public Inquiry, Executive Summary. Available online: https://assets.publishing.service.gov.uk/government/uploads/system/uploads/attachment_data/file/279124/0947.pdf (accessed on 23 March 2021).
12. Department of Health. *High-Quality Care for All: NHS Next Stage Review Final Report. CM 7432*; The Stationary Office: London, UK, 2008. Available online: https://www.gov.uk/government/publications/high-quality-care-for-all-nhs-next-stage-review-final-report (accessed on 20 March 2020).
13. Rose, L. Better Leadership for Tomorrow NHS Leadership Review. 2015. Available online: https://assets.publishing.service.gov.uk/government/uploads/system/uploads/attachment_data/file/445738/Lord_Rose_NHS_Report_acc.pdf (accessed on 30 June 2021).
14. Department of Health; NHS Improvement. Developing People—Improving Care. National Improvement and Leadership Development Board. Available online: https://improvement.nhs.uk/documents/542/Developing_People-Improving_Care-010216.pdf (accessed on 20 March 2021).
15. Kline, R. Leadership in the NHS. *BMJ Lead.* **2019**, *3*, 129–132. [CrossRef]
16. NHS Leadership Academy. Leadership Framework—A Summary. Available online: https://www.leadershipacademy.nhs.uk/wp-content/uploads/2012/11/NHSLeadership-Framework-LeadershipFramework-Summary.pdf (accessed on 18 March 2021).
17. NHS Leadership Academy. Healthcare Leadership Model. In *The Nine Dimensions of Leadership Behaviour*; NHS Leadership Academy: England, UK, 2013. Available online: https://www.leadershipacademy.nhs.uk/wp-content/uploads/2014/10/NHSLeadership-LeadershipModel-colour.pdf (accessed on 21 August 2020).
18. Royal Pharmaceutical Society. Leadership Development Framework. January 2015. Available online: https://www.rpharms.com/resources/frameworks/leadership-development-framework (accessed on 1 April 2021).
19. Royal Pharmaceutical Society. The Pharmacy Contribution to Antimicrobial Stewardship. September 2017. Available online: https://www.rpharms.com/recognition/all-our-campaigns/policy-a-z/antimicrobial-stewardship (accessed on 1 April 2021).
20. International Pharmaceutical Federation (FIP) Development Goals. 2020. Available online: https://www.fip.org/fip-development-goals (accessed on 20 May 2021).
21. NHS Health Education England. Improving Global Health through Leadership. Development Programme. Available online: https://www.hee.nhs.uk/our-work/global-engagement/improving-global-health-through-leadership-development-programme-0 (accessed on 28 May 2021).
22. Faculty of Medical Leadership and Management. Chief Pharmaceutical Officer's Clinical Fellow Scheme. Available online: https://www.fmlm.ac.uk/CFS-pharmacy (accessed on 28 May 2021).
23. Briggs, K.; Briggs Myers, I. The Myers-Briggs Type Indicator. 2015. Available online: https://www.myersbriggs.org/my-mbti-personality-type/mbti-basics/thinking-or-feeling.htm (accessed on 20 March 2021).
24. NHS Leadership Academy. The Edward Jenner Programme. Available online: https://www.leadershipacademy.nhs.uk/programmes/the-edward-jenner-programme/ (accessed on 14 April 2021).
25. Tyler, N.; Collares, C.; Byrne, G.; Byrne-Davis, L. Measuring the outcomes of volunteering for education: Development and pilot of a tool to assess healthcare professionals' personal and professional development from international volunteering. *BMJ Open* **2019**, *9*, e028206. [CrossRef] [PubMed]
26. Bertrum, D. Likert Scales. Available online: http://poincare.matf.bg.ac.rs/~{}kristina/topic-dane-likert.pdf (accessed on 21 August 2020).
27. Royal Pharmaceutical Society (RPS) Faculty Peer Assessment Tool. Available online: https://www.rpharms.com/development/credentialing/faculty/10-week-plan (accessed on 26 February 2020). Used with permission from the Royal Pharmaceutical Society.
28. NHS Health Research Authority. Is My Study Research Decision Tool. Available online: http://www.hra-decisiontools.org.uk/research/result7.html (accessed on 16 June 2021).
29. West, M.; Armit, K.; Loewenthal, L.; Eckert, R.; West, T.; Lee, A. Leadership and Leadership Development in Health Care. 2015. Available online: https://www.kingsfund.org.uk/sites/files/kf/field/field_publication_file/leadership-leadership-development-health-care-feb-2015.pdf (accessed on 24 May 2017).
30. Kluger, A.N.; DeNisi, A. The effects of feedback interventions on performance: A historical review, a meta-analysis, and a preliminary feedback intervention theory. *Psychol. Bull.* **1996**, *119*, 254–284. [CrossRef]
31. Seifert, C.F.; Yukl, G.; Mcdonald, R.A. Effects of multisource feedback and a feedback facilitator on the influence behavior of managers toward subordinates. *J. Appl. Psychol.* **2003**, *88*, 561–569. [CrossRef] [PubMed]
32. MacPhail, A.; Young, C.; Ibrahim, J.E. Workplace-based clinical leadership training increases willingness to lead. *Leadersh. Health Serv.* **2015**, *28*, 100–118. [CrossRef] [PubMed]
33. Bhandari, A.; Wagner, T. Self-reported utilization of health care services: Improving measurement and accuracy. *Med. Care Res. Rev.* **2006**, *63*, 217–235. [CrossRef] [PubMed]
34. Mianda, S.; Voce, A. Developing and evaluating clinical leadership interventions for frontline healthcare providers: A review of the literature. *BMC Health Serv. Res.* **2018**, *18*, 747. [CrossRef] [PubMed]

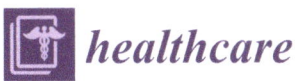

Article

A Comparison of Nursing and Pharmacy Students' Perceptions of an Acute Care Simulation

Jill Pence [1], Shannon Ashe [1], Georges Adunlin [2] and Jennifer Beall [2,*]

[1] College of Health Sciences, Samford University, Birmingham, AL 35229, USA; jnpence@samford.edu (J.P.); sashe@samford.edu (S.A.)
[2] McWhorter School of Pharmacy, Samford University, Birmingham, AL 35229, USA; gadunlin@samford.edu
* Correspondence: jwbeall@samford.edu

Abstract: Patient outcomes are improved when healthcare professionals work collaboratively. In order for future professionals to have these entry-level skills, students from different disciplines must work together in scenarios simulating patient care. This paper provides an overview of a large-scale, acute care simulation involving students of different disciplines, including nursing and pharmacy. A survey using the validated Student Perceptions of Interprofessional Clinical Education Revised (SPICE-R2) tool was administered to students participating in the simulation prior to and within 1 week of the simulation. There were between-group statistically significant differences on two items on the pre-simulation survey and two items on the post-simulation survey. Student participants reported more positive perceptions after the simulation on every item except for "During their education, health professional students should be involved in teamwork with students from other health professions to understand their perspective roles". The authors concluded that an interprofessional acute care simulation allowed students in both professions to recognize the value of a team approach to patient care.

Keywords: interprofessional; simulation; acute care; nursing; pharmacy; students; standardized patients; high fidelity; SPICE-R2

1. Introduction

Providing patient-centered care and improving patient outcomes are this century's primary focuses in medicine. Following the call to action by the Institute of Medicine (IOM) in 1999 to improve patient care through interprofessional practice and collaboration, the World Health Organization (WHO) provided a framework for action supporting this mission in 2010 [1]. Further, the Interprofessional Educational Collaborative (IPEC) was founded by the WHO to identify how to instill these important skills in future generations of healthcare professionals [2]. The objective was that integrated, well-structured, interprofessional education experiences would guide students to effectively communicate and collaborate with other health professionals after graduation.

Studies over the past decade have been slowly showing that the pillars of interprofessional education (IPE) (values and ethics, roles and responsibilities, communication, and teamwork) are gained through IPE [3,4]. Various processes have been utilized to promote these skills, with the most evidence-based initiatives coming through simulation-based training (SBT) [4]. SBT provides learners with the opportunity to utilize the desired skills as well as to review the effectiveness of their skills and decide a direction for future actions [5]. When utilized in IPE, SBT provides a safe, clinical-like environment for students to utilize, refine, and enhance the skills necessary for effective interprofessional collaboration with learners from other health professions [6].

Current studies in simulation-based IPE typically involve two to three disciplines working in a single clinical environment, such as nursing and medical students in an emergency department [7]. Most of the studies show increases in students' self-efficacy, understanding of roles and responsibilities, and attitudes towards working in healthcare teams [3]. Limitations of current studies of IPE are that the professions are connected through phone and electronic communications [8,9]. Uniquely, in this study, the activity permitted students from multiple disciplines to directly interact with each other in patient care. Additionally, there were multiple patient cases in a variety of interrelated scenarios concurrently to provide situational reality, an additional limitation of the current research [10,11]. The unique setting of the activity produced synchronous interdisciplinary collaboration of professional students in a large-scale scenario, similar to hospital-based clinical interactions.

There is a need to allow students from varied health profession programs to participate in a realistic, in-depth interprofessional simulation optimizing the IPEC competencies of communication, collaboration, and teamwork to achieve positive patient outcomes. Therefore, the purpose of this study was to compare nursing and pharmacy students' perceptions of interprofessional clinical education before and after the activity.

2. Materials and Methods

2.1. Study Design and Setting

A total of 250 students from six health science programs at a small, private university in southeastern United States participated in a simulation-based IPE. The recruitment to participate in the cross-sectional study was limited to undergraduate nursing and professional pharmacy students due to profession-specific experiential education requirements. The university's institutional review board approved this study.

2.2. Sample Size Determination

A total of 129 pharmacy and 140 nursing students participated in the IPE simulation. A target sample size for each group of students was calculated with the Qualtrics sample size calculator (https://www.qualtrics.com/blog/calculating-sample-size/ (accessed on 1 April 2022)), specifying a confidence level of 95% and a margin of error of 5%. Based on the criteria, ideal sample sizes of 97 pharmacy and 103 nursing students were determined adequate for the study. Attendance for the simulation was mandatory for pharmacy and nursing students as part of a required course. However, participation in the study via completion of the surveys was voluntary.

2.3. Interprofessional Education Experience

This activity took place in the fall of 2018 at a college of health sciences at a small, private university in southeastern United States. It involved 250 students from six health science programs: undergraduate nursing, respiratory therapy, pharmacy, physical therapy, nurse anesthesia, and social work. There were close to 50 faculty who participated as facilitators, resources for team members, and pre-debriefing facilitators. Additional personnel included manikin operators, runners, unit support personnel, and event coordinators, who were all filled by simulation personnel and volunteers from the participating programs.

The event took place over two consecutive days, which were each divided into two 4 h shifts. Each shift consisted of a 30 min pre-briefing; a 3 h patient care experience, including patient rounds; and a 30 min debriefing. Students were divided among the four shifts and then subdivided into seven teams, each covering a patient group/unit together.

The teams included students from each of the participating health profession disciplines. The patient units included four medical–surgical teams, one emergency room team, one ICU team, one labor and delivery team, one pediatric team, and one home care team. A total of 25 patient cases were written and filled by standardized patients (SPs) and high-fidelity manikins, with family members and support partners throughout. A total of 29 SPs and 5 manikins were utilized.

Each team was given a pre-assignment of watching orientation videos of the overall experience, event flow, and processes. Pre-briefing included unit orientation, team building, and reports on the patients on their respective units. Each patient case unfolded over the course of the day with a "shift change" in the middle of the day, where the morning shift reported to the evening shift, and the patient care continued. Students experienced processes such as patient admission, discharge, transfer, and medication dispensing, as well as tasks such as IV and catheter placement, physical therapy sessions, and bedside counseling. Patient charts were developed in an electronic health record that all students had access to, allowing for continuity of care regardless of patient location or team member utilization. Patient cases were scripted so that all materials would be included. If a team member wanted to do something that was not scripted, it was the role of the faculty resource member in that area to allow the student to discuss the rationale and why it may not be a priority. Test results were kept at a central location and were given based on a timed-release schedule (i.e., CT scan results = 15 min wait).

The simulation was paused midway through each shift for a patient rounds simulation. While patient rounds were facilitated by a faculty member, they were student-led, allowing the students to collaborate and develop a plan together. A structured debriefing session was held at the end of the shift, focusing on the objectives relating to the IPEC competencies previously mentioned.

2.4. Assessment

Students from each of the participating disciplines were asked to complete the Student Perceptions of Interprofessional Clinical Education Revised (SPICE-R2) survey prior to and within 1 week of simulation. The SPICE-R2 is a validated tool examining students' attitudes toward interprofessional teams and the team approach to care of patients. It uses a five-point Likert scale and is composed of ten items across three factors (also known as subscales) [12]. The subscales include:

- Interprofessional teamwork and team-based practice (four items);
- Roles and responsibilities for collaborative practice (three items);
- Patient outcomes from collaborative practice (three items).

The SPICE-R2 items and factors are indicated in Table 1.

Table 1. SPICE-R2 items and factors.

1.	Working with students from different disciplines enhances my education [a]
2.	My role within an interprofessional team is clearly defined [b]
3.	Patient/client satisfaction is improved when care is delivered by an interprofessional team [c]
4.	Participating in educational experiences with students from different disciplines enhances my ability to work on an interprofessional team [a]
5.	I have an understanding of the courses taken by, and training requirements of, other health professionals [b]
6.	Healthcare costs are reduced when patients/clients are treated by an interprofessional team [c]
7.	Health professional students from different disciplines should be educated to establish collaborative relationships with one another [a]
8.	I understand the roles of other health professionals within an interprofessional team [b]
9.	Patient/client-centeredness increases when care is delivered by an interprofessional team [c]
10.	During their education, health professional students should be involved in teamwork with students from different disciplines in order to understand their respective roles [a]

Factors: [a] = interprofessional teamwork and team-based practice (T); [b] = roles and responsibilities for collaborative practice (R); [c] = patient outcomes from collaborative practice (O).

Because individual identifiers were not used for the pre- and post-simulation surveys, paired responses were not feasible. Other disciplines (physical therapy, respiratory therapy, and social work) also participated in the simulation, but there were not comparable numbers of participants from these disciplines to allow for comparison with nursing and pharmacy student responses. For that reason, the current study compared the perceptions of nursing and pharmacy students only.

2.5. Statistical Analysis

Individual identifiers were not used for the pre- and post-simulation assessments; therefore, there was no way to pair the responses and use tests designed for paired responses. We tested responses on the SPICE-R2 for normality with the Shapiro–Wilk test and used a histogram to identify major asymmetries, revealing non-normal distribution. An independent samples t-test was used to test for group differences (i.e., nursing vs. pharmacy) in self-reported prior experience with IPE activity on the pre- and post-test SPICE-R2 instrument. The Mann–Whitney U test was used to compare the scores on each of the SPICE-R2 items between nursing and pharmacy students. The Wilcoxon signed-rank test was used to determine whether there was a significant difference between the pre-test and post-test scores. The level of significance was alpha ≤ 0.05.

3. Results

3.1. Demographics

The participants in the study consisted of senior-level baccalaureate nursing students and third-year pharmacy students. Although there were undergraduate and graduate students, their clinical knowledge levels were similar due to program design and clinical experience. The study did not achieve the calculated sample size of 97 pharmacy and 103 nursing students.

In Table 2, prior exposure and participation in IPE and perception of the IPE simulation are reported.

Table 2. Prior experience with IPE (POST) and post-simulation perceptions.

Demographic Variable	Pharmacy Students ($n = 51$)	Nursing Students ($n = 83$)
Previous experience with IPE		
Yes	25 (49%)	49 (59%)
No	26 (51%)	34 (41%)
I believe this was a valuable learning experience		
Yes	49 (96%)	82 (99%)
No	2 (4%)	1 (1%)
Overall, I enjoyed the simulation		
Yes	46 (90%)	76 (92%)
No	5 (10%)	7 (8%)

A total of 134 students completed the post-IPE simulation survey. Of those, 51 were pharmacy students, and 83 were nursing students. While 49% of the pharmacy students reported previous experience with IPE, 41% of nursing students reported having no prior experience with IPE. The students' perceptions were positive following the IPE simulation, with the vast majority of pharmacy students (96%) and nursing students (99%) indicating that the IPE simulation activity was a valuable learning experience. The vast majority of pharmacy students (90%) and nursing students (92%) indicated that they enjoyed the IPE simulation.

3.2. Evaluating Pre- and Post-Simulation Scores

Table 3 shows the results of the Mann–Whitney U test conducted.

Table 3. Comparison of between-group differences in average scores pre- and post-simulation.

SPICE-R2 Items Number	Between-Group Pre-Simulation Averages [a]			Between-Group Post-Simulation Averages [a]		
	Pharmacy Students ($n = 52$) Pre-Simulation Mean (SD)	Nursing Students ($n = 136$) Pre-Simulation Mean (SD)	p-Value	Pharmacy Students ($n = 51$) Post-Simulation Mean (SD)	Nursing Students ($n = 83$) Post-Simulation Mean (SD)	p-Value
1	4.71 (0.49)	4.61 (0.69)	0.634	4.84 (0.36)	4.66 (0.73)	0.167
2	4.59 (0.60)	4.33 (0.76)	**0.023 ***	4.64 (0.52)	4.46 (0.84)	0.375
3	4.82 (0.43)	4.75 (0.61)	0.553	4.90 (0.30)	4.79 (0.57)	0.317
4	4.73 (0.48)	4.61 (0.64)	0.309	4.78 (0.46)	4.69 (0.65)	0.606
5	4.01 (0.91)	3.88 (1.15)	0.834	4.50 (0.54)	4.21 (1.08)	0.482
6	4.71 (0.53)	4.16 (0.91)	**0.000 ***	4.82 (0.47)	4.43 (0.87)	**0.002 ***
7	4.84 (0.36)	4.77 (0.53)	0.461	4.90 (0.30)	4.83 (0.53)	0.538
8	4.36 (0.59)	4.30 (0.82)	0.842	4.60 (0.60)	4.49 (0.80)	0.536
9	4.80 (0.39)	4.69 (0.57)	0.276	4.92 (0.27)	4.75 (0.57)	**0.050 ***
10	4.80 (0.39)	4.76 (0.49)	0.720	4.88 (0.32)	4.74 (0.58)	0.142

* Results demonstrating statistical significance ($p < 0.05$) appear in bold.

Some notable pre- and post-test between-group differences were observed. In the pre-simulation, significant differences were observed between groups for two items relating to "My role within an interprofessional team is clearly defined" (Table 3, Item 2) and "Healthcare costs are reduced when patients/clients are treated by an interprofessional team" (Table 3, Item 6). On Item 2, the pre-simulation average score of pharmacy students was significantly higher (M = 4.59, SD ± 0.60) than that of nursing students (M = 4.33, SD ± 0.76), $p = 0.023$. On Item 6, the pre-simulation average score of pharmacy students was also significantly higher (M = 4.71, SD ± 0.53) than that of nursing students (M = 4.16, SD ± 0.91), $p = 0.000$. A mean score increase was noted on all survey items on the SPICE-R2 in the post-simulation. Between the two items that demonstrated significant differences in the pre-simulation, only one ("Healthcare costs are reduced when patients/clients are treated by an interprofessional team" (Table 3, Item 6)) remained significant post-simulation. Specifically, the Item 6 post-simulation score of pharmacy students remained significantly higher (M = 4.82, SD ± 0.47) than that of nursing students (M = 4.43, SD ± 0.87), $p = 0.002$. Statistically significant increases were observed on one other item ("Patient/client-centeredness increases when care is delivered by an interprofessional team" (Table 3, Item 9)), with pharmacy students scoring higher (M = 4.92, SD ± 0.27) than nursing students scored (M = 4.75, SD ± 0.57), $p = 0.050$.

As previously indicated, the SPICE-R2 instrument contains 10 items and 3 factors focused on interprofessional teamwork and team-based practice, roles and responsibilities for collaborative practice, and patient outcomes from collaborative practice. The analysis comparing the mean scores for SPICE-R2 factors pre- and post-simulation was completed using the Wilcoxon signed-rank test, and the results are presented in Table 4. Effect sizes are reported using Cohen's d [13]. We considered values of 0.2 as small, 0.5 as medium, and 0.8 and higher as large effect sizes [13].

Table 4. Comparison of pre- to post-test factor scores.

Factors	Pharmacy Students					Nursing Students				
	Pre (SD)-$n = 52$	Post (SD)-$n = 51$	Difference [a]	p-value	D [b]	Pre (SD)-$n = 136$	Post (SD)-$n = 83$	Difference [a]	p-value	d [b]
T	4.77 (0.39)	4.86 (0.35)	0.09	0.210	0.24	4.69 (0.51)	4.78 (0.56)	0.090	0.226	0.17
R	4.32 (0.57)	4.54 (0.54)	0.22	**0.047 ***	0.39	4.17 (0.78)	4.42 (0.83)	0.250	**0.025 ***	0.31
O	4.78 (0.34)	4.90 (0.30)	0.12	0.061	0.37	4.54 (0.56)	4.71 (0.60)	0.170	**0.034 ***	0.29

Pharmacy students (pre-$n = 52$; post-$n = 51$); nursing students (pre-$n = 136$; post-$n = 83$); [a] Cohen's d (0.2 as small, 0.5 as medium, and 0.8 and higher as large); [b] Cohen's d standardized effect size. SD: standard deviation. * Results demonstrating statistical significance ($p < 0.05$) appear in bold.

Among the nursing students, statistically significant increases in mean scores were noted for the roles and responsibilities for collaborative practice (M = 4.42, SD ± 0.83, $p = 0.025$) and patient outcomes from collaborative practice factors (M = 4.71, SD ± 0.60, $p = 0.034$) in the post-simulation. Among the pharmacy students, there was a statistically significant increase in mean score for the roles and responsibilities for collaborative practice factor within the SPICE-R2 instrument in the post-simulation (M = 4.54, SD ± 0.54, $p = 0.047$). Among the pharmacy students, the effect-size values for the three factors ranged from 0.24 to 0.39, indicating small effects. Among the nursing students, the effect-size values for the three factors ranged from 0.17 to 0.31, also indicating small effect sizes.

4. Discussion

The study results indicate that there were baseline differences observed between groups for Items 2 ("My role within an interprofessional team is clearly defined") and 6 ("Healthcare costs are reduced when patients/clients are treated by an interprofessional team") of the SPICE-R2 instrument. After the simulation, these differences remained for Item 6 and were also observed for Item 9 ("Patient/client-centeredness increases when care is delivered by an interprofessional team"). Scores increased in both groups between every item except Item 10 ("During their education, health professional students should be involved in teamwork with students from other health professions to understand their respective roles in the nursing student group"). There were also changes in factor scores from pre- to post-simulation experience. Significant changes were observed for factor R (roles and responsibilities for collaborative practice).

A literature search revealed two studies that were published comparing nursing and pharmacy students' perceptions of an interprofessional simulation that used SPICE instruments [14,15]. In our study, there was an increase in mean score overall for all students as well as for individual scores from pre-test to post-test. No significant difference was seen based on discipline between pre-test and post-test. Similarly, a study of nursing and pharmacy students showed an increase in perceptions of healthcare teams following an acute care experience [14]. Fusco and Foltz-Ramos investigated the change in perceptions of interprofessional practice in nursing and pharmacy students before and after a high-fidelity simulation experience. The SPICE-R tool was used for this study. There were no decreases in median or interquartile range scores from pre-test to post-test for either discipline. Another study by Muzyk and colleagues investigated attitudes of nursing and pharmacy students in an interprofessional substance use disorder course [15]. The SPICE-R2 instrument was used, and results were reported by subscales. Similarly to our study, there were statistically significant differences between pre- and post-course surveys in the subscale of roles and responsibilities; however, the results are presented with nursing and pharmacy students combined.

Evaluating simulation-based IPE is reliant on the goals and objectives to be assessed. Currently, there are multiple tools available to measure student objectives, and all focus on some, if not all, of the tenants of IPE as described by IPEC in 2016 [3]. The SPICE-R2 instrument focuses on the student perceptions of roles and responsibilities of interprofessional groups, teamwork and team-based practice, and patient outcomes [12]. Modifications to the initial instrument were designed to enable use by professions outside of medicine and pharmacy. In previous studies, nursing and medical students improved their perceptions of interprofessional practice and role stereotypes [16]. Lockeman and colleagues developed a quasi-experimental pre-test–post-test study to explore whether a series of simulation experiences promoted changes in perceptions of IPE among medical and nursing students. The SPICE-R2 survey was used, as it was used in the current study. Utilizing the SPICE-R2 to identify the baseline of and changes in students' understanding of roles and responsibilities, as well as teamwork and collaboration, provided insight into a healthcare team's role in the dynamic patient care that is a hospital setting.

Overall, most student respondents reported that this simulation activity was a valuable learning experience and that they enjoyed it. There were increases in average scores from pre- to post-simulation survey results in all items for pharmacy students and in all but one of the items for nursing students. The results of this assessment will be used for an ongoing evaluation of the simulation activity and to implement necessary changes for a more effective experience.

Limitations of the current study include a lower than desirable response rate on the surveys, including a drop in responses from pre- to post-simulation surveys. As mentioned previously, the numbers of students from other disciplines who participated in the simulation were not compared to allow the comparison of nursing and pharmacy student responses. Because individual identifiers were not used, paired responses between pre- and post-simulation surveys were not feasible. Future research should be performed to compare perceptions of acute care simulations across various academic institutions to strengthen the current literature.

5. Conclusions

The interprofessional acute care simulation allowed students in both professions to recognize the value of a team approach to patient care. The simulation activity demonstrated the impact that IPE plays in ensuring that nursing and pharmacy students complete their educational training with the skills and competencies needed not only to be effective healthcare providers but also to be efficient members of a healthcare team. As academic institutions seek to bridge health disciplines, this study demonstrated an IPE activity that can help achieve this goal.

Author Contributions: Conceptualization, J.P. and S.A.; methodology, J.P. and S.A.; formal analysis, G.A.; investigation, J.P. and S.A.; resources, J.P. and S.A.; data curation, J.P. and G.A.; writing—original draft, J.P., S.A., G.A. and J.B.; writing—reviewing and editing, J.P., S.A., G.A. and J.B.; visualization, J.P., S.A., G.A. and J.B.; supervision, J.P. and S.A.; project administration, J.P., S.A. and J.B. All authors have read and agreed to the published version of the manuscript.

Funding: This research received no external funding.

Institutional Review Board Statement: The study was conducted according to the guidelines of the Declaration of Helsinki and approved by the Institutional Review Board of Samford University (EXMT-N-19-F, approved 15 October 2019).

Informed Consent Statement: Informed consent was waived due to anonymity of survey responses.

Conflicts of Interest: The authors declare no conflict of interest.

References

1. World Health Organization. *Framework for Action on Interprofessional Education and Collaborative Practice*; World Health Organization: Geneva, Switzerland, 2010.
2. Interprofessional Education Collaborative. *Core Competencies for Interprofessional Collaborative Practice*; Interprofessional Education Collaborative: Washington, DC, USA, 2016; Available online: https://ipec.memberclicks.net/assets/2016-Update.pdf (accessed on 21 April 2021).
3. Visser, C.L.F.; Ket, J.C.F.; Croiset, G.; Kusurkar, R.A. Perceptions of residents, medical and nursing students about interprofessional education: A systematic review of the quantitative and qualitative literature. *BMC Med. Educ.* **2017**, *17*, 1–13. [CrossRef] [PubMed]
4. Herath, C.; Zhou, Y.; Gan, Y.; Nakandawire, N.; Gong, Y.; Lu, Z. A comparative study of interprofessional education in global health care. *Medicine (Baltimore)* **2017**, *96*, e7336–e7343. [CrossRef] [PubMed]
5. INACSL Standards Committee. INACSL standards of best practice: Simulation design. *Clin. Simul. Nurs.* **2016**, *12*, S5–S12. [CrossRef]
6. Palaganas, J.C.; Epps, C.; Raemer, D.B. A history of simulation-enhanced interprofessional education. *J. Interprof. Care* **2014**, *28*, 110–115. [CrossRef] [PubMed]
7. Jakobsen, R.B.; Gran, S.F.; Grimsmo, B.; Arntzen, K.; Fosse, E.; Frich, J.C.; Hjortdahl, P. Examining participant perceptions of an interprofessional simulation-based trauma team training for medical and nursing students. *J. Interprof. Care* **2018**, *32*, 80–88. [CrossRef] [PubMed]
8. Weir-Mayta, P.; Green, S.; Abbott, S.; Urbina, D. Incorporating IPE and simulation experiences into graduate speech-language pathology training. *Cogent Med.* **2020**, *7*, 1847415. [CrossRef]
9. Lairamore, C.; Reed, C.C.; Damon, Z.; Rowe, V.; Baker, J.; Griffith, K.; VanHoose, L. A peer-led interprofessional simulation experience improves perceptions of teamwork. *Clin. Simul. Nurs.* **2019**, *34*, 22–29. [CrossRef]

10. Burford, B.; Greig, P.; Kelleher, M.; Merriman, C.; Platt, A.; Richards, E.; Davidson, N.; Vance, G. Effects of a single interprofessional simulation session on medical and nursing students' attitudes toward interprofessional learning and professional identity: A questionnaire study. *BMC Med. Educ.* **2020**, *20*, 1–11. [CrossRef] [PubMed]
11. Bourke, S.L.; Cooper, S.; Lam, L.; McKenna, L. Undergraduate Health Professional Students' Team Communication in Simulated Emergency Settings: A Scoping Review. *Clin. Simul. Nurs.* **2021**, *60*, 42–63. [CrossRef]
12. Zorek, J.A.; Fike, D.S.; Eickhoff, J.C.; Engle, J.A.; MacLaughlin, E.J.; Dominguez, D.G.; Seibert, C.S. Refinement and validation of the student perceptions of physician-pharmacist interprofessional clinical education instrument. *Am. J. Pharm. Educ.* **2016**, *80*, 1–8. [CrossRef] [PubMed]
13. Cohen, J. *Statistical Power Analysis for the Behavioral Sciences*, 2nd ed.; L. Erlbaum Associates: Hillsdale, NJ, USA, 1988; pp. 20–26.
14. Fusco, N.; Foltz-Ramos, K. Measuring changes in pharmacy and nursing students' perceptions following an interprofessional high-fidelity simulation experience. *J. Interprof. Care* **2018**, *32*, 648–652. [CrossRef] [PubMed]
15. Muzyk, A.; Mullan, P.; Andolsek, K.; Derouin, A.; Smothers, Z.; Sanders, C.; Holmer, S. A pilot interprofessional course on substance use disorders to improve students' empathy and counseling skills. *Am. J. Pharm. Educ.* **2020**, *84*, 438–444. [CrossRef] [PubMed]
16. Lockeman, K.S.; Appelbaum, N.P.; Dow, A.W.; Orr, S.; Huff, T.A.; Hogan, C.J.; Queen, B.A. The effect of an interprofessional simulation-based education program on perceptions and stereotypes of nursing and medical students: A quasi-experimental study. *Nurse Educ. Today* **2017**, *58*, 32–37. [CrossRef] [PubMed]

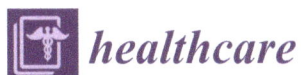

Article

Community Pharmacists' Opinions towards Poor Prescription Writing in Jazan, Saudi Arabia

Saad Saeed Alqahtani [1,2]

1. Department of Clinical Pharmacy, College of Pharmacy, Jazan University, Jazan 45142, Saudi Arabia; ssalqahtani@jazanu.edu.sa
2. Pharmacy Practice Research Unit, College of Pharmacy, Jazan University, Jazan 45142, Saudi Arabia

Abstract: Avoidance of medication errors is imperative for the safe use of medications, and community pharmacists are uniquely placed to identify and resolve the errors that may arise due to poorly handwritten prescriptions. **Purpose:** To explore the opinion and attitudes of community pharmacists towards poor prescription writing and their suggestions to overcome this concern. **Methods:** A cross-sectional, self-administered survey was conducted among the community pharmacists in the Jazan region, Saudi Arabia. Descriptive analysis and chi-square test were used at 5% p-value ($p > 0.05$) as the significance level. **Results:** The response rate for the survey was 78.66%, and 140 community pharmacists agreed to participate. Among the study subjects, the majority (73.57%) had a bachelor's degree. Nearly three-fourths (3/4) of the pharmacists (72.29%) chose to send the patient back to the prescriber when they found difficulty in interpreting the information from an illegible prescription. As many as 80.71% of the pharmacists believed that poorly handwritten prescriptions were the cause of actual errors when dispensing medications. The most commonly encountered problem due to poorly handwritten prescriptions was the commercial name of medicine, which was reported by around two-thirds (67.86%) of the pharmacists. The use of e-prescription was suggested by 72.86% of the pharmacists as a probable solution to encounter this problem. **Conclusion:** Our findings highlight the belief and attitudes of community pharmacists in the region and their opinions to solve this impending problem of poor prescription writing. Continuous professional development courses can be adopted to tackle the problem. Additionally, health authorities can work on incorporating and facilitating the use of e-prescription in the community sector, which can be a boon to physicians, pharmacists, and patients. Proper and extensive training is however needed before the implementation of e-prescribing.

Keywords: e-prescription; prescription writing; Jazan; Saudi Arabia; prescription errors

Citation: Alqahtani, S.S. Community Pharmacists' Opinions towards Poor Prescription Writing in Jazan, Saudi Arabia. *Healthcare* **2021**, *9*, 1077. https://doi.org/10.3390/healthcare9081077

Academic Editor: Georges Adunlin

Received: 20 June 2021
Accepted: 17 August 2021
Published: 21 August 2021

Publisher's Note: MDPI stays neutral with regard to jurisdictional claims in published maps and institutional affiliations.

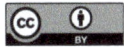

Copyright: © 2021 by the author. Licensee MDPI, Basel, Switzerland. This article is an open access article distributed under the terms and conditions of the Creative Commons Attribution (CC BY) license (https://creativecommons.org/licenses/by/4.0/).

1. Introduction

The community pharmacist is usually the first point of contact for people due to their easy accessibility. They dispense medications as stated in the prescription and are licensed to prescribe over-the-counter drugs [1]. Nowadays, community pharmacists also contribute professionally through a wide range of activities that concern patient care from the optimization of drug therapy to promote health awareness and to educate people on the prevention of diseases. All this is not to mention their essential role in providing rational drug information and to counsel patients about drug safety and cost-effectiveness [2]. One of the primary tasks of a pharmacist is to verify the legality, safety, and appropriateness of the prescription and to ensure accurate dispensing of the medication before deciding to hand it over to the patients with directions of use and counselling [1].

The WHO's Guide to Good Prescribing states "A prescription is an instruction from a prescriber to a dispenser" [3]. The word *prescription* stems from the Latin language, wherein *pre-* translates as "before" and *scribe-* translated for writing [4]. A written prescription is the physician's/prescriber's order to the dispenser, usually for a pharmacist to prepare and/or dispense the specified medication to that patient [5]. Almost all interactions between a doctor and a patient end with prescription writing [6], therefore making it imperative that the prescriber should always ensure the legibility and unambiguity of the written order, including the date and sign. This facilitates clear communication between health care professionals. Moreover, an ideal prescription should also present ample information to allow the dispenser (in most cases the pharmacist) to identify any errors before dispensing [5].

A medication error can be defined as an unwanted event that may lead to inappropriate use of medications and potentially be harmful to the patients [7,8]. According to world estimates, the cost of medication errors is around 42 billion US dollars [9]. These medication errors are often preventable if identified at the right time [7]. Although medication errors occur at different stages such as writing, transcribing, and administration, illegible handwriting appears to be the predominant cause of these errors [10].

Bobb et al. (2004), Delgado Silveira et al. (2007), and Aljadhey et al. (2013) reported that the point of prescribing medication is usually linked to a high incidence of medication errors, which in turn is the leading cause of adverse drug events [11–13]. More importantly, the illegibility of prescriptions leads to a greater chance of errors, whether or not the written order is complete and accurate. Illegible prescription is one of the factors that can increase the risk of medication errors regardless of the accuracy and completeness of the prescription [14]. Analysis of self-reporting was done by Knudsen et al. (2007) in community pharmacies, and they found a positive correlation between dispensing errors and illegible handwriting [15].

A study by Hartel et al. (2011) evaluated and noted significant variation in the legibility and quality of the handwriting of prescribers and concluded that there are differences in the ability of pharmacists to read these written orders [16]. Additionally, Brits et al. (2017) demonstrated in their study that community pharmacists were not better than nurses or physicians in reading the prescription, and they attributed this to the lack of direct work associated with the doctors [17]. In a similar Saudi study done by Albarrak et al. (2014), pharmacists with less experience found difficulty in reading 21.6% of prescriptions as opposed to experienced pharmacists (2%) [18]. Winslow et al. (1997) reported that 20% of prescriptions had poor handwriting and could not be understood [19]. In a study done in Saudi Arabia by Irshaid et al. (2005), around 64% of medication orders were illegible [20]. Calligaris et al. (2009), after evaluating the prescriptions in an Italian hospital confirmed that 24% of them were illegible [10].

In view of the above evidence, critically addressing the illegibility problem in medication orders is the need of the hour. The current study aimed at exploring the attitude of the community pharmacists towards poor prescriptions in the Jazan region of Saudi Arabia. We also investigated the prescription-related problems due to poor handwriting and suggestions. Lastly, we aimed to garner suggestions from the community pharmacists about improving the quality of handwritten prescriptions.

2. Methodology

2.1. Ethics Approval

The study was approved by the Institutional Research Review and Ethics Committee (IRREC) of the Faculty of Pharmacy, Jazan University, KSA. The study protocol was in accordance with principles and guidelines laid out in the Declaration of Helsinki and the International Council on Harmonization Good Clinical Practice. All pharmacists were asked to complete a written consent form prior to the start of the survey.

2.2. Study Design and Area

This was a cross-sectional, structured, self-administered survey of the belief, attitudes, and suggestions of pharmacists about poor prescription writing in the Jazan province of Saudi Arabia. Jazan is a province located in the Southwestern part of the Kingdom with a total population of 1,535,167 (2016), and the city of Jazan serves as its administrative headquarter [21].

2.3. Study Population and Sample Size

The questionnaire (Supplementary Materials) was distributed among licensed pharmacists working in community pharmacies in different areas of Jazan province, and the data were gathered through an anonymous, self-administered questionnaire. The selection of licensed pharmacists working in both independent and chain pharmacies was done randomly. After obtaining their consent, the questionnaire was delivered to them and was collected the next day by a research assistant. A total of 140 community pharmacists agreed to enroll in the study from the Jazan province.

2.4. Data Collection Tool

The questionnaire was face-validated by a five-member expert panel prior to the study. The panel comprised one English language expert, one psychologist, two practicing community pharmacists, and one academic pharmacist. The two practicing community pharmacists were excluded from the study. The questionnaire was in the English language and included the demographic information of the respondents along with their education level and ownership details. The community pharmacists were further asked about the number of prescriptions filled by them per day and the number of poorly written prescriptions received per day. The respondents were also asked for their opinion about handwritten prescriptions, their related errors, and the action to be taken.

The second part of the questionnaire was designed to identify the most common prescription-related problem that arises due to poor handwritten prescriptions. The last part of the questionnaire explored the measures that were suggested by the pharmacists to minimize the errors due to illegible prescriptions.

2.5. Statistical Analysis

The items in the questionnaire were first coded and then entered into Microsoft Excel. The data were then analyzed on STATA (Version 15.0 software, Stata Corp LP, College Station, TX, USA), and descriptive analysis (frequencies and percentages) was performed for all variables included in the study. Chi-square test was employed for categorical data and significance was considered if the *p*-value was less than 0.05 (5% *p*-value)

3. Results

3.1. Demographic Data

Out of 178 community pharmacists approached for the study, 140 (78.66 %) consented for enrollment in this study. The mean age of participants was 31.9 years. More than half of the respondents were found to be less than 30 years (62.75%) and had less than 10 years of experience (62.06%), with the mean experience as 8.5 years. Regarding the level of education, around three-fourths of pharmacists (73.57%) held a Bachelor's of Pharmacy degree. Nearly all of the respondents (97.13%) were working as employees in the private sector. The detailed demographic data are presented in Table 1.

3.2. Prescriptions

A total number of 2762 prescriptions (mean: 19.58 prescriptions per pharmacist) were dispensed by all the responding pharmacists. The number of prescriptions dispensed on a daily basis were stratified into two groups: <50 and $\geq$50. The majority of community pharmacists (92.41%) were found to fill less than 50 prescriptions on daily basis. As many as 93.79% of community pharmacists reported that they received around 30 poor handwritten prescriptions per day (Table 1).

Table 1. Baseline data of the study subjects.

Variable	n = 140	%
Age		
>30 years	54	38.57
≤30 years	86	61.43
Years of experience		
<10 years	90	64.29
≥10 years	50	35.71
Education Level		
B. Pharm	103	73.57
Pharm. D	37	26.43
Pharmacy Ownership		
Employee	136	97.13
Owner	4	2.85
Average prescriptions filled per day		
<50	130	92.86
≥50	10	7.14
Average number of poor handwritten prescriptions received per day		
<30	132	94.29
≥30	8	5.71

3.3. Response of the Pharmacists

When community pharmacists were asked about their response upon receiving an illegible prescription, nearly three-fourths (72.29%) of the pharmacists preferred to return the patient back to the physician when they could not interpret the information from the prescription. Around 93% of the pharmacists responded that they would never tell the patient that the medication was not available when they were not able to read the name of the medication. We only found a significant association between the experience of the pharmacist and the variable "I cannot read the prescription" ($p = 0.008$) (Table 2). No association was found between the educational degree of the pharmacist and their response to poor prescriptions.

Table 2. Comparison between the experience of the pharmacists and the response of the pharmacist.

Response of the Pharmacist	<10 Years		≥10 Years		p Value
	Yes	No	Yes	No	
Tell the patient this medication is not available.	4	86	7	43	0.092
Return the patient back to the physician.	69	21	42	8	0.419
I cannot read the prescription.	33	57	7	43	0.008 *

* $p < 0.05$.

3.4. Belief of the Pharmacists

About 60% of the pharmacists believed that poorly written prescriptions are increasing. In addition, the majority of pharmacists (80.71%) thought that actual errors when dispensing medications were due to the poor handwriting in the prescription. Sixty percent of the community pharmacists had the belief that the community pharmacist should not dispense the medication based on diagnosis without consulting the physician (Figure 1).

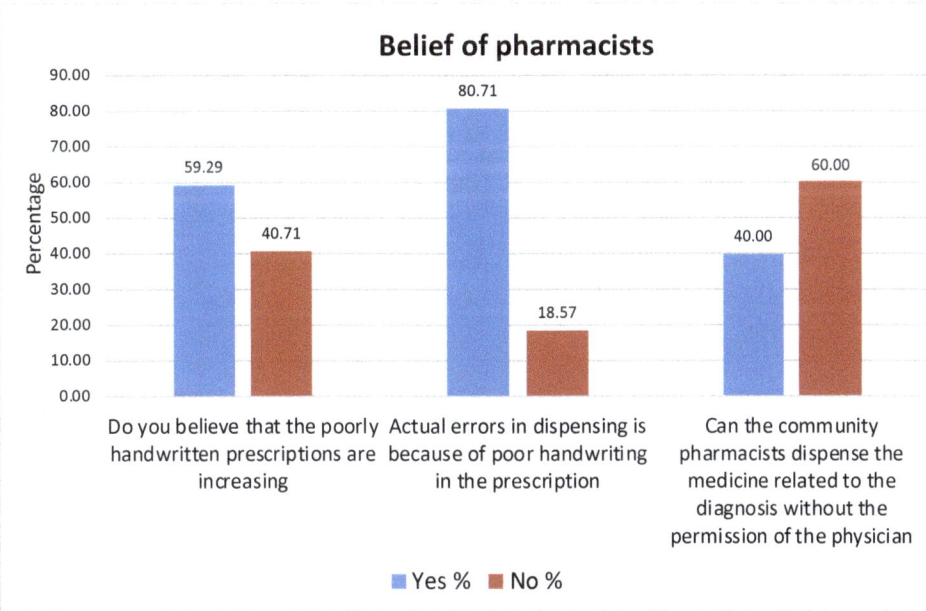

Figure 1. Beliefs of pharmacists of poorly handwritten prescriptions.

3.5. Prescription-Related Problems Due to Poor Handwriting

Around two-thirds (67.86%) of the respondents reported that the name of the trade medicine was the common prescription problem encountered due to poor handwriting followed by dose of the medication (49.29%). Of the nine items that were asked, the patient's name was the least reported (8.57%) to be a problem due to illegible handwriting (Figure 2).

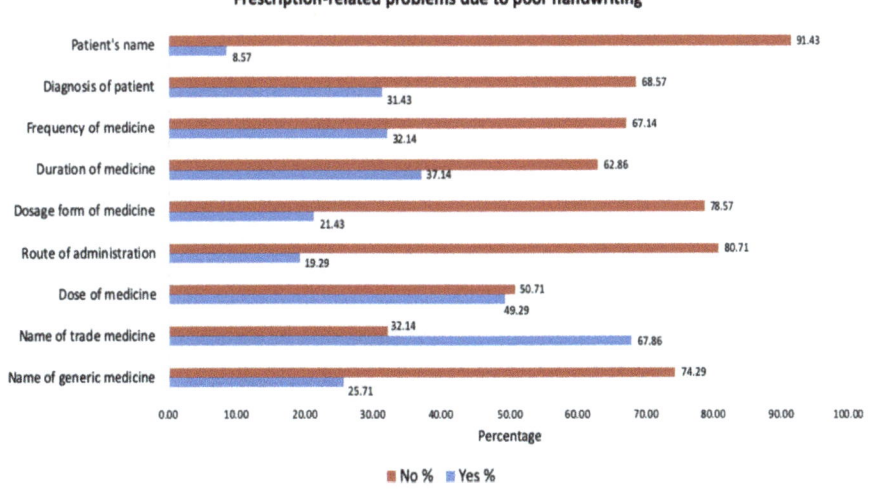

Figure 2. Problems encountered due to poor handwritten prescriptions.

3.6. Actions Suggested by the Community Pharmacists

Around three-fourths (72.86%) of the respondents suggested the use of e-prescription, and this only had a significant association with the educational degree of the pharmacist (p-value = 0.002) (Table 3). Most of the community pharmacists (90.27%) did not think that decimal numbers should be avoided when writing the dose of medications. Additionally, more than three-fourths (78.57%) did not suggest writing in capital letters, followed by two-thirds (66.43%) who did suggest the need for introducing a structured prescription form. There was no association between any of the actions suggested by the pharmacists and their experience. However, there was a significant association (p = 0.002) between the educational degree of the respondents and the suggestion to use e-prescriptions (Table 4).

Table 3. Actions suggested by pharmacists to overcome problems due to poor handwriting in prescriptions.

Suggestions by Pharmacists	Yes	No	Yes %	No %
Write in capital letters	30	110	21.43	78.57
Avoid abbreviations	64	76	45.71	54.29
Avoid the trade name of the medicine	57	83	40.71	59.29
Avoid the decimal number	13	127	9.29	90.71
Use e-prescription	102	37	72.86	26.43
Introducing a structured prescription form	47	93	33.57	66.43

Table 4. Comparison between the educational degree of the pharmacists and their suggestions to improve the prescriptions.

Suggestions by Pharmacists	B.Pharm		Pharm D		p-Value
	Yes	No	Yes	No	
Write in capital letters	21	83	9	27	0.711
Avoid abbreviations	48	56	16	20	1.0
Avoid trade name of the medicine	41	63	16	20	0.740
Avoid the decimal number	10	94	3	33	1.0
Use e-prescription	84	20	19	17	0.002 *
Introducing a structured prescription form	58	46	23	13	0.513

* $p < 0.05$.

4. Discussion

The present study is the first of its type to evaluate the attitude and belief of the pharmacists about poorly handwritten prescriptions in the Jazan region of Saudi Arabia. Poorly written prescriptions can cause errors that can lead to some serious consequences for the patient. An appropriately written prescription is a result of not only the effort by a prescriber to minimize errors but also to strive to achieve better prescribing [22]. Lopes et al. had reported that most medications errors reported in community pharmacies are due to poorly handwritten prescriptions [23]. In our study, nearly 80% of the pharmacists preferred to return the prescription to the physician for review. This seems to be the right decision by the pharmacists, as the prescribing physician can re-write the prescription or clarify the concern related to the prescription. This will prevent any unwanted dispensing error and will also be a reminder to the physician to be more legible. Moreover, the experience of the community pharmacist had a statistically significant association (p = 0.008) with the response "I cannot read the prescription". This seems to be logical as community pharmacists who are experienced will not respond that they cannot read the prescription, as this response would affect the confidence and trust between the patient and the pharmacist.

Nearly 80% of our respondents believed that the actual errors in dispensing are because of poor handwriting. A recent study done by Al-Arifi in Central Saudi Arabia reported that around 55% of the community pharmacists had a perception that dispensing errors are most common, and poor handwriting was identified as one of the major causes [24].

An earlier study by Knudsen et al. in Denmark also identified handwritten prescriptions as one of the four causes for the increase in dispensing errors [25].

In our study, nearly 68% reported that trade medicine was a major problem in poorly written prescriptions. This is consistent with many studies where the use of the trade name of the medicine was one of the main contributors to the prescription errors [10,24,25]. Moreover, nearly half (49.29%) of the respondents opined that the dose of the medication was also a concern in illegible prescriptions. This is much higher than the observations of Knudsen et al., who reported errors in dosages of 37.4%.

Community pharmacists in our study were also asked for their suggestions to improve the quality of prescriptions. The majority of them (72.86 %) suggested the use of e- prescriptions as a solution to the problems arising due to poor handwriting. There was a statistically significant association ($p = 0.002$) between the educational degree of the pharmacist and their suggestion to use e-prescription (Table 3). No significant association was found between the years of experience as a pharmacist and the suggestion to use e-prescription. The use of electronic prescribing can be a viable alternative that could reduce the incidence of prescribing errors. Various studies have shown that e-prescription smoothens the dispensing process compared to handwritten prescriptions due to their better completeness, clarity, and legibility [25–27]. However, the implementation of e-prescriptions seems to be a problem in the community pharmacy settings in Saudi Arabia. Although major hospitals and specialist centers in Saudi Arabia practice e-prescribing [28], there is still a need for implementation in public health centers and the private health sector. Along with the challenges pertaining to implementation, e-prescribing is not void of its own share of limitations.

The present study highlights the responses of the community pharmacists and prescription-related problems due to poor handwriting in the Jazan region of Saudi Arabia. The data from this study can be used as baseline data to elicit further research into the barriers to e-prescribing in private physician practice and integration with the community pharmacies. However, our study had its own share of limitations. The results from our study cannot be generalized, as we used a convenience random sampling technique and the data pertain to a single province in Saudi Arabia. It would be of great benefit to conduct a similar nationwide survey as the results would then be generalizable and will aid the healthcare authorities in making impactful decisions. Additionally, only descriptive analysis was performed due to the small sample size. The study could not investigate the pharmacist-dependent factors such as work stress, lack of time, and workload, which may have affected the response of the pharmacist upon receiving an illegible prescription.

5. Conclusions

Our findings concluded the belief and attitudes of the community pharmacists in the Jazan region of Saudi Arabia and their opinions to solve this impending problem of poor prescription writing. Electronic medical records, structured prescription forms, and educational training are some of the reasonable solutions for the current problem; however, this research intends to seek the attention of the health care authorities about the issues faced by community pharmacists due to poor prescription writing. Healthcare authorities should take the initiative to provide training workshops on proper prescription writing, as this would not only benefit physicians and pharmacists but also help safeguard patient safety. Future research can be targeted at recognizing the barriers in implementing e-prescribing as well as the use of printed prescriptions as it can highlight the roadblocks in the path of implementing a safe prescribing and dispensing environment.

Supplementary Materials: The following are available online at https://www.mdpi.com/article/10.3390/healthcare9081077/s1, Community Pharmacists' opinions towards poor prescription writing in Jazan, Saudi Arabia.

Funding: The author declares that no funding was received for conducting the present study.

Institutional Review Board Statement: The study was conducted according to the guidelines of the Declaration of Helsinki, and approved by the Institutional Research Review and Ethics Committee (IRREC) of the Faculty of Pharmacy, Jazan University, KSA (protocol code REC41/1-053).

Informed Consent Statement: Informed consent was obtained from all subjects involved in the study.

Data Availability Statement: Data sharing not applicable.

Acknowledgments: I would like to acknowledge Abdulaziz Shunaymir, Essa Mayan, Mohammed Tohary, and Abdullah Hakami (students of the College of Pharmacy, Jazan University, KSA) for their help in data collection for the study. In addition, I would like to acknowledge Otilia Banji and Mamoon H. Syed (faculty members of the clinical pharmacy department at Jazan University, KSA) for their support, review, and guidance during this work.

Conflicts of Interest: The author declares that there is no conflict of interest regarding the publication of this paper.

References

1. World Health Organization. *The Legal and Regulatory Framework for Community Pharmacies in the WHO European Region*; WHO Regional Office for Europe: Copenhagen, Denmark, 2019.
2. Beney, J.; Bero, L.; Bond, C.M. Expanding the roles of outpatient pharmacists: Effects on health services utilisation, costs, and patient outcomes. *Cochrane Database Syst. Rev.* **2000**, *3*, CD000336. [CrossRef]
3. De Vries, T.P.; Henning, R.H.; Hogerzeil, H.V.; Fresle, D.A. *Guide To Good Prescribing*; WHO: Geneva, Switzerland, 1994.
4. Panchbhai, A. Rationality of Prescription Writing. *Indian J. Pharm. Educ. Res.* **2014**, *47*, 7–15. [CrossRef]
5. Lofholm, P.W.; Katzung, B.G. *Rational Prescribing & Prescription Writing, Basic and Clinical Pharmacology*, 12th ed.; Tata MacGraw-Hill: Mumbai, India, 2012; pp. 1140–1141.
6. Dyasanoor, S.; Urooge, A. Insight into Quality of Prescription Writing—An Institutional Study. *J. Clin. Diagn. Res.* **2016**, *10*, ZC61–ZC64. [CrossRef]
7. Cerio, A.A.P.; Mallare, N.A.L.B.; Tolentino, R.M.S. Assessment of the Legibility of the Handwriting in Medical Prescriptions of Doctors from Public and Private Hospitals in Quezon City, Philippines. *Procedia Manuf.* **2015**, *3*, 90–97. [CrossRef]
8. Assiri, G.A.; Shebl, N.A.; Mahmoud, M.A.; Aloudah, N.; Grant, L.; Aljadhey, H.; Sheikh, A. What is the epidemiology of medication errors, error-related adverse events and risk factors for errors in adults managed in community care contexts? A systematic review of the international literature. *BMJ Open* **2018**, *8*, e019101. [CrossRef] [PubMed]
9. Aitken, M.; Gorokhovich, L. Advancing the Responsible Use of Medicines: Applying Levers for Change. Available online: http://pharmanalyses.fr/wp-content/uploads/2012/10/Advancing-Responsible-Use-of-Meds-Report-01-10-12.pdf (accessed on 18 June 2021).
10. Calligaris, L.; Panzera, A.; Arnoldo, L.; Londero, C.; Quattrin, R.; Troncon, M.G.; Brusaferro, S. Errors and omissions in hospital prescriptions: A survey of prescription writing in a hospital. *BMC Clin. Pharmacol.* **2009**, *9*, 9. [CrossRef]
11. Bobb, A.; Gleason, K.; Husch, M.; Feinglass, J.; Yarnold, P.R.; Noskin, G.A. The epidemiology of prescribing errors: The potential impact of computerized prescriber order entry. *Arch. Intern. Med.* **2004**, *164*, 785–792. [CrossRef]
12. Delgado, S.E.; Soler, V.M.; Pérez, M.C.; Delgado, T.L.; Bermejo, V.T. Prescription errors after the implementation of an electronic prescribing system. *Farm. Hosp.* **2007**, *31*, 223–230.
13. Aljadhey, H.; Mahmoud, M.A.; Mayet, A.; Alshaikh, M.; Ahmed, Y.; Murray, M.D.; Bates, D.W. Incidence of adverse drug events in an academic hospital: A prospective cohort study. *Int. J. Qual. Health Care* **2013**, *25*, 648–655. [CrossRef] [PubMed]
14. Mendonça, J.M.D.; Lyra, D.P.; Rabelo, J.S.; Siqueira, J.S.; Balisa-Rocha, B.J.; Gimenes, F.; Bonjardim, L.R. Analysis and detection of dental prescribing errors at Primary Health Care Units in Brazil. *Pharm. World Sci.* **2010**, *32*, 30–35. [CrossRef] [PubMed]
15. Knudsen, P.; Herborg, H.; Mortensen, A.R.; Knudsen, M.; Hellebek, A. Preventing medication errors in community pharmacy: Root-cause analysis of transcription errors. *Qual. Saf. Health Care* **2007**, *16*, 285–290. [CrossRef] [PubMed]
16. Hartel, M.J.; Staub, L.P.; Röder, C.; Eggli, S. High incidence of medication documentation errors in a Swiss university hospital due to the handwritten prescription process. *BMC Health Serv. Res.* **2011**, *11*, 199. [CrossRef] [PubMed]
17. Brits, H.; Botha, A.; Niksch, L.; Terblanché, R.; Venter, K.; Joubert, G. Illegible handwriting and other prescription errors on prescriptions at National District Hospital, Bloemfontein. *S. Afr. Fam. Pr.* **2017**, *59*, 52–55. [CrossRef]
18. Albarrak, A.I.; Al Rashidi, E.A.; Fatani, R.K.; Al Ageel, S.I.; Mohammed, R. Assessment of legibility and completeness of handwritten and electronic prescriptions. *Saudi Pharm. J.* **2014**, *22*, 522–527. [CrossRef]
19. Winslow, E.H.; Nestor, V.A.; Davidoff, S.K.; Thompson, P.G.; Borum, J.C. Legibility and completeness of physicians' handwritten medication orders. *Heart Lung* **1997**, *26*, 158–164. [CrossRef]
20. Irshaid, Y.M.; Al Homrany, M.; A Hamdi, A.; Adjepon-Yamoah, K.K.; A Mahfouz, A. Compliance with good practice in prescription writing at outpatient clinics in Saudi Arabia. *East. Mediterr. Health J.* **2006**, *11*, 922–928.
21. General Authority for Statistics. Demography Survey. Available online: https://www.stats.gov.sa/sites/default/files/en-demographic-research-2016_2.pdf (accessed on 18 June 2021).

22. Velo, G.P.; Minuz, P. Medication errors: Prescribing faults and prescription errors. *Br. J. Clin. Pharmacol.* **2009**, *67*, 624–628. [CrossRef]
23. Fadare, J.O.; Agboola, S.M.; Alabi, R.A. Quality of prescriptions in a tertiary care hospital in south west Nigeria. *J. Appl. Pharm. Sci.* **2013**, *3*, 81–84.
24. Rambhade, S.; Shrivastava, A.; Rambhade, A.; Chakarborty, A.; Patil, U. A survey on polypharmacy and use of inappropriate medications. *Toxicol. Int.* **2012**, *19*, 68–73. [CrossRef]
25. Motulsky, A.; Winslade, N.; Tamblyn, R.; Sicotte, C. The impact of electronic prescribing on the professionalization of community pharmacists: A qualitative study of pharmacists' perception. *J. Pharm. Pharm. Sci.* **2008**, *11*, 131–146. [CrossRef]
26. Garfield, S.; Hibberd, R.; Barber, N. English community pharmacists' experiences of using electronic transmission of prescriptions: A qualitative study. *BMC Health Serv. Res.* **2013**, *13*, 435. [CrossRef] [PubMed]
27. Odukoya, O.; A Chui, M. Retail pharmacy staff perceptions of design strengths and weaknesses of electronic prescribing. *J. Am. Med. Inform. Assoc.* **2012**, *19*, 1059–1065. [CrossRef] [PubMed]
28. Qureshi, N.; Al-Bedah, A.M.; Koenig, H.G. Handwritten to Electronic Prescriptions: Emerging Views and Practices, Saudi Arabia. *Br. J. Med. Med. Res.* **2014**, *4*, 4607–4626. [CrossRef]

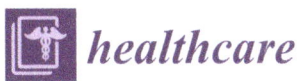

Article

Pharmacy Student Perceptions of a Virtual Pharmacogenomics Activity

Darrow Thomas [1], John A. Soldner [2], Cheryl D. Cropp [3] and Jennifer Beall [4,*]

[1] Central Alabama Veterans Health Care System, 215 Perry Hill Rd, Montgomery, AL 36109, USA; Dgerrell@ymail.com
[2] Department of Genetics, The University of Alabama at Birmingham, 720 20th Street South, Birmingham, AL 35294, USA; jsoldner@uab.edu
[3] Department of Pharmaceutical, Social, and Administrative Sciences; Samford University McWhorter School of Pharmacy, 800 Lakeshore Drive, Birmingham, AL 35229, USA; ccropp@samford.edu
[4] Department of Pharmacy Practice; Samford University McWhorter School of Pharmacy, 800 Lakeshore Drive, Birmingham, AL 35229, USA
* Correspondence: jwbeall@samford.edu; Tel.: +1-205-726-2534

Abstract: Pharmacogenomics (PGx) utilizes a patient's genome to guide drug treatment and dosing. The Accreditation Council for Pharmacy Education (ACPE) included PGx as a critical content area. Pharmacists are increasingly involved in providing this service, which necessitates training. Second-year pharmacy students at Samford University McWhorter School of Pharmacy have didactic training in the principles of PGx and managing drug therapy using PGx data. A clinical skills lab activity was developed to reinforce these principles and allow students to navigate resources to develop and communicate recommendations for drug therapy. The activity was initially planned as synchronous, but transitioned to asynchronous when students began remote learning in the spring of 2020 due to the COVID-19 pandemic. The investigators sought students' perceptions of the PGx lab activity and the delivery of its content via a virtual format. This study gathered data from an anonymous, voluntary student survey through Samford University's course management system, Canvas, in the spring of 2020 soon after completion of the virtual PGx learning activity. The investigators' goal is to obtain the information and insights obtained from the students who participated in the PGx lab activity to provide guidance for the improvement of their PGx lab activity and for other schools of pharmacy to deliver a PGx lab activities using nontraditional teaching methodologies.

Keywords: pharmacogenomics; learning activity; pharmacy education; asynchronous learning; virtual learning; student survey

1. Introduction

Pharmacogenomics (PGx) studies the relationship between a patient's genetic variations and how those variations impact the response to medication [1]. This field has developed rapidly since the completion of the Human Genome Project in 2003 [2]. President Barack Obama launched the Precision Medicine Initiative in 2016 to advance medicine from a population-focused approach to a patient-focused one [3].

Patients can now receive a report on their pharmacogenetic variants through direct-to-consumer products, such as 23andMe® [4]. Resources, such as PGx information in drug labeling, are available for those pharmacists who use PGx to manage medication therapy [5]. Online resources are also available including the Clinical Pharmacogenetics Implementation Consortium (CPIC®) and The Pharmacogenomics Knowledgebase (PharmGKB) [1,6–8].

While there is support for the field and resources available, its implementation into curricula and practice has not been as swift. The 2007–2008 Argus Commission released updated policy statements on biotechnology, which included personalized medicine [9]. The statements were that pharmacy curricula must address advances in these fields, to include genetics/genomics, and that faculty development is needed to prepare them to lead and contribute to this field. In 2015, the American Society of Health-System Pharmacists published a position statement on the role of pharmacists in PGx [10]. This statement originated from the belief that PGx testing can improve outcomes related to medications and delineate pharmacists' responsibilities and functions in this field. Additionally, the Accreditation Council for Pharmacy Education (ACPE) included PGx as one of the content areas "viewed as central to a contemporary, high-quality pharmacy education" [11].

PGx and its applications are viewed as important and beneficial to patients, yet confidence in its application remains lacking. In a survey of health sciences and other university students, Siamoglou and colleagues found that the students held positive attitudes towards PGx and its benefits on disease management, drug efficacy, and reduction of adverse effects [12]. Zawiah and colleagues found strong support from pharmacy and medical students of PGx testing to help to decrease adverse events, optimize drug dosing and improve drug efficacy [13]. The majority of these students did not agree that they were competent to discuss PGx information with other providers, or that they could accurately apply PGx test results. The authors concluded that there is a need to improve knowledge and better prepare pharmacy and medical students to apply PGx in practice.

Samford University McWhorter School of Pharmacy is a private school in the Southeastern United States. A PGx activity was developed as part of a required skills lab course. This lab course is the third in a six-course sequence that allows for the teaching, practice, and assessment of various skills. The activity was intended to be delivered in-person for its second iteration in the spring of 2020; however, it transitioned to an asynchronous virtual activity with the transition to remote learning due to the COVID-19 pandemic.

The purpose of this study is to determine students' perceptions of a PGx lab activity and its delivery through a virtual format.

2. Materials and Methods

The principles of PGx and management of drug therapy using PGx data are taught in the didactic curriculum during the fall semester of the second year. A clinical skills lab activity was developed for the following semester in the spring of the second year to reinforce these principles and allow students to navigate PGx information resources to develop and communicate recommendations for drug therapy. Upon completion of the PGx virtual learning activity, each student was expected to (1) learn to navigate pharmacogenomics-related databases; (2) demonstrate an awareness of the use and impact of pharmacogenomics within pharmacy and the health care system; and (3) effectively communicate pharmacogenomics-related pharmacotherapy and drug information recommendations using relevant pharmacogenomics-related databases.

The introduction to the PGx lab activity was conceptualized as a three-part activity (visualized in Figure 1). Part I was designed to give the students a 60 min, self-guided introduction to navigate through the most widely used databases for PGx information and guidelines, specifically, CPIC (https://cpicpgx.org/; accessed on 31 January 2022) and PharmGKB (https://www.pharmgkb.org/; accessed on 31 January 2022). Students were also exposed to several other PGx databases, specifically ClinVar (https://www.ncbi.nlm.nih.gov/clinvar/; accessed on 31 January 2022), Online Mendelian Inheritance in Man (OMIM; https://www.omim.org/; accessed 31 January 2022, PharmacoDB (https://pharmacodb.pmgenomics.ca/; accessed on 31 January 2022), and other genomic and precision medicine websites, including "All of Us" (https://allofus.nih.gov; accessed on 31 January 2022) and the "Alabama Genomic Health Initiative" (https://hudsonalpha.org/the-aghi/; accessed on 31 January 2022), through a short series of practice exercises. Students gained experience in navigation and search functions unique to each database by completing exercises that required them to search for a specific gene and/or other pre-determined phenotype and report their findings.

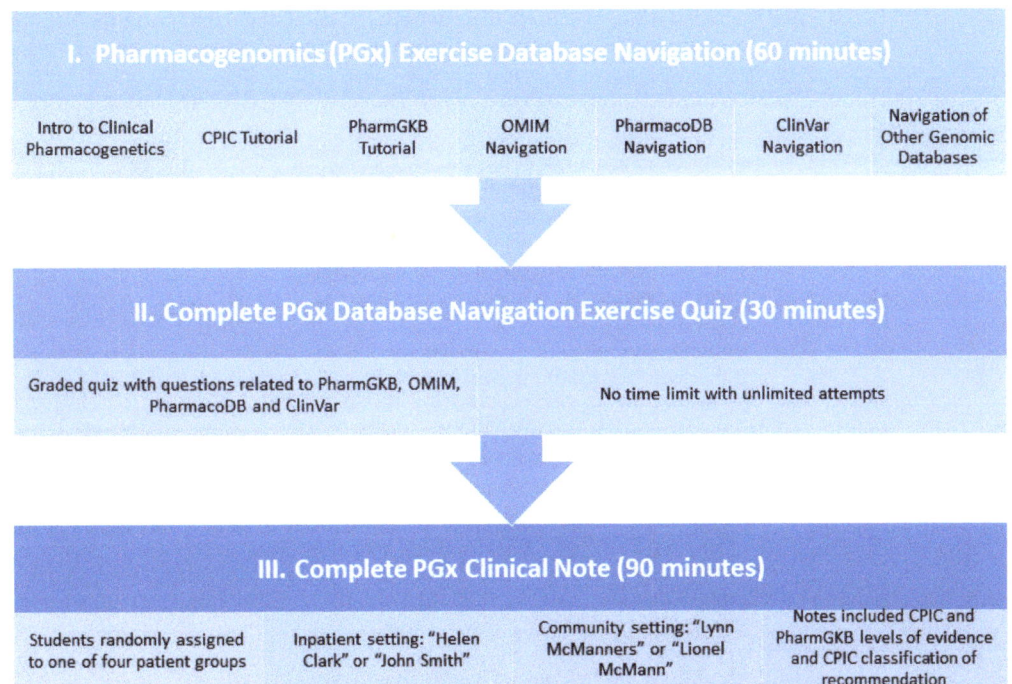

Figure 1. Flowchart and timing of virtual PGx learning activity.

For Part II of the assignment, students took a graded quiz (constructed to take 30 min to complete) with an unlimited time and number of attempts to assess their familiarity with the websites introduced in Part I. Part III of the virtual PGx learning activity consisted of patient cases that challenged the students to utilize the PGx databases. The students evaluated a patient scenario identifying potential gene–drug interactions based on the patient's genomic profile and evidence-based recommendations. Patient scenarios included two potentially actionable gene-drug interactions, a primary and a secondary, and several other non-genetic medication therapy errors commensurate with their level of didactic training. Part III patient cases were divided into inpatient and community settings to allow for communication adaptability to the target audience. The inpatient scenario allowed for pharmacist-to-physician exchange, while the outpatient scenario included a pharmacist-to-patient appropriate conversation. Four patient cases were constructed for each setting and given different patient names (inpatient: "Helen Clark" or "John Smith"; community: "Lynn McManners" or "Lionel McMann"). Each case included a primary drug with a potential actionable gene–drug paring and a secondary gene–drug interaction. The primary drug was defined as the drug that the predominance of the scenario was built around. The secondary drug was uniform across all four patient cases, but the genomic profile (i.e., patient genotypes) relative to that drug differed within each case. The students were given a history of present illness, past medical history, medication summary, and follow-up for each case. The patient's PGx "genotype profile" and medication-related questions were included in the follow-up section. Specifically, students were tasked to provide written recommendations that included the patient's PGx background information, potential gene–drug interactions and recommendations for their resolution, and any other recommendations for drug-related problems. The students had to provide support for their recommendations and to include the CPIC and level, PharmGKB levels of evidence, and the CPIC classification of recommendation. An anonymous, voluntary survey was sent to all students to capture their perceptions soon after completing the PGx virtual learning activity. This survey was sent through Samford University's course management system, Canvas, and was available for ten days. The students were not provided with an incentive to participate in the survey. The survey asked for free-text responses to the following questions:

1. What did you learn from this pharmacogenomics (PGx) assignment?
2. What were your strengths during this learning activity?
3. What were your areas for improvement during this learning activity?
4. What did you like best about this PGx assignment?
5. What did you like least about this PGx assignment?
6. What recommendation(s) do you have for changing this PGx assignment?
7. What did you learn about the clinical application of pharmacogenomics from this learning activity?
8. If this learning activity is taught in the future, do you think it should be taught live (in person), synchronously (online instruction in real time), asynchronously (online instruction not in real time) or hybrid (blend of live and asynchronous)?
9. Please provide any additional comments about this assignment and/or suggestions for improving pharmacogenomics instruction at the McWhorter School of Pharmacy.

Survey responses were collected, and themes were identified among the responses.

3. Results

3.1. Survey Response

A total of 31 out of 113 students participated in the survey, giving a response rate of 27%. The study was conducted in accordance with the Declaration of Helsinki. The University's Institutional Review Board approved this study as exempt since student responses were collected anonymously with no identifying information. The investigators gathered the student survey results and identified themes among the responses using content analysis for the purposes of improving teaching and learning in the virtual environment and as a guidance for other schools of pharmacy in the delivery of PGx lab activities using nontraditional teaching methodologies.

3.2. Themes and Supporting Quotes

Table 1 presents the major themes identified from each survey question, along with student comments that support these themes.

Table 1. Survey question themes and supporting quotes.

Survey Question	Theme(s)	Student Comments
1. What did you learn from this PGx assignment?	Databases and information	"I learned how to use databases to access pharmacogenomic drug interactions." "I learned what pharmacogenomics databases were available and how to use them." "I learned to be able to proficiently navigate the PGx databases, and how to read and interpret the CPIC guidelines." "How to use various PGx resources and how to access information on various drug–gene interactions."
2. What were your strengths during this learning activity?	Navigate websites	"My strength was conducting the search for the genes and drug interactions. It was easy for me to navigate the websites needed to complete the assignment." "I feel that my strengths in this activity were being able to navigate and find the other guidelines that were needed to make recommendations and be able to critically think about what drug(s) could be optimized for the patient." "Finding research on the CPIC website to figure out if patient needs to take different medication based on their genotyping."

Table 1. *Cont.*

Survey Question	Theme(s)	Student Comments
3. What were your areas for improvement during this learning activity?	Long, time, note, video, websites	"The note was a little confusing and I was unsure of exactly what to do." "I could improve upon my knowledge of PGx. Most of the information was unfamiliar to me." "Need to familiarize with websites more." "I feel as though the lab could have been explained more. It was also really long considering this time of online learning." "It took me twice as long as lab normally lasts to complete this activity."
4. What did you like best about this PGx assignment?	Patient, guidelines, recommendations, databases	"Learning about CYP metabolism and applying new information to a patient case." "Learning that there is evidence behind why some drugs work for some people but not all even though the disease state may be the same." "I enjoyed learning about all the databases I can utilize when treating a patient." "I liked the case scenario. It is definitely a situation that we would encounter as practicing pharmacists and this practice would help develop the skills to properly respond when it does occur." "I enjoyed the puzzle aspect of the assignment. I liked following the clues of the genetic testing results to guidelines to making recommendations that could benefit the patient in multiple ways."
5. What did you like least about this PGx assignment?	Quiz, time, answers, instructions	"It was extremely long and I was confused by the directions." "Having minimal guidance throughout the lab and having to figure out/troubleshoot problems on my own. This was very discouraging because the lab took me twice as long due to this." "I felt very unprepared and confused about the instructions, it was very lengthy." "I thought the length due to the number of medications he/she was taking and genes that were looked at." "This took an extended amount of time. I would suggest that next year this be given in January or February when there is a lull in lab activities. We have so much going on right now, and even if we were not living and learning under quarantine, we would still be stressed with the last exams of our two major classes around this time and finals looming. It's great learning experience. I just wish it had been when I was not so busy and stressed. Additionally, the Canvas quiz was not really necessary in my opinion. We have enough background knowledge on CYP enzymes and polymorphisms by spring of P2 year to just do the assignment without it."
6. What recommendation(s) do you have for changing this PGx assignment?	Instructions, time, note, lab	"Instructions on navigating the website should be clearer to cut back on time performing web searches." "A review of terminology before the lab. In class assignment and in groups." "If there is a way to incorporate this assignment with EHR Go I think it would improve the delivery of this assignment." "It was difficult as an online module. I believe many issues would be resolved by in person instruction like the lab was initially planned." "I would try to make the assignment just a bit shorter. And perhaps make the instructions a little more clear like if we needed to include recommendations on therapy that was not one of the results of the genome analysis."
7. What did you learn about the clinical application of PGx from this learning activity?	Important, certain, medications, different genes, patients	"It helped me integrate pharmacogenomics into an MTM like scenario." "I learned that it is important for some medications to do genetic testing before prescribing a medication because it may not work at all in the patient, or it may need a dose adjustment due to certain mutations in genes." "I learned that individualized medicine is a necessary development and understanding that patients may vary in their metabolizing capability is important in tailoring their pharmacotherapy." "I learned about different resources that can be used to help modify treatment for patients based on their specific genes."

Table 1. Cont.

Survey Question	Theme(s)	Student Comments
8. Please provide any additional comments about this assignment and/or suggestions for improving PGx instruction at the McWhorter School of Pharmacy.	Time, example, semester	"I would have enjoyed an example note." "If you could have the guest speaker there during lab that is a clinical pharmacist working in pharmacogenomics to help navigate the different websites, that would be a great experience." "I would like to see more pharmacogenomics explicitly included in the curriculum."

3.3. Student Preference for Delivery Format

Figure 2 presents student responses to survey Question #8, which asked "If this learning activity is taught in the future, do you think it should be taught live (in person), synchronously (online instruction in real time), asynchronously (online instruction not in real time) or hybrid (blend of live and asynchronous)?".

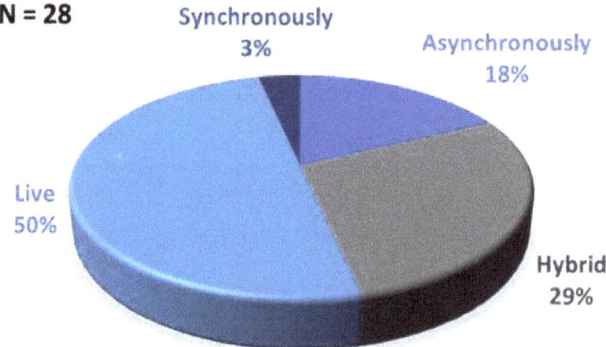

Figure 2. Responses to how should this learning activity be taught in the future (Question #8).

4. Discussion

Student responses revealed that there were things learned from this PGx activity, and suggested areas for improvement related to logistics. In general, students responded that they learned about the PGx databases and guidelines related to drug–gene interactions, and how PGx can be used in practice. Students also mentioned logistical challenges related to the time it took to complete the learning activity and a desire for clearer instructions and/or examples.

This virtual PGx learning activity took place in the spring of 2020, four weeks after the students began virtual learning during the COVID-19 pandemic. During this time, communication was erratic, and testing procedures were in flux. It is possible that the students would have experienced a smoother experience if, at the time, the faculty were more familiar with virtual learning and had developed communication techniques that translate well for virtual learners. Overall, this PGx learning activity represents a novel example of how to create an asynchronous, simulated PGx activity in a virtual learning environment.

There have been other studies that gauged student perceptions of a PGx activity, and of a PGx course. Patel and colleagues investigated students' knowledge and perceptions of applying pharmacogenetics in a patient encounter using simulation [14]. Perception questions included confidence in their own as well as their team's abilities to perform clinical activities using pharmacogenetic results. The results of the perception question related to their individual confidence improved in the post-simulation survey. Powers and colleagues investigated changes in knowledge, confidence, and skills of third-year pharmacy students in clinical pharmacogenetics following a laboratory session [15]. A confidence survey was administered to the students prior to and after the lecture upon which the session was based, and then again at the end of the semester. The post-lecture and post-lab results demonstrated statistically significant increases in confidence, and there were also significant increases in the post-lecture to post-lab results. Assem et al. surveyed pharmacy students before and after an intervention, whereby the students were given the opportunity to receive their PGx test results [16]. They reported increased confidence on each of the items related to conducting PGx counselling, and increased usefulness on each of the items relate to PGx testing.

Remsberg and colleagues investigated student perceptions of a pharmacogenomics course [17]. The pre-/post-course surveys asked students to rate confidence in their abilities to educate and manage patients using pharmacogenomics. The results of the post-course survey suggested that the course improved their confidence in their ability to educate and manage patients using pharmacogenomics. Marcinak and colleagues investigated the effectiveness of a required pharmacogenomics course, including perceived comfort and ability to apply the content in a clinical setting [18]. There were statistically significant increases in the items gauging perceived comfort and ability from the pre- to post-course surveys.

Coriolan and colleagues investigated perceptions and attitudes toward pharmacogenomics in pharmacy students from eight schools who were nearing graduation [19]. In contrast to other studies presented, this one did not investigate a specific learning experience, but rather perceptions from their overall training in pharmacogenomics. Given that there were multiple schools involved, the amount of pharmacogenomic content in their curricula varied from none to a required course. Responses related to clinical relevance were generally in agreement that pharmacogenomics is integral to the profession of pharmacy as well as to the practice of pharmacists.

These studies primarily investigated the students' confidence in their abilities in pharmacogenomics. Comparing these to the current study, we did not specifically address confidence, and this was not one of the themes identified in student responses. Students did report, however, learning how to use resources needed to evaluate pharmacogenomic information and manage interactions. The students also reported learning the importance of pharmacogenomics in patient care.

Along with determining students' perceptions of the lab activity, this current study also sought to determine students' perceptions of the virtual format specifically. As schools move into a time where a variety of delivery methods are an option, it was important to gage the students' preferences for delivery formats as there are times when each option is feasible. The majority of students in this study chose live delivery as opposed to hybrid, asynchronous, or synchronous. Themes emerged from the question of what students liked least about the assignment that indicated frustration with instructions and the time it took to complete the lab. This information can be useful for determining which types of content or processes are more conducive to certain delivery formats, as well as ways to improve an activity that would be delivered virtually.

The strengths of the current study are that qualitative methods allow respondents to give context to their responses as compared to quantitative results. Additionally, questions gathered various aspects of students' preferences as well as what they learned. Lastly, information regarding format for teaching the activity in the future can be useful. The limitations include a lower response rate, and the overall timing of the activity. In the spring of 2020, the investigators were novices at developing and implementing virtual activities so there are elements of the frustrations expressed by respondents that may no longer be applicable as we have gained experience in this.

Future iterations of this activity could include modifications to instructions and timing of the activity to allow it to be more conducive to a virtual format. This would help to determine whether the virtual format was based on logistics or whether the activity is truly best delivered in person.

Author Contributions: Conceptualization, D.T.; methodology, D.T., C.D.C., J.A.S., and J.B.; formal analysis, C.D.C.; investigation, C.D.C.; resources, D.T., C.D.C., J.A.S., and J.B.; data curation, C.D.C.; writing—original draft preparation, D.T., C.D.C., J.A.S., and J.B.; writing—review and editing, D.T., C.D.C., J.A.S., and J.B.; visualization, C.D.C. and J.B.; supervision, D.T., C.D.C., J.A.S., and J.B.; project administration, C.D.C. and J.B. All authors have read and agreed to the published version of the manuscript.

Funding: This research received no external funding.

Institutional Review Board Statement: The study was conducted according to the guidelines of the Declaration of Helsinki and approved by the Institutional Review Board of Samford University (EXMT-P-20-F; approved 13 October 2020).

Informed Consent Statement: Informed consent was waived due to the anonymity of the survey responses.

Conflicts of Interest: The authors declare no conflict of interest.

References

1. PharmGKB. What Is Pharmacogenomics? Available online: https://www.pharmgkb.org/ (accessed on 13 December 2021).
2. The Human Genome Project. National Human Genome Research Institute. Updated 22 December 2020. Available online: https://www.genome.gov/human-genome-project (accessed on 13 December 2021).
3. FACT SHEET: President Obama's Precision Medicine Initiative. The White House President Barack Obama. Published 30 January 2015. Available online: https://obamawhitehouse.archives.gov/the-press-office/2015/01/30/fact-sheet-president-obama-s-precision-medicine-initiative (accessed on 13 December 2021).
4. 23andMe. 23andMe Pharmacogenetics Reports: What You Should Know. Available online: https://www.23andme.com/test-info/pharmacogenetics/ (accessed on 13 December 2021).
5. U.S. Food & Drug Administration. Table of Pharmacogenomic Biomarkers in Drug Labeling. Updated 20 August 2021. Available online: https://www.fda.gov/drugs/science-and-research-drugs/table-pharmacogenomic-biomarkers-drug-labeling (accessed on 13 December 2021).
6. Whirl-Carrillo1, M.; Huddart1, R.; Gong, L.; Sangkuhl, K.; Thorn, C.F.; Whaley, R.; Klein, T.E. An evidence-based framework for evaluating pharmacogenomics knowledge for personalized medicine. *Clin. Pharmacol. Ther.* **2021**. online ahead of print. [CrossRef] [PubMed]
7. Clinical Pharmacogenetics Implementation Consortium. Stanford University and St. Jude Children's Research Hospital. Website. 21 April 2020. Available online: https://cpicpgx.org (accessed on 13 December 2021).
8. Relling, M.V.; Klein, T.E. CPIC: Clinical Pharmacogenetics Implementation Consortium of the Pharmacogenomics Research Network. *Clin. Pharmacol. Ther.* **2011**, *89*, 464–467. [CrossRef] [PubMed]
9. Wells, B.G.; Beck, D.E.; Draugalis, J.R.; Kerr, R.A.B.; Maine, L.L.; Plaza, C.M.; Speedie, M.K. Report of the 2007–2008 Argus Commission: What Future Awaits Beyond Pharmaceutical Care? *Am. J. Pharm. Educ.* **2008**, *72*, S8. [CrossRef]
10. American Society of Health-System Pharmacists. ASHP statement on the pharmacist's role in clinical pharmacogenomics. *Am. J. Health-Syst. Pharm.* **2015**, *72*, 579–581. [CrossRef] [PubMed]
11. Accreditation Council for Pharmacy Education. Accreditation Standards and Key Elements for the Professional Degree Program in Pharmacy Leading to the Doctor of Pharmacy Degree ("Standards 2016"). Published 2 February 2015. Available online: https://www.acpe-accredit.org/pdf/Standards2016FINAL.pdf (accessed on 13 December 2021).
12. Siamoglou, S.; Koromina, M.; Politopoulou, K.; Samiou, C.G.; Papadopoulou, G.; Balasopoulou, A.; Kanavos, A.; Mitropoulou, C.; Patrinos, G.P.; Vasileiou, K. Attitudes and awareness toward pharmacogenomics and personalized medicine adoption among health sciences trainees: Experiences from Greece lessons for Europe. *OMICS* **2021**, *25*, 190–199. [CrossRef] [PubMed]
13. Zawiah, M.; Yousef, A.M.; Al-Ashwal, F.Y.; Abduljabbar, R.; Al-Jamei, S.; Hayat Khan, A.; Alkhawaldeh, B. Pharmacogenetics: A perspective and preparedness of Pharm-D and medical students in Jordan. *Pharmacogenet. Genom.* **2021**, *31*, 125–132. [CrossRef] [PubMed]
14. Patel, R.V.; Chudow, M.; Vo, T.T.; Serag-Bolos, E.S. Evaluation of pharmacy students' knowledge and perceptions of pharmacogenetics before and after a simulation activity. *Curr. Pharm. Teach. Learn.* **2018**, *10*, 96–101. [CrossRef] [PubMed]
15. Powers, K.E.; Buffington, T.M.; Contaifer, D., Jr.; Wijesinghe, D.S.; Donohoe, K.L. Implementation of an active-learning laboratory on pharmacogenetics. *Am. J. Pharm. Educ.* **2019**, *83*, 6605. [CrossRef] [PubMed]
16. Assem, M.; Broeckel, U.; MacKinnon, G.E. Personal DNA testing increases pharmacy students' confidence and competence in pharmacogenomics. *Am. J. Pharm. Educ.* **2021**, *85*, 8249. [CrossRef] [PubMed]
17. Remsberg, C.M.; Bray, B.S.; Wright, S.K.; Ashmore, J.; Kabasenche, W.; Wang, S.; Lazarus, P.; Daoud, S.S. Design, implementation, and assessment approaches within a pharmacogenomics course. *Am. J. Pharm. Educ.* **2017**, *81*, 11. [CrossRef] [PubMed]

18. Marcinak, R.; Paris, M.; Kinney, S.R.M. Pharmacogenomics education improves pharmacy student perceptions of their abilities and roles in its use. *Am. J. Pharm. Educ.* **2018**, *82*, 6424. [CrossRef]
19. Coriolan, S.; Arikawe, N.; Moscati, A.; Zhou, L.; Dym, S.; Donmez, S.; Garba, A.; Falbaum, S.; Loewy, Z.; Lull, M.; et al. Pharmacy students' attitudes and perceptions towards pharmacogenomics education. *Am. J. Health Syst. Pharm.* **2019**, *76*, 836–846. [CrossRef] [PubMed]

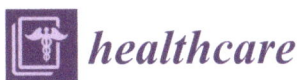

Article

Pharmacy Students' Attitudes and Perceptions toward Financial Management Education

Georges Adunlin [1,*] and Kevin Pan [2]

[1] Department of Pharmaceutical, Social and Administrative Sciences, McWhorter School of Pharmacy, Samford University, 800 Lakeshore Drive, Birmingham, AL 35229, USA

[2] Department of Economics, Finance and Quantitative Analysis, Brock School of Business, Samford University, 800 Lakeshore Drive, Birmingham, AL 35229, USA; kpan@samford.edu

* Correspondence: gadunlin@samford.edu

Abstract: (1) Background: Pharmacy-related financial management training and education are an integral part of the pharmacy curriculum. This study aims to evaluate pharmacy students' perceptions toward financial management education, their attitudes on its clinical relevance, and their ability to use financial management knowledge in introductory and advanced pharmacy practice experiences. (2) Methods: An online survey was sent to third- and fourth-year pharmacy students. The survey assessed the following three themes: perceptions toward financial management education; attitudes toward the clinical relevance of financial management education; and the student's ability to use knowledge of financial management in practice. Descriptive statistics were used to summarize the data. (3) Results: The overall response rate for the survey was 60% (139/233). Overall, the study showed a positive perception and attitude toward financial management education. Results indicate that pharmacy students were confident in their ability to use financial management knowledge in pharmacy practice. (4) Conclusions: This survey found an overall optimism in financial management education's role in pharmacy practice and the ability to obtain financial management competencies in professional pharmacy training. With the evolving practice requirements, pharmacy schools should adapt their financial management curricula with relevant skills to prepare students to become effective entrepreneurs, innovators, and practice leaders.

Keywords: financial management; pharmacy management; business; entrepreneurship; pharmacy students; perception; attitudes; ability

Citation: Adunlin, G.; Pan, K. Pharmacy Students' Attitudes and Perceptions toward Financial Management Education. *Healthcare* **2022**, *10*, 683. https://doi.org/10.3390/healthcare10040683

Academic Editor: Tracy Comans

Received: 31 December 2021
Accepted: 28 March 2022
Published: 5 April 2022

Publisher's Note: MDPI stays neutral with regard to jurisdictional claims in published maps and institutional affiliations.

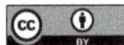

Copyright: © 2022 by the authors. Licensee MDPI, Basel, Switzerland. This article is an open access article distributed under the terms and conditions of the Creative Commons Attribution (CC BY) license (https://creativecommons.org/licenses/by/4.0/).

1. Introduction

Financial management plays an important role in every business enterprise ranging from manufacturing, logistics, to healthcare [1]. Without funding and proper planning, organizing, directing, and controlling of its financial activities, a healthcare organization would not be profitable, grow, or likely survive [1]. In today's rapidly changing healthcare environment, financial management plays a critical role in helping providers and institutions to identify new sources of revenue, find innovative ways to reduce spending and manage long-term investments. Other key aspects of financial management in healthcare include managing contracts to prevent costly mistakes and ensuring regulatory compliance, establishing sound risk-management strategies related to patient safety, and securing sufficient day-to-day financing [1].

In recent decades, the role of pharmacists in the United States has evolved along with the healthcare needs of the population [2–4]. The role of pharmacists has extended beyond medication distribution to screenings and consultations [5,6]. In addition to dispensing medications and ensuring patient safety, today's pharmacists must deliver a range of progressive profit-driven services [7,8], leading them to take on a more significant managerial and entrepreneurial role [9]. The pharmacist is also being given more responsibility in patient care, such as in vaccination services [10,11]. With the release of the Center for Advancement of Pharmacy Education (CAPE) Educational Outcomes 2013 [12], and the National Association of Boards of Pharmacy Curriculum Outcomes Assessment (PCOA) content areas and sub-areas [13], the essentials for practice and care and pharmacy practice management have received a new emphasis in pharmacy education. The CAPE subdomain 2.2 addresses financial management and emphasizes medication-use systems management, (Manager)-Manage patient healthcare needs using human, financial, technological, and physical resources to optimize the safety and efficacy of medication use systems [14]. Within the PCOA Social/Behavioral/Administrative Sciences content areas for the 2016–2017 administration, the specific topics related to financial management include economic and humanistic outcomes of healthcare delivery (Section 3.3) and pharmacy practice management (Section 3.4). The Accreditation Council for Pharmacy Education (ACPE) standard broadly addresses aspects of financial management under practice management and underlines the application of sound management principles (including operations, information, resource, fiscal, and personnel) and quality metrics to advance patient care and service delivery within and between various practice settings.

With the rapid change in the healthcare landscape, opportunities for expanding and implementing new services and programs, and the high costs of pharmaceuticals, it is crucial to prepare pharmacy students with literacy in business, management, and finance-related topics relevant to their practices [15,16]. In the context of pharmacy, financial management is commonly associated with independent pharmacy ownership. However, financial management and its associated skills are important in developing clinical pharmacy services in a wide range of practice settings. It could be argued that financial-management competency should be one of the most fundamental of all skills for pharmacists, since all problems faced by pharmacy organizations and their solutions relate to questions related to how to manage financial resources [17–19]. However, the topic occupies an uncertain place within pharmacy programs. It does not enjoy the same breadth of course offerings.

In some schools or colleges of pharmacy, the number of credit hours spent on financial management-related topics is unclear because financial management education is not taught as a separate course. Instead, financial management is incorporated into other courses. There is also a divergence in the content of financial management education, the primary cause of which is perhaps that "financial management" has no singular definition, especially within pharmacy programs [20]. There is a need to confirm whether financial management education and training that pharmacy students are receiving generates a good perception, nurtures positive attitudes, and delivers satisfactory competencies in core areas of financial management. Therefore, this study sought to evaluate third- and fourth-year pharmacy students' perceptions toward financial management education, their attitudes on its clinical relevance, and their ability to use financial management knowledge in their introductory and advanced pharmacy practice experiences. Perception is the awareness of something which is related to previous knowledge [21]. Perception becomes more skillful with practice and experience, and individual's perception influences opinion, judgment, and understanding of a situation. Attitude is a learned tendency or readiness to evaluate things or react to some ideas or situations in certain ways, either consciously or unconsciously [22]. In typical educational practice, the terms 'abilities' and 'aptitudes' are used interchangeably to denote an individual's potential for acquiring and applying new knowledge or skills [22].

2. Materials and Methods

2.1. Course Description

Financial Management is a required 3-credit-hour semester course in the pharmacy curriculum at Samford University McWhorter School of Pharmacy. It is taught in the Fall semester of the second academic year of didactic coursework. The course is scheduled for weekly 3 h classroom sessions over a 15-week semester calendar. The class meets each week for 2 h on Tuesdays and 1 h on Thursdays. The course catalog description is "Financial

Management addresses concepts related to the fiscal management of pharmacy services at the system, pharmacy, and patient-level in various practice settings. Emphasizes decision-making related to the evaluation, procurement, and utilization of financial resources to maximize the value of the organization and to optimize patient care." The course is organized into three main sections, including an overview of financial management, managing money in pharmacy, and managing pharmacy products and services. The topics covered are listed in Table 1. In the course, all modules are built within the following framework:

- Description and learning objectives;
- PowerPoint lecture;
- Reading and/or listening assignments;
- Reading comprehension questions and/or activities;
- Class discussion questions;
- Additional resources.

Table 1. Course Sections and Topics.

Course Section	Topics
Course Section 1: Overview of Financial Management	<ul><li>Management and Management Functions</li><li>Innovation and Entrepreneurship</li><li>Strategic Planning to Achieve Results</li><li>Justifying, Planning, Developing, and Evaluating Clinical Pharmacy Services</li><li>Risk Management in Contemporary Pharmacy Practice</li><li>Pharmacy Business & Staff Planning</li><li>Legal Aspects of Starting and Managing a Pharmacy Business</li><li>Writing a Pharmacy Business Plan</li></ul>
Course Section 2: Managing Money in Pharmacy	<ul><li>Principles of Accounting</li><li>Financial Statement Analysis and Ratio Analysis</li><li>Budgeting</li><li>Break-even Analysis</li></ul>
Course Section 3: Managing Pharmacy Products and Services	<ul><li>Purchasing and Inventory Management</li><li>Pricing Pharmacy Products and Services</li><li>Pharmacy Merchandising</li><li>Pharmacy Customer Service</li><li>Marketing Strategies, Advertising, and Promotion</li><li>Value-Added Services</li></ul>

In addition to didactic lectures, and guest speakers' presentations, pharmacy students work individually to develop a pharmacy business plan that details a business idea—in this case, a new or expanded pharmacy service or product. This project represents the synthesis, and demonstrates the application, of the knowledge acquired during the course. The students are also presented with case studies and simulation exercises in which they are required to devise strategies and make decisions to ensure the success of a pharmacy organization. Two textbooks are required in this course [23,24]. Journal articles and other readings are assigned for some specific lectures. These practical resources focus on applying knowledge to develop an in-depth understanding of financial management ideas, issues, and concepts.

2.2. Study Design, Population, and Samples

A cross-sectional survey was administered to the previous two cohorts enrolled in the course, consisting of third- and fourth-year students. These two cohorts were surveyed with the hypothesis that fourth-year students have a more positive opinion due to their exposure to real-world experience with financial aspects of pharmacy during their advanced pharmacy practice experiences (APPEs), commonly referred to as "rotations". The third-year students participated in the class in the fall of 2020, while the fourth-year students took the class in the fall of 2019. The total number of students enrolled in the third year was 119, while the number of students enrolled in the fourth year was 114. Therefore, an ideal sample size of 146 participants in total was calculated a priori to achieve an effect size of 0.20, with a power of 0.80 at the alpha level of 0.05 [25,26]. The survey was conducted and managed using Qualtrics XM (Qualtrics, Provo, UT, USA), an online survey-development platform. The survey was delivered via a link through the classes' mailing lists. To obtain responses that were as truthful as possible, the survey was made anonymous, thus, students were not prompted to provide any identifying information that would reveal their identity. The survey was open for 3 weeks (7–28 November 2021), with two email communications, including the initial survey launch and one reminder.

2.3. Survey Instrument

The survey questionnaire was created by modifying various surveys found in the literature [27–29]. While most of the survey questions were adapted and modified from previous literature to apply to financial management, a few were developed by the author. A draft version of the survey was distributed to two faculty members within the school of pharmacy in which the study was conducted, and two other faculty members at two other schools of pharmacy to assess its readability and content validity. The survey was also pretested among a group of four randomly selected pharmacy students that were not part of the study population to test clarity, relevance, acceptability, and time to completion (i.e., face validity). Modifications were made as required in terms of language comprehension, font size, and question organization before distributing the final survey to the students. A major modification included consistency with the use of the term 'pharmacy financial management' throughout the survey. This was suggested to prevent any confusion and indicate to the student that the survey assessment was strictly based on the instructions received within the course. Another major alteration was made in the ability section of the survey, where each statement was associated with a specific financial management subtopic to facilitate students' comprehension of these statements.

The final structured survey consisted of a total of 19 questions that could be completed within 5 min. The survey included seven demographic questions and 12 statements divided into three sections asking the students about their level of agreement in terms of their perception attitudes towards financial management education, and their ability to use such knowledge in practice. The participants indicated their level of agreement with the statements using a five-item Likert- type scale. Answers included "strongly disagree", "disagree", "neither agree nor disagree", "agree", and "strongly agree".

2.4. Data Analysis

Descriptive statistics were used to summarize the data. Incomplete surveys were only included in the analysis if they contained full responses for all the 12 statements on perception, attitude, and ability as well as partial responses to the demographic questions. Therefore, the number of respondents for each question varied. Data were analyzed using SPSS Statistics for Windows, Version 28.01 (IBM SPSS Statistics for Windows, Version 28.0. Armonk, NY, USA: IBM. Corp).

3. Results

3.1. Demographic Characteristics

Of the 233 students eligible to complete the survey, 139 (60%) students completed the survey, which included 77 third-year students and 62 fourth-year students. The demographic characteristics of respondents are summarized in Table 2.

The demographic characteristics of the third-year students and the fourth-year students are shown in Table 2. To compare the frequency distributions of the two years, a Chi-Square test of independence was used. For gender, third-year students included 72.7% female and fourth-year students included 56.5% female; there was no statistical significance in the difference between third-year and fourth-year (p-value = 0.090). For age, most of the third-year respondents (64.9%) were younger than 25 years, while 46.8% of fourth-year respondents were younger than 25 years; there was a statistical significance in the difference between third-year and fourth-year at the significance level of 0.05 (p-value = 0.032). This was not surprising, since fourth-year students are expected to be one year older than third-year students. For the highest degree achieved before pharmacy school, there was no statistical significance in the difference between third-year and fourth-year students (p-value = 0.321). In terms of prior business courses, 58.7% of third-year and 73.2% of fourth-year had taken business-related courses prior to pharmacy school; therefore, there was no statistical significance in the difference between third-year and fourth-year (p-value = 0.156). Lastly, for postgraduate plans, for third-year, 56.6% chose hospital pharmacy, 17.4% chose community pharmacy, 6.5% chose pharmaceutical industry, and 19.6% undecided; for fourth-year, 39.0% chose hospital pharmacy, 36.6% chose community pharmacy, 22.0% chose pharmaceutical industry, and 2.4% were undecided. There is a statistical significance in the difference between third-year and fourth-year students, with a p-value of 0.003 at a significance level of 0.01, according to a Chi-square test. For postgraduate plans, since some cells have values less than 5, to test the difference between third-year and fourth-year students, we also applied Fisher's exact test (IBM SPSS (Armonk, NY, USA: IBM. Corp.)), which can be applied when cell values are less than 5. Fisher's exact test confirms that there was statistical significance, with a p-value of 0.002. The difference between third-yead and fourth-year postgraduate plans was not surprising, since fourth-year students had more experience in clinical rotations than third-year students, and therefore might change their career choices.

Table 2. Demographic characteristics of Third- and fourth-year Pharmacy Student Respondents.

Characteristics	Overall (n = 139) Frequency (Percentage)	Third-Year (n = 77) Frequency (Percentage)	Fourth-Year (n = 62) Frequency (Percentage)	Chi-Square p-Value of Third-Year vs. Fourth-Year
Gender	(n = 139)	(n = 77)	(n = 62)	
Female	91 (65.5)	56 (72.7)	35 (56.5)	
Male	47 (33.8)	21 (27.3)	26 (41.9)	0.090
Prefer not to answer	1 (0.7)	0 (0)	1 (1.6)	
Age	(n = 139)	(n = 77)	(n = 62)	
<25 years old	79 (56.8)	50 (64.9)	29 (46.8)	0.032 *
≥25 years	60 (43.4)	27 (35.1)	33 (53.2)	
Highest degree achieved before pharmacy school	(n = 139)	(n = 77)	(n = 62)	
High school diploma	47 (33.8)	22 (28.6)	25 (40.3)	
Associate degree	16 (11.5)	11 (14.3)	5 (8.1)	0.321
Bachelor's degree	67 (48.2)	40 (51.9)	27 (43.5)	
Master's degree	9 (6.5)	4 (5.2)	5 (8.1)	
Taken business-related courses prior to pharmacy school	(n = 87)	(n = 46)	(n = 41)	
Yes	57 (65.5)	27 (58.7)	30 (73.2)	0.156
No	30 (34.5)	19 (41.3)	11 (26.8)	
Postgraduate plans	(n = 87)	(n = 46)	(n = 41)	
Hospital pharmacy	42 (48.3)	26 (56.5)	16 (39.0)	0.003 **
Community pharmacy	23 (26.4)	8 (17.4)	15 (36.6)	(Fisher's exact test
Pharmaceutical industry	12 (13.8)	3 (6.5)	9 (22.0)	p-value = 0.002 **) +
Undecided	10 (11.5)	9 (19.6)	1 (2.4)	

* p-value < 0.05; ** p-value < 0.01; + For postgraduate plans, since some cells have values less than 5, to test the difference between third-year and fourth-year, we also applied Fisher's exact test (IBM SPSS) which evaluates the statistical significance of the difference between third-year and fourth-year.

3.2. Perception of the Clinical Relevance of Pharmacy Financial Management Education

Table 3 shows students' perception of the clinical relevance of pharmacy financial management education. Four questions were used to assess the perception of the clinical relevance of pharmacy financial management education among the survey respondents. Most respondents agreed that financial management is an integral part of the pharmacy profession (n = 66, 46.2%), they may encounter financial management-related questions during their practice as pharmacists (n = 63, 44.1%) and that financial management competencies are useful for effective pharmacy practice in today's health care environment ($n = 66$, 46.2%). More than half of the respondents ($n = 72$, 50.3%) agreed that financial management competencies are useful skills and functions that pharmacists can use to manage aspects of pharmacy operations. The responses were stratified according to the professional year program and by business-related courses received prior to enrolling in pharmacy school (see Appendix A).

Table 3. Perception of the clinical relevance of pharmacy financial management education ($n = 139$).

Statement	Strongly Agree n (%)	Agree n (%)	Neither Agree nor Disagree n (%)	Disagree n (%)	Strongly Disagree n (%)
Financial management is an integral part of the pharmacy profession.	47 (32.9)	66 (46.2)	15 (10.5)	12 (8.4)	3 (2.1)
I may encounter financial management-related questions during my practice as a pharmacist.	41 (28.7)	63 (44.1)	20 (14.0)	15 (10.5)	4 (2.8)
Financial management competencies are useful for effective pharmacy practice in today's health care environment.	42 (29.4)	66 (46.2)	16 (11.2)	15 (10.5)	4 (2.8)
Financial management competencies are useful skills and functions that pharmacists can use to manage aspects of pharmacy operations using appropriate data and procedures and/or improve clinical processes and patient care.	47 (32.9)	72 (50.3)	8 (5.6)	13 (9.1)	3 (2.1)

3.3. Attitudes toward Pharmacy Financial Management Education

Table 4 shows students 'attitudes toward pharmacy financial management education. Most of the respondents agreed that financial management has been a relevant part of their Doctor of Pharmacy curriculum ($n = 57$, 40.1%), financial management should be covered in detail for all colleges and schools of pharmacy ($n = 58$, 40.8%) and that final-year (fourth-year) pharmacy students should be required to have a substantial knowledge of financial management prior to graduation ($n = 54$, 38.0%). The majority also agreed that they intend to read more about financial management, especially in terms of how it influences their practice and/or specialty post-graduation ($n = 52$, 36.6%). The responses were stratified according to the professional year program and business-related courses received prior to enrolling in pharmacy school (see Appendix B).

3.4. Ability to Use Pharmacy Financial Management Knowledge in Practice

Table 5 shows students' the ability to use pharmacy financial management knowledge in practice. Most of the respondents agreed that they were able to manage pharmacy operations ($n = 64$, 46.0%) and manage value-added pharmacy services ($n = 66$, 47.5%). More than half of the respondents agreed that they are able to manage people ($n = 74$, 53.2%), and manage money ($n = 75$, 54.0%). The responses were stratified according to the professional year program and business-related courses received prior to enrolling in pharmacy school (see Appendix C).

Table 4. Attitudes toward pharmacy financial management education ($n = 139$).

Statement	Strongly Agree n (%)	Agree n (%)	Neither Agree nor Disagree n (%)	Disagree n (%)	Strongly Disagree n (%)
Financial management has been a relevant part of my Doctor of Pharmacy curriculum.	28 (19.7)	57 (40.1)	23 (16.2)	22 (15.5)	12 (8.5)
Financial management should be covered in detail for all colleges and schools of pharmacy.	38 (26.8)	58 (40.8)	22 (15.5)	18 (12.7)	6 (4.2)
Final-year (P4) pharmacy students should be required to have substantial knowledge of financial management prior to graduation.	27 (19.0)	54 (38.0)	26 (18.3)	28 (19.7)	7 (4.9)
Post-graduation, I intend to read more about financial management, especially about how it influences my practice and/or specialty.	34 (23.9)	52 (36.6)	16 (11.3)	28 (19.7)	12 (8.5)

Table 5. Ability to use pharmacy financial management knowledge in practice ($n = 139$).

Statement	Strongly Agree n (%)	Agree n (%)	Neither Agree nor Disagree n (%)	Disagree n (%)	Strongly Disagree n (%)
Managing operations: I am able to apply management knowledge related to strategic planning, business planning, operations management, quality, and risk management in typical situations within a pharmacy organization.	28 (20.1)	64 (46.0)	2 (17.3)	18 (12.9)	5 (3.6)
Managing people: I am able to apply management knowledge related to organizational structure and behavior, human resources management functions, performance appraisal systems, and leadership.	28 (20.1)	74 (53.2)	17 (12.2)	16 (11.5)	4 (2.9)
Managing money: I am aware of the underlying principles that guide budgetary and financial management within a pharmacy organization.	28 (20.1)	75 (54.0)	17 (12.2)	15 (10.8)	4 (2.9)
Managing value-added services: I am able to apply management knowledge related to evaluating the market for and implementing value-added pharmacy services.	29 (20.9)	66 (47.5)	23 (16.5)	17 (12.2)	4 (2.9)

4. Discussion

This study is one of several that have been conducted in recent years to discuss financial management and business education in pharmacy [15,30–32]. However, it is one of the few of its kind used to assess United States pharmacy students' perceptions and attitudes toward financial management education, and their ability to use their knowledge of financial management in practice. Overall, the study showed a positive perception and attitude toward financial management education. Most of the participants reported being able to use pharmacy financial management in their practice.

Pharmacy students are exposed to financial management and business-related coursework and experiential learning opportunities more than ever before, both within and outside their pharmacy programs [30,33–35]. Several trends in pharmacy have influenced this growth, including the expanding role of pharmacists and responsibilities within healthcare organizations, changes in accreditation standards, and educational outcomes that emphasize a wider range of skills relevant to pharmacists. These trends reflect broader economic conditions and shifts in the healthcare system which affect pharmacy practice [36]. Other important factors are changes in pharmacy practice models and patients' expectations and knowledge, as well as the rapid development of technology in the medication-use process [37–39].

In the context of United States pharmacy education, courses and programs that deliver financial management skills, knowledge, and experiences to students are very diverse in terms of key objectives, lecture or credit hours provided, and the professional year in which the financial management course is offered [20]. Given that financial management provides an integrated set of concepts and applications, drawing from entrepreneurship, finance, business, accounting, marketing, and management, pharmacy programs can also vary considerably in terms of their desired outcomes [35,40]. Certain pharmacy programs focus on business management (concentrating on accounting, financial statements, and financial statement analysis) [34,41], while others focus on entrepreneurship, innovation, and creativity to develop new opportunities for pharmacists [20]. On a more pragmatic level, program requirements diverge. Several programs emphasize experiential learning and extra-curricular activities that may or may not be tied to a specific course and credit hours, while others involve a specific sequence of courses for credit [42]. These experiential learning and extra-curricular activities are designed to expose pharmacy students to real business by means of company and pharmacy visits, teaching cooperation, practical training, and providing entrepreneurship-in-residence programs. The entrepreneurship-in-residence programs typically provide pharmacy students with opportunities to engage with accomplished entrepreneurs from the business community. The coaching sessions offered by those entrepreneurs in residence allow pharmacy students to learn about the business environment, beyond the formal curriculum and classroom setting. Even though some programs provide a few hours of instructions on financial management as part of a required course, they do however offer in-depth instruction on financial management as part of an elective course [33,43,44]. Some features distinguish financial management in pharmacy education from other pharmacy courses and influence its structure, emphasis, and outcomes. In many instances, business, finance, and management-related topics are not part of the prerequisite academic work required for entry into pharmacy programs at several institutions. Second, the business environment in which a pharmacy program operates can also play an important role in the ability to leverage important resources to develop a comprehensive and engaging financial management course.

The lesson learned while undertaking this work call for a redesign of the financial management course to include an experiential component. In the previous financial management course structure, students learned a great deal about financial management and acquired a lot of information, but were not provided exposure and hands-on experience outside of the classroom. To overcome this limitation, two courses have been included in the new pharmacy curriculum 'Practice- and Team-Ready Curriculum' to provide access to more hands-on experience. In the new curriculum, the Financial Management course is offered in the second year of the program, and a Management, Innovation, Leadership, and Entrepreneurship (MILE) course is offered in the fourth year. These courses are designed to advance pharmacy students who develop entrepreneurial skills in both didactic and experiential work. The MILE course aims to provide pharmacy students with management, innovation, leadership, intrapreneurial, and entrepreneurial knowledge, tools, and skills to allow them to participate effectively in the creation and growth of high-impact pharmaceutical business ventures. Students will have an opportunity to develop their ideas in a team-based setting, identify needs, assess opportunities, and cultivate a lasting competitive advantage when creating innovative products and services with the potential for implementation/commercialization.

Overall, the aim of this work was not to draw representative conclusions regarding all United States pharmacy students, but instead to understand how pharmacy students' perspective of financial management education could inform curriculum development. Moreover, it was not the immediate purpose of this study to be prescriptive about course content in financial management, as the findings provide information about student respondents' perception and attitude toward the financial management course taught in their schools of pharmacy. This information can be useful to curriculum committees interesting in making changes to their curriculum. Having knowledge of what other schools or colleges of pharmacy cover in their financial management courses may have some utility. As a next step, we will assess the breadth, depth, and perceived importance of financial management instruction and the level of faculty development in this area in schools and colleges of pharmacy in the United States.

Certain limitations of this study should be considered in the interpretation of the results, their generalization to other educational contexts, and comparison with other studies. The survey responses were conducted from a sample consisting of student pharmacists at one academic institution, which may limit its generalizability and may influence study findings. The survey was dependent upon voluntary subject participation which made it particularly vulnerable to sampling bias. Because of the cross-sectional nature of the study, there is a possibility of self-report bias. While student respondents were asked about experiences that would have taken place within a relatively recent period, recall bias may have occurred. This issue should be addressed in future work using other study designs including using quasi-experimental or repeated measure designs. Since this study was not longitudinal, it would be presumptuous to draw conclusions about changes in students' perceptions, attitudes, and abilities over time.

5. Conclusions

This study has clear educational implications. With ever-increasing pressure to reduce healthcare spending and improve patient outcomes, the need for pharmacists skilled in both the clinical and business aspects of pharmacy is warranted. With so many pharmacy career pathways that require business skills and the growing interest in entrepreneurship, pharmacy students need to be offered the opportunity to access essential financial management training without adding additional time to their degree. Regardless of how pharmacy programs incorporate financial management, curricula must remain dynamic and respond to changes in the healthcare landscape. Future studies should clarify which teaching strategies are suitable for financial management education, as well as the amount of financial management education that is best suited to achieve competency in the pharmacy field.

Author Contributions: Conceptualization, G.A.; methodology, GA.; formal analysis, G.A. and K.P.; investigation, G.A.; data curation, G.A.; writing—original draft preparation, G.A.; writing—review and editing, G.A. and K.P.; visualization, G.A. and K.P.; project administration, G.A. All authors have read and agreed to the published version of the manuscript.

Funding: This research received no external funding.

Institutional Review Board Statement: The study was conducted according to the guidelines of the Declaration of Helsinki and approved by the Institutional Review Board of Samford University (EXMT-P-22-S-1).

Informed Consent Statement: Subjects' participation in the survey was voluntary and was considered their consent to take part in the study.

Data Availability Statement: The data presented in this study are available upon request from the corresponding author.

Conflicts of Interest: The author declares no conflict of interest.

Appendix A. Perception Tables

Table A1. Perception of the clinical relevance of pharmacy financial management education by professional pharmacy year (N = 139).

Statement	Strongly Agree		Agree		Neither Agree nor Disagree		Disagree		Strongly Disagree	
	3rd Year	4th Year	3rd Year	4th Year	3rd Year	4th Year	3rd Year	4th Year	3rd Year	4th Year
Financial management is an integral part of the pharmacy profession.	25 (32.47)	30 (32.26)	40 (51.95)	26 (41.94)	9 (11.69)	5 (8.06)	2 (2.60)	9 (14.52)	1 (1.30)	2 (3.23)
I may encounter financial management-related questions during my practice as a pharmacist.	24 (31.17)	16 (25.81)	37 (48.05)	25 (40.32)	9 (11.69)	10 (16.13)	5 (6.49)	9 (14.52)	2 (2.60)	2 (3.23)
Financial management competencies are useful for effective pharmacy practice in today's health care environment.	23 (29.87)	18 (29.03)	43 (55.84)	22 (35.48)	5 (6.49)	10 (16.13)	5 (6.49)	9 (14.52)	1 (1.30)	3 (4.84)
Financial management competencies are useful skills and functions that pharmacists can use to manage aspects of pharmacy operations using appropriate data and procedures and/or improve clinical processes and patient care.	26 (33.77)	20 (32.26)	42 (54.55)	29 (46.77)	3 (3.90)	4 (6.45)	5 (6.49)	7 (11.29)	1 (1.30)	2 (3.23)

Table A2. Perception of the clinical relevance of pharmacy financial management education (N = 139) by business related courses prior to pharmacy school (N = 139).

Statement	Strongly Agree		Agree		Neither Agree nor Disagree		Disagree		Strongly Disagree	
	Yes	No	Yes	No	Yes	No	Yes	No	Yes	No
Financial management is an integral part of the pharmacy profession.	23 (40.35)	3 (10.00)	22 (38.60)	20 (66.67)	5 (8.77)	4 (13.33)	6 (10.53)	2 (6.67)	1 (1.75)	1 (1.33)
I may encounter financial management-related questions during my practice as a pharmacist.	20 (35.09)	4 (13.33)	23 (40.35)	17 (56.67)	6 (10.53)	4 (13.33)	8 (14.04)	3 (10.00)	0 (0.00)	2 (6.67)
Financial management competencies are useful for effective pharmacy practice in today's health care environment.	20 (35.09)	7 (23.33)	25 (43.86)	14 (46.67)	4 (7.02)	4 (13.33)	7 (12.28)	3 (10.00)	1 (1.75)	2 (6.67)
Financial management competencies are useful skills and functions that pharmacists can use to manage aspects of pharmacy operations using appropriate data and procedures and/or improve clinical processes and patient care.	21 (36.84)	6 (20.00)	28 (49.12)	19 (63.33)	2 (3.51)	1 (3.33)	5 (8.77)	2 (6.67)	1 (1.75)	2 (6.67)

Appendix B. Attitudes Tables

Table A3. Attitudes toward pharmacy financial management education by professional pharmacy year (N = 139).

Statement	Strongly Agree		Agree		Neither Agree nor Disagree		Disagree		Strongly Disagree	
	3rd Year	4th Year	3rd Year	4th Year	3rd Year	4th Year	3rd Year	4th Year	3rd Year	4th Year
Financial management has been a relevant part of my Doctor of Pharmacy curriculum.	16 (20.78)	12 (19.35)	32 (41.56)	24 (38.71)	15 (19.48)	7 (11.29)	9 (11.69)	12 (19.35)	5 (6.49)	7 (11.29)
Financial management should be covered in detail for all colleges and schools of pharmacy.	22 (28.57)	15 (24.19)	35 (45.45)	23 (37.10)	11 (14.29)	10 (16.13)	6 (7.79)	11 (17.74)	3 (3.90)	3 (4.84)
Final-year (P4) pharmacy students should be required to have substantial knowledge of financial management prior to graduation.	16 (20.78)	11 (17.14)	29 (37.66)	24 (38.71)	16 (20.78)	9 (14.52)	13 (16.88)	14 (22.58)	3 (3.90)	4 (6.45)
Post-graduation, I intend to read more about financial management, especially about how it influences my practice and/or specialty.	19 (24.68)	15 (24.19)	29 (37.66)	22 (35.48)	9 (11.69)	6 (9.68)	13 (16.88)	14 (22.58)	7 (9.09)	5 (8.06)

Table A4. Attitudes toward pharmacy financial management education by business related courses prior to pharmacy school (N = 139).

Statement	Strongly Agree		Agree		Neither Agree nor Disagree		Disagree		Strongly Disagree	
	Yes	No	Yes	No	Yes	No	Yes	No	Yes	No
Financial management has been a relevant part of my Doctor of Pharmacy curriculum.	15 (26.32)	1 (3.33)	23 (40.35)	13 (43.33)	7 (12.28)	6 (20.00)	9 (15.79)	4 (13.33)	3 (5.26)	6 (20.00)
Financial management should be covered in detail for all colleges and schools of pharmacy.	20 (35.09)	3 (10.00)	23 (40.35)	13 (43.33)	4 (7.02)	7 (23.33)	9 (15.79)	3 (10.00)	1 (1.75)	4 (13.33)
Final-year (P4) pharmacy students should be required to have substantial knowledge of financial management prior to graduation.	18 (31.58)	1 (3.33)	19 (33.33)	11 (36.67)	11 (19.30)	7 (23.33)	7 (12.28)	8 (26.67)	2 (3.51)	3 (10.00)
Post-graduation, I intend to read more about financial management, especially about how it influences my practice and/or specialty.	19 (33.33)	4 (13.33)	20 (35.09)	11 (36.67)	6 (10.53)	5 (16.67)	10 (17.54)	4 (13.33)	2 (3.51)	6 (20.00)

Appendix C. Ability Tables

Table A5. Ability to use pharmacy financial management knowledge in practice by professional pharmacy year (N = 139).

Statement	Strongly Agree		Agree		Neither Agree nor Disagree		Disagree		Strongly Disagree	
	3rd Year	4th Year	3rd Year	4th Year	3rd Year	4th Year	3rd Year	4th Year	3rd Year	4th Year
Managing operations: I am able to apply management knowledge related to strategic planning, business planning, operations management, quality, and risk management in typical situations within a pharmacy organization.	17 (17 (22.08)	11 (17.74)	37 (48.05)	27 (43.55)	12 (15.58)	12 (19.35)	9 (11.69)	9 (14.52)	2 (2.60)	3 (4.84)
Managing people: I am able to apply management knowledge related to organizational structure and behavior, human resources management functions, performance appraisal systems, and leadership.	16 (20.78)	12 (19.35)	43 (55.84)	31 (50.00)	9 (11.69)	8 (12.90)	7 (9.09)	9 (14.52)	2 (2.60)	2 (3.23)
Managing money: I am aware of the underlying principles that guide budgetary and financial management within a pharmacy organization.	16 (20.78)	12 (19.35)	44 (57.14)	31 (50.00)	10 (12.99)	7 (11.29)	5 (6.49)	10 (16.13)	2 (2.60)	2 (3.23)
Managing value-added services: I am able to apply management knowledge related to evaluating the market for and implementing value-added pharmacy services.	16 (20.78)	13 (20.97)	40 (51.95)	26 (41.94)	10 (12.99)	13 (20.97)	8 (10.39)	9 (14.52)	3 (3.90)	1 (1.61)

Table A6. Ability to use pharmacy financial management knowledge in practice by business related courses prior to pharmacy school (N = 139).

Statement	Strongly Agree		Agree		Neither Agree nor Disagree		Disagree		Strongly Disagree	
	Yes	No	Yes	No	Yes	No	Yes	No	Yes	No
Managing operations: I am able to apply management knowledge related to strategic planning, business planning, operations management, quality, and risk management in typical situations within a pharmacy organization.	16 (28.07)	1 (3.33)	22 (38.60)	14 (46.67)	11 (19.30)	7 (23.33)	7 (12.28)	7 (23.33)	1 (1.75)	1 (3.33)
Managing people: I am able to apply management knowledge related to organizational structure and behavior, human resources management functions, performance appraisal systems, and leadership.	17 (29.82)	2 (6.67)	26 (45.61)	17 (56.67)	6 (10.53)	6 (20.00)	8 (14.04)	4 (13.33)	0 (0.00)	1 (3.33)
Managing money: I am aware of the underlying principles that guide budgetary and financial management within a pharmacy organization.	17 (29.82)	1 (3.33)	28 (49.12)	19 (63.33)	5 (8.77)	6 (20.00)	7 (12.28)	3 (10.00)	0 (0.00)	1 (3.33)
Managing value-added services: I am able to apply management knowledge related to evaluating the market for and implementing value-added pharmacy services.	17 (29.82)	2 (6.67)	25 (43.86)	15 (50.00)	8 (14.04)	6 (20.00)	6 (10.53)	6 (20.00)	1 (1.75)	1 (3.33)

References

1. Gapenski, L.C.; Pink, G.H. *Understanding Healthcare Financial Management*; Health Administration Press Chicago: Chicago, IL, USA, 2007.
2. Blouin, R.A.; Adams, M.L. The role of the pharmacist in health care: Expanding and evolving. *N. C. Med. J.* **2017**, *78*, 165–167. [CrossRef] [PubMed]
3. Lott, B.E.; Anderson, E.J.; Zapata, L.V.; Cooley, J.; Forbes, S.; Taylor, A.M.; Manygoats, T.; Warholak, T. Expanding pharmacists' roles: Pharmacists' perspectives on barriers and facilitators to collaborative practice. *J. Am. Pharm. Assoc.* **2021**, *61*, 213–220.e1. [CrossRef] [PubMed]
4. Strand, M.A.; Mager, N.A.D.; Hall, L.; Martin, S.L.; Sarpong, D.F. Pharmacy contributions to improved population health: Expanding the public health roundtable. *Prev. Chronic Dis.* **2020**, *17*, E113. [CrossRef] [PubMed]
5. Majercak, K.R. Advancing pharmacist prescribing privileges: Is it time? *J. Am. Pharm. Assoc.* **2019**, *59*, 783–786. [CrossRef] [PubMed]
6. Gonzalvo, J.D.; Kenneally, A.M.; Pence, L.; Walroth, T.; Schmelz, A.N.; Nace, N.; Chang, J.; Meredith, A.H. Reimbursement outcomes of a pharmacist-physician co-visit model in a Federally Qualified Health Center. *J. Am. Coll. Clin. Pharm.* **2021**, *4*, 667–673.
7. Reyes, L.D.; Hong, J.; Lin, C.; Hamper, J.; Kroon, L. Community pharmacists' motivation and barriers to providing and billing patient care services. *Pharmacy* **2020**, *8*, 145. [CrossRef]
8. Strand, M.A.; Eukel, H.; Burck, S. Moving opioid misuse prevention upstream: A pilot study of community pharmacists screening for opioid misuse risk. *Res. Soc. Adm. Pharm.* **2019**, *15*, 1032–1036. [CrossRef]
9. Dong, B.J.; Lopez, M.; Cocohoba, J. Pharmacists performing hepatitis C antibody point-of-care screening in a community pharmacy: A pilot project. *J. Am. Pharm. Assoc.* **2017**, *57*, 510–515.e2. [CrossRef]
10. Schmit, C.D.; Penn, M.S. Expanding state laws and a growing role for pharmacists in vaccination services. *J. Am. Pharm. Assoc.* **2017**, *57*, 661–669. [CrossRef]
11. Beal, J.L.; Kadakia, N.N.; Reed, J.B.; Plake, K.S.I. Pharmacists' impact on older adults' access to vaccines in the United States. *Vaccine* **2020**, *38*, 2456–2465. [CrossRef]
12. Medina, M.S.; Plaza, C.M.; Stowe, C.D.; Robinson, E.T.; DeLander, G.; Beck, D.E.; Melchert, R.B.; Supernaw, R.B.; Roche, V.F.; Gleason, B.L. Center for the Advancement of Pharmacy Education 2013 educational outcomes. *Am. J. Pharm. Educ.* **2013**, *77*, 162. [CrossRef] [PubMed]
13. National Association of Boards of Pharmacy. The Pharmacy Curriculum Outcomes Assessment®(PCOA®). Available online: https://nabp.pharmacy/programs/pcoa/ (accessed on 14 February 2022).
14. Center for the Advancement of Pharmacy Education (CAPE) 2013 Educational Outcomes. 2013 Panel. Available online: https://www.isu.edu/media/libraries/pharmacy/documents/office-of-experiential-education/CAPEoutcomes.pdf (accessed on 14 February 2022).
15. Rollins, B.L.; Broedel-Zaugg, K.; Reiselman, J.; Sullivan, D. Assessment of pharmacy students' perceived business management knowledge: Would exclusion of business management topics be detrimental to pharmacy curricula? *Curr. Pharm. Teach. Learn.* **2012**, *4*, 197–201. [CrossRef]
16. Mospan, C.M. Management education within pharmacy curricula: A need for innovation. *Curr. Pharm. Teach. Learn.* **2017**, *9*, 171–174. [CrossRef] [PubMed]
17. Titman, S.; Keown, A.J. *Financial Management: Principles and Applications*; Pearson Education, Inc.: New York, NY, USA, 2018.
18. Wilson, A.L. *Financial Management for Health-System Pharmacists*; ASHP: Bethesda, MA, USA, 2008.
19. Herist, K.N.; Rollins, B.L.; Perri, M. *Financial Analysis in Pharmacy Practice*; Pharmaceutical Press: London, UK, 2011.
20. Afeli, S.A.; Adunlin, G. Curriculum content for innovation and entrepreneurship education in US pharmacy programs. *Ind. High. Educ.* **2021**, *35*, 953–957. [CrossRef]
21. Efron, R. What is perception? In *Proceedings of Boston Colloquium for the Philosophy of Science 1966/1968*; Springer: Dordrecht, The Netherlands, 1969; pp. 137–173.
22. The United Nations Educational, Scientific and Cultural Organization. Glossary of Curriculum Terminology. Available online: http://www.ibe.unesco.org/en/glossary-curriculum-terminology (accessed on 14 February 2022).
23. Zgarrick, D.P.; Desselle, S.P.; Moczygemba, L.R.; Greg, A. *Pharmacy Management Essentials for All Practice Settings*, 5th ed.; McGraw Hill: New York, NY, USA, 2020.
24. Chisholm-Burns, M.A.; Vaillancourt, A.M.; Shepherd, M. *Pharmacy Management, Leadership, Marketing, and Finance (Book Only)*; Jones & Bartlett Publishers: Burlington, MA, USA, 2012.
25. Polit, D.F.; Beck, C.T. *Nursing Research: Principles and Methods*; Lippincott Williams & Wilkins: Philadelphia, PA, USA, 2004.
26. Qualtrics[XM]. Calculating Sample Size: A Quick Guide (Calculator Included). Available online: https://www.qualtrics.com/blog/calculating-sample-size/ (accessed on 22 December 2021).
27. Murphy, J.E.; Green, J.S.; Adams, L.A.; Squire, R.B.; Kuo, G.M.; McKay, A. Pharmacogenomics in the curricula of colleges and schools of pharmacy in the United States. *Am. J. Pharm. Educ.* **2010**, *74*, 7. [CrossRef]
28. Muzoriana, N.; Gavi, S.; Nembaware, V.; Dhoro, M.; Matimba, A. Knowledge, attitude, and perceptions of pharmacists and pharmacy students towards pharmacogenomics in Zimbabwe. *Pharmacy* **2017**, *5*, 36. [CrossRef]

29. Coriolan, S.; Arikawe, N.; Moscati, A.; Zhou, L.; Dym, S.; Donmez, S.; Garba, A.; Falbaum, S.; Loewy, Z.; Lull, M. Pharmacy students' attitudes and perceptions toward pharmacogenomics education. *Am. J. Health-Syst. Pharm.* **2019**, *76*, 836–845. [CrossRef]
30. Amin, K.A.; Hoffmaster, B.S.; Misko, B.L. Prioritizing financial knowledge and skills within the doctor of pharmacy curriculum. *Curr. Pharm. Teach. Learn.* **2021**, *13*, 953–957. [CrossRef]
31. Mattingly, T.J.; Abdelwadoud, M.; Mullins, C.D.; Eddington, N.D. Pharmapreneur–Defining a Framework for Entrepreneurship in Pharmacy Education. *Am. J. Pharm. Educ.* **2019**, *83*, 7548. [CrossRef]
32. Slavcev, R.A.; Tjendra, J.; Korenevsky, A.; Boran, V.; Kanji, N. Pharmacy Investment Club: Fostering financial management skills from beyond the classroom. *Can. Pharm. J. Rev. Pharm. Can.* **2013**, *146*, 143–145. [CrossRef]
33. Chui, M.A. An elective course in personal finance for health care professionals. *Am. J. Pharm. Educ.* **2009**, *73*, 6. [CrossRef] [PubMed]
34. Augustine, J.; Slack, M.; Cooley, J.; Bhattacharjee, S.; Holmes, E.; Warholak, T.L. Identification of key business and management skills needed for pharmacy graduates. *Am. J. Pharm. Educ.* **2018**, *82*, 6364. [CrossRef] [PubMed]
35. Gatwood, J.; Hohmeier, K.; Farr, G.; Eckel, S. A comparison of approaches to student pharmacist business planning in pharmacy practice management. *Am. J. Pharm. Educ.* **2018**, *82*, 6279. [CrossRef] [PubMed]
36. Dolovich, L.; Austin, Z.; Waite, N.; Chang, F.; Farrell, B.; Grindrod, K.; Houle, S.; McCarthy, L.; MacCallum, L.; Sproule, B. Pharmacy in the 21st century: Enhancing the impact of the profession of pharmacy on people's lives in the context of health care trends, evidence and policies. *Can. Pharm. J. Rev. Pharm. Can.* **2019**, *152*, 45–53. [CrossRef]
37. Cobaugh, D.J.; Thompson, K.K. Embracing the role of artificial intelligence in the medication-use process. *Am. J. Health-Syst. Pharm.* **2020**, *77*, 1915–1916. [CrossRef]
38. Cortes, D.; Leung, J.; Ryl, A.; Lieu, J. Pharmacy Informatics: Where Medication Use and Technology Meet. *Can. J. Hosp. Pharm.* **2019**, *72*, 320. [CrossRef]
39. Livet, M.; Easter, J. Optimizing medication use through a synergistic technology testing process integrating implementation science to drive effectiveness and facilitate scale. *J. Am. Pharm. Assoc.* **2019**, *59*, S71–S77. [CrossRef]
40. Rollins, B.L.; Gunturi, R.; Sullivan, D. A pharmacy business management simulation exercise as a practical application of business management material and principles. *Am. J. Pharm. Educ.* **2014**, *78*, 62. [CrossRef]
41. Hicks, C.; Siganga, W.; Shah, B. Enhancing pharmacy student business management skills by collaborating with pharmacy managers to implement pharmaceutical care services. *Am. J. Pharm. Educ.* **2004**, *68*, BD1–BD7. [CrossRef]
42. Cohn, M. *Pharmacy School to Foster More Entrepreneurial Spirit*; The Baltimore Sun: Baltimore, MA, USA, 2017.
43. Wilhoite, J.; Skelley, J.W.; Baker, A.; Traxler, K.; Triboletti, J. Students' Perceptions on a Business Plan Assignment for an Ambulatory Care Pharmacy Elective. *Am. J. Pharm. Educ.* **2019**, *83*, 6789. [CrossRef]
44. Bullock, K.C.; Horne, S. A Didactic Community Pharmacy Course to Improve Pharmacy Students' Clinical Skills and Business Management Knowledge. *Am. J. Pharm. Educ.* **2019**, *83*, 6581. [CrossRef] [PubMed]

MDPI
St. Alban-Anlage 66
4052 Basel
Switzerland
Tel. +41 61 683 77 34
Fax +41 61 302 89 18
www.mdpi.com

Healthcare Editorial Office
E-mail: healthcare@mdpi.com
www.mdpi.com/journal/healthcare

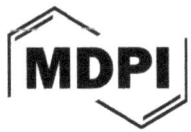

www.ingramcontent.com/pod-product-compliance
Lightning Source LLC
LaVergne TN
LVHW070453100526
838202LV00014B/1718